Sexually Transmitted Diseases in Homosexual Men

Diagnosis, Treatment, and Research

Sexually Transmitted Diseases in Homosexual Men

Diagnosis, Treatment, and Research

Edited by

David G. Ostrow, M.D., Ph.D.
Howard Brown Memorial Clinic
Northwestern University Medical School and
Lakeside Veterans Administration Medical Center
Chicago, Illinois

Terry Alan Sandholzer
San Francisco, California

and

Yehudi M. Felman, M.D., M.A., M.Phil., F.A.C.P.
State University of New York
Downstate Medical School
Brooklyn, New York, and
Bureau of Venereal Disease Control
New York City Health Department
New York, New York

Plenum Medical Book Company
New York and London

Library of Congress Cataloging in Publication Data

Main entry under title:

Sexually transmitted diseases in homosexual men.

Includes bibliographies and index.
1. Venereal diseases. 2. Homosexuals, Male—Diseases. I. Ostrow, David G.,
1947–   . II. Sandholzer, Terry Alan, date–   . III. Felman, Yehudi. IV. Title:
Sexually transmitted diseases in homosexual men. [DNLM: 1. Homosexuality. 2.
Venereal diseases. WC 140 S798]
RC200.1.S7 1983   616.95′1′008041   83-10957
ISBN-13: 978-1-4684-1166-9   e-ISBN-13: 978-1-4684-1164-5
DOI: 10.1007/978-1-4684-1164-5

© 1983 Plenum Publishing Corporation
Softcover reprint of the hardcover 1st edition 1983
233 Spring Street, New York, N.Y. 10013

Plenum Medical Book Company is an imprint of Plenum Publishing Corporation

Contributors

HERAND ABCARIAN, M.D., F.A.C.S. ● Chairman, Section of Colon and Rectal Surgery, Cook County Hospital, and Associate Professor of Surgery, University of Illinois College of Medicine at Chicago, Chicago, Illinois 60612

YEHUDI M. FELMAN, M.D., M.A., M.Phil., F.A.C.P. ● Clinical Professor of Dermatology and Lecturer in Preventive Medicine and Community Health, State University of New York, Downstate Medical School, Brooklyn, New York 11203

ALEXANDER A. FISHER, M.D. ● Clinical Professor, Department of Dermatology, New York University Postgraduate Medical School, New York, New York 10003

TERENCE C. GAYLE, M.D. ● Resident in Psychiatry, Department of Psychiatry and Behavioral Sciences, University of Washington, Seattle, Washington 98195

KING K. HOLMES, M.D., Ph.D. ● Division of Infectious Diseases, Seattle Public Health Hospital, and Professor of Medicine, University of Washington at Seattle, Seattle, Washington 98144

STEVE B. KALISH, M.D. ● Instructor, Department of Medicine, Section of Infectious Disease, Northwestern University Medical School, Chicago, Illinois 60611

HOWARD I. MAIBACH, M.D. ● Professor of Dermatology, University of California School of Medicine, San Francisco, California 94143

KENNETH H. MAYER, M.D. ● Research Fellow, Departments of Medicine, and Microbiology and Molecular Genetics, Harvard Medical School, and

Research Director and Staff Physician, Fenway Community Health Center, Boston, Massachusetts 02115

JAMES A. NIKITAS, M.D. ● Clinical Assistant Professor of Dermatology, New York Medical College, Metropolitan Hospital Center, Valhalla, New York 10595

ALFRED OBERMAIER, M.S.S.E. ● Tucson Gay Health Project, Tucson, Arizona 85703

MILTON ORKIN, M.D. ● Clinical Professor, Department of Dermatology, University of Minnesota Medical School, Minneapolis, Minnesota 55422

DAVID G. OSTROW, M.D., Ph.D. ● Coordinator, Biological Psychiatry Program, Lakeside Veterans Administration Medical Center, and Associate Professor of Psychiatry and Community Medicine, Northwestern University Medical School, Chicago, Illinois 60611; and Director of Research, Howard Brown Memorial Clinic, Chicago, Illinois 60616

JOHN P. PHAIR, M.D. ● Professor of Medicine and Head, Section of Infectious Disease, Northwestern University Medical School, Chicago, Illinois 60611

TERRY ALAN SANDHOLZER ● Writer and Lecturer, San Francisco, California 94117

DANIEL C. WILLIAM, M.D. ● Instructor in Clinical Medicine, Columbia University College of Physicians and Surgeons, New York, New York 10032; and Staff Physician, St. Luke's–Roosevelt Hospital Center, New York, New York 10019

Preface

This book is intended to educate the primary health care provider about sexually transmitted and related diseases as they present in homosexually active men. But why a book discussing sexually transmitted diseases (STDs) in this population only? Surely STDs are not limited to homosexual males. The relatively high rates of incidence of many of these diseases among homosexually active men, however, and the large number of associated diagnostic and treatment problems have necessitated the collection into one volume of the information that is particularly relevant to the primary health care of this population.

A book dealing with current trends in the diagnosis and treatment of sexual diseases can, by nature of the task, be neither encyclopedic nor all-encompassing. In this volume, the choice of disease entities and the amount of material included on each are based on consideration of the amount of current information and the relative degree of uniqueness of a given problem in homosexual men, rather than the absolute frequency of the disease. There is, therefore, a considerable amount of material on hepatitis B and gonococcal infections, reflecting the recent explosion of research and clinical investigation in these two areas. In contrast, little is said about nonspecific urethritis, chancroid, and lymphogranuloma venereum. In the case of nonspecific urethritis, although it is extremely common in homosexual men, little progress has been made in diagnosis or therapy. Incidence of chancroid and lymphogranuloma venereum in homosexual males is not considered to be widespread, so these diseases are included only as part of discussions of the differential diagnosis of other high-incidence STDs, such as syphilis.

While scientific progress continues to be made, new and resurgent disease entities are challenging the health care provider in the 1980s. In fact, the rapid pace with which new information is accumulated, the constant recognition of new diseases that are thought to be sexually transmitted, and the frequent appearance of new therapeutic modalities all make the preparation of an up-to-date monograph extremely difficult. We have tried, therefore, to include as much current information as possible, with the hope that this information will be still valid at the time of publication. In an attempt to overcome the inherent time lag involved in the writing and publication of this work, we have included in many of the chapters sections highlighting current research activities. Our readers are invited to contribute comments about the content of the volume as well as any ideas regarding subjects that they feel should be addressed in future editions.

It is customary in a Preface to thank those persons who have contributed to the work and to explain why the authors have written on a particular subject. A brief history of this project will, we hope, serve both purposes. The idea for this volume on STDs written for an audience of primary care practitioners originated from discussions among the medical directors of several community clinics serving predominantly homosexual male populations. Beginning in 1975 in Chicago, these discussions were facilitated by the organization by Walter Lear, M.D., Chairperson of the Gay Caucus of the American Public Health Association (APHA), of a Venereal Disease Task Force of that caucus. Much of the energy and enthusiasm of that group's activities came from the rapid growth in size and number of gay-community-sponsored STD clinics in major metropolitan centers during the mid-1970s. In 1976, the Gay Caucus and the American Venereal Disease Association (AVDA) sponsored a symposium at the APHA annual meeting on STDs in homosexual men that included contributions from the Los Angeles Gay Community STD Clinic, the New York Gay Men's Health Project, and the Howard Brown Memorial Clinic of Chicago. In the course of the preparation of those papers, the discussion that followed their presentation, and the commentary following their publication in the *Journal of the American Venereal Disease Association* (now the *Journal of Sexually Transmitted Diseases*) it became increasingly clear that lack of knowledge within the health care professions regarding the myriad STD problems endemic in the homosexual male population was a major barrier to improving health care services to this community.

The medical directors of several of the major gay community STD clinics met during the 1977 APHA meeting in Washington, D.C., to plan a monograph that would specifically address this need. The preface to what was then titled *Providing Health Care for Gay Men* included the following passage:

> Gay men have a variety of unique medical problems that are related primarily to their sexual lifestyle and these problems have not been formally addressed by medical education. Traditional health care education has not addressed the issue of human sexuality completely, and certainly not the area of homosexuality and the health care needs of homosexual and bisexual men. In part as a result of the lack of facilities and programs to meet these needs (beginning in the early 1970s), gay communities in many of the major American cities have formed their own community-sponsored health care facilities. As a result of this development, and the large and ever-growing use of these facilities, a significant amount of experience, expertise,

and information relating to the health care needs of the gay male population has accumulated. As the medical directors of three such clinics and as persons concerned with the need to both integrate the information accumulated in our experiences working with these clinics, and to help redirect the mainstream health care delivery system to better meet the specific needs of the gay male community, we have decided to write this book.

The goal of this book is to help eliminate the need for separate health care facilities for gay persons. To do this, we hope to provide a framework to assist the primary health care provider in dealing more effectively with the unique problems and needs of the gay or bisexual male patient. Within this context, we hope to diminish the significant and understandable anxieties that many providers have in dealing with an historically uncomfortable area in medicine. As a result of improved awareness, we hope to someday return the responsibility of care to where it belongs, namely the mainstream of the American health care system.

Many changes have occurred in the six years since the above was written. Perhaps most important has been the change in focus and stature of the gay community health care clinics. As a result of their overwhelming success in focusing attention on the unmet health care needs of homosexual men, and by virtue of their demonstrating that community-sponsored and -organized clinics could do much to innovate in this area, these clinics have matured into major centers of delivery for specialized health care. The clinics have progressed from working largely independently to the undertaking of collaborative health care delivery programs with local public health agencies. Even more dramatic has been the recognition that, as specialized health care delivery systems working in an area with many unresolved diagnostic and treatment dilemmas, the gay community clinics are in an ideal position to perform research. This recognition, in turn, has led to the establishment of collaborative research partnerships among the various clinics, the Centers for Disease Control (CDC) in Atlanta, and prominent university-affiliated researchers in the areas of STDs, microbiology, and vaccine development. In particular, as Director of the CDC's Venereal Disease Control Program between 1975 and 1982, Paul Wiesner, M.D., enthusiastically supported the increasingly important role of gay-community-sponsored clinics in the clinical research programs of the CDC. Other CDC personnel who have contributed significantly to the work described in this volume include Mr. Joseph Miller, William Darrow, Ph.D., Sumner Thompson, M.D., Gladys Reynolds, Ph.D., Harold Jaffe, M.D., and Donald Francis, M.D., Ph.D.

In recognition of the growing body of knowledge emanating from such collaborative research projects, the Howard Brown Memorial Clinic and the Infectious Diseases Training Program of the University of Chicago jointly sponsored the first "Current Aspects of STDs" (CASTDS I) symposium in June 1979. At that symposium, seventeen papers were presented by research groups from five of the gay community venereal disease clinics, the Venereal Disease Control and Hepatitis Research Programs of the CDC, and four major university medical centers. Recognizing that they had much valuable information to contribute to this volume, we invited people working in major university medical centers to contribute chapters in their major areas of interest. This book, like the clinics themselves, has evolved from a local project into a collaborative effort involving individuals and organizations throughout the United States working at local clinics, major medical centers, city departments of health, and the Centers for Disease Control.

The National Coalition of Gay STD Services (NCGSTDS) was formed at the time of CASTDS I. The Coalition has grown to include as members virtually all of the clinics, counseling services, and referral organizations delivering STD diagnosis, treatment, or referral services to gay communities throughout the United States and Canada. In addition, the Coalition includes many individual members with an interest in the area of STD work and concerned citizens interested in aiding the gay community's efforts to combat STDs. Acting as a clearinghouse for information regarding STDs for the medical, scientific, and gay communities, the Coalition publishes a quarterly newsletter, which greatly facilitates this communication. In July 1983, the Coalition sponsored the third CASTDS in Seattle. The major topics covered at CASTDS III included prophylaxis against viral and bacterial STDs, improved treatments for enteric infections, and an update on the acquired immunodeficiency syndrome (AIDS).

It is that last subject which provides the most compelling justification for the appearance of a monograph on homosexually related STDs at this time. Whatever the cause(s) of AIDS (and as of this writing no etiology has been established), it is clearly the most serious syndrome to enter the category of STDs since the discovery of antibiotics. It has transformed the entire field of venereology from one focusing on infectious agents and chemotherapies to one focusing on cellular immunology and the host's response to infection or carcinogenic processes. As persons working in the field of public health, we bemoan the addition of immunologic, neoplastic, and opportunistic disease entities to the repertoire of sexually transmitted or related diseases. The immense interest in and rapid proliferation of information about this new disease syndrome led us to add an entire section to this book, which includes a chapter on Kaposi's sarcoma and other neoplastic conditions, a consideration of the diagnosis and treatment of opportunistic infections, and a review of the information regarding the safety and possible role of volatile nitrites in immune dysfunction.

In August 1982, the National Gay Task Force, the National Gay Health Education Foundation, and the National Gay Health Coalition organized an "AIDS Forum" at the Dallas Gay Leadership Conference, which led to the formation of a national AIDS network to coordinate community responses to this problem. We can only hope that the cause(s) of the AIDS epidemic will be discovered before many more persons have died and that preventive measures will be adopted by both health care providers and consumers. The primary health care provider can, by focusing on the role of basic health care services, gain a thorough understanding of his/her patient's sexual practices and other major disease risk factors. We feel that this book provides a conceptual basis for a grass-roots-level response by health care providers to the AIDS phenomenon.

Finally, it is a pleasure to acknowledge other persons who have contributed to this project. All of the staff and volunteers of the Howard Brown Memorial Clinic have contributed generously of their time to the work of the clinic, which in turn has enabled us to learn about the problems discussed here. Mr. Norman Altman, Hepatitis Research Project Coordinator between 1977 and 1982, helped in the collection and analysis of the epidemiologic data contained in the chapters on gonorrhea and hepatitis. Mr. Ralph Burke, Director of Chicago's Venereal Disease Control Program between 1972 and 1981, worked diligently to coordinate the efforts of the Howard Brown Memorial Clinic and the gay community in STD prevention and research with the City of Chicago's own programs. Ms. Laura Coats performed the arduous task of typing the many drafts of each chapter and kept smiling throughout. Messrs. William Fairweather and Robert Dowey prepared the figures and diagrams. And Mrs. Marian Shelby patiently read the entire manuscript in an attempt to provide clarity and stylistic consistency. Still, responsibility for any inaccuracies or inconsistencies must remain with the editors and individual contributors.

A complete listing of all the persons who have contributed either directly or indirectly to the collection of the information included in this work would take many pages. And yet, without the dedication of those persons, the study of STDs would still be in the dark ages, and all of the information regarding the diagnosis and treatment of homosexual male patients would not fill a single page. Therefore, this book is respectfully dedicated to all the men and women in the health care delivery system who are working so diligently on the diagnosis and treatment of sexually transmitted diseases.

David G. Ostrow
Chicago, Illinois

Terry Alan Sandholzer
San Francisco, California

Yehudi M. Felman
Brooklyn, New York

Contents

I. General Considerations

II. Bacterial Sexually Transmitted Diseases

III. Enterically Transmitted Diseases

IV. Anal Disorders

V. Dermatologic Disorders

VI. Acquired Immune Disorders

16. Kaposi's Sarcoma and Other Rare Malignancies in Homosexual Men

YEHUDI M. FELMAN, DAVID G. OSTROW, AND
TERRY ALAN SANDHOLZER

VII. A Special Consideration

General Considerations

General Considerations

Factors Affecting the Incidence and Management of Sexually Transmitted Diseases in Homosexual Men

TERRY ALAN SANDHOLZER

According to Kinsey, between 4% and 10% of the adult white male population practice homosexuality exclusively for a significant portion of their lives.[1] This population is held responsible for at least a third of the national cases of infectious syphilis[2] and a high, although unknown, number of cases of gonorrhea. Further, among homosexual men, a continuously increasing incidence of hepatitis A and B,[3,4] shigellosis and giardiasis,[5] and herpes[6] has been reported. Since 1981, a totally new set of diseases relating to immune deficiency dysfunction has been linked to patterns of homosexual male behavior. These epidemics and near-epidemics of heretofore low-incidence diseases within the homosexual male population are causing anxious concern among the health care professionals most responsible for their control and present a challenge to existing clinical protocols, medical curricula, attitudes toward homosexuality and sexually transmitted diseases (STDs), and health care funding policies.

THE SCOPE OF THE PROBLEM

Each year, on a worldwide basis, over 250 million persons are infected with gonorrhea and over 50 million persons are infected with syphilis, as esti-

TERRY ALAN SANDHOLZER ● San Francisco, California 94117.

mated by the World Health Organization.[7] Webster claims that only 10% of all gonorrhea infections[8] and only 12% of the cases of infectious syphilis[9] are reported. In the United States in 1977, about 25,000 cases of infectious syphilis were reported to the Centers for Disease Control (CDC) in Atlanta.[7] Because these figures reflect only reported cases, the true incidence is probably much higher. The CDC estimate nearly 3 million cases of gonorrhea in the United States in 1977 and 400,000 cases of syphilis that required treatment.

For syphilis, the statistics are considered somewhat more accurate than those for gonorrhea concerning homosexual male incidence. Evidence from New York City, for example, indicates that syphilis is epidemic in homosexual males while it has decreased in the heterosexual population. In New York City in 1977, 55% of the primary, secondary, and early latent syphilis cases that were reported occurred in homosexual males. Moreover, while there was a decrease of 15% in the overall number of cases of infectious syphilis, a greater than 15% increase occurred within the homosexual male community. Extrapolation of existing data yields an estimation that homosexual men may account for as many as 50% of the reported cases of syphilis in large cities and about a third of the cases nationally.[2] The homosexual male is said to be at ten times greater risk of contracting syphilis than the heterosexual male.[11,12]

The actual incidence of gonococcal infections in homosexual men is not known. About 600,000 of all reported cases (60%) occur in men, and this may indicate a larger homosexual male than heterosexual incidence.[10]

The true national incidence of these two diseases can only be extrapolative for many reasons. Most states have reporting laws for cases of gonorrhea and syphilis and national figures reflect the degree of compliance. Each state total is based upon reports of positive findings from laboratories, public venereal disease (VD) clinics, hospitals, emergency rooms, and physicians in the private sector. Weekly, monthly, and quarterly reports are sent to the CDC for national computation and then to the World Health Organization for international inclusion.

Private physicians, who treat at least 80% of all STDs,[8] tend to underreport cases of gonorrhea and syphilis, particularly gonorrhea. The reason is that bacteriologic confirmation, which often requires the aid of an outside laboratory and thus increases the chance of entering the case into national computation, is rarely done. For the male presenting with urethral gonorrhea the private practitioner can diagnose the disease by the patient's painful discharge, confirm its presence in the office by a gram stain smear, and treat the patient on his first visit.

A large reservoir exists of asymptomatic men with STDs who are undetected carriers of disease. On the other side, the individual repeatedly infected with STDs skews existing data and probably represents a sizable proportion of STD patients in the population at large.[13] Consequently, not only are national statistics an estimate at best, but sexual contacts of infected individuals and their sexual contacts in turn remain at large to infect still others, and asymptomatic carriers remain undetected for long periods of time.

Of epidemiologic significance is that physicians often acquiesce in the patient's request to remain anonymous to board of health contact tracers. The patient, through ignorance or misinformation, many times believes that contact tracing will eventually reveal his homosexuality to employer or family (if he lives at home with parents or wife) and fears the consequences (e.g., loss of job, family turmoil) if this disclosure is made. The physician, who could explain the confidentiality of contact tracing, often does not, perhaps honoring the patient's plea for anonymity with at most a casual suggestion that the patient tell his sexual partner to "get checked." Also, for the physician who grants this request there is one less form to complete. In this way, an indeterminate number of cases are again lost to national computation.

Interestingly, there are reports from irate patients of some unscrupulous physicians who, in effect, blackmail the homosexual male who presents with an STD. These physicians have charged exorbitant fees for treatment of gonorrhea in return for a guarantee that there would be no report to board of health "authorities."[14] These two examples of why STDs are not reported represent misguided sympathies and unprincipled practices, both of which undermine the control of STDs and demonstrate a thorough lack of understanding of the importance of epidemiologic concerns.

Several factors have been implicated in the epidemics of STDs among homosexual men. Perhaps leading the list is gay liberation, which began nationally in the late 1960s and which allowed a structured, political viability to an oppressed minority. The liberation movement has allowed and encouraged homosexual men and women to express their sexuality openly and to overcome fear of social and political censure for their preference. Increasingly through the 1970s meeting places of all types sprang up to accommodate this freedom. Bars, discos, and bathhouses as well as nonsexually oriented meeting places opened to obviate the need for clandestine sexual activity. Homosexual men were free to be sexually active, and with this freedom were subject to the same consequences—except unwanted pregnancies and abortions—as the entire sexually active population, regardless of sexual orientation.

Charges of promiscuity directed at the entire homosexual male population can no more be documented than similar charges directed at heterosexual or bisexual individuals. The anonymity of the sexual partners of many members of the "single" homosexually active male population, however, does contribute to STD incidence, since contact tracing to interrupt the cycle of transmission is rendered almost impossible. Also, the particular sexual practices of anilinction, fellatio, and anal intercourse by homosexual men are the major risk factors toward the spread of infection. According to Vaisrub,[15] homosexual men are at this greater risk since during sexual activity each partner's penile epithelium and urethral mucosa are exposed to deep-seated pathogens in any body orifice. Being excellent transmitters of infection, the penis and urethra are responsible for transferring these pathogens, especially during ejaculation.

Another important aspect of the high STD incidence in homosexual men is improper or overlooked diagnosis as a result of lack of professional training in STDs and poor physician–patient communications. Failure by the physician to obtain a sexual practices history unites with a failure by the patient to reveal his sexual preference and practices to compound underreporting. This lack of communication on both sides of the examination table reveals the regrettable cycle of poor physician attitudes toward sexuality and homosexuality, guilt by the patient, and a lack of information and education in both parties concerning STDs. In the physician–patient relationship, the results are sometimes unfortunate and expensive.

SEX EDUCATION

While little is known about the attitudes of individual physicians concerning human sexuality, some evidence exists of their education and knowledge of the subject. Courses in human sexuality in medical schools, which would by definition have to include instruction on sexual dysfunction, homosexuality, heterosexuality, and bisexuality, are not commonly taught and are rarely compulsory.

Pauly[16] claims that 83% of physicians have no formal training in human sexuality and suggests that medical educators consider sexual intercourse necessary only for procreation. Masters and Johnson[17] report that physicians know no more (or less) than other college graduates and that they are biased by the same misconceptions and fallacies concerning sexuality as are nonmedical persons. Ernest Jones[18] has written, "I have often wondered why sexual topics are often euphemistically termed 'medical questions' since doctors receive no technical instruction whatsoever concerning them." A lack of instruction necessarily affects attitudes. As James and Lord[19] state, "the ability of the doctor to distinguish between his own personal ideological or moral viewpoint and an opinion based on actual and available information may determine whether or not a patient is led incorrectly to feel abnormal and hence guilty."

STD EDUCATION

Coupled with the lack of instruction in human sexuality is the gross lack of training physicians in the United States receive in the management of STDs. In the United States, according to Harris,[20] "a major contributory factor in the failure to reduce the incidence of infectious syphilis has been the professional ignorance of the medical profession." Harris ascribes this failure to the "wave of complacency" of a postpenicillin era that relegated syphilis to a minor position. Webster[8] concurs that "general practitioners have not received adequate training in control of [STDs] and are not easily able to obtain laboratory facilities for diagnostic procedures" and that "there is therefore a tendency to treat empirically without making an accurate diagnosis." Reviewing the curricula of medical schools in the United States for the Pan-American Health Organization, Webster reports that "teaching about venereal diseases was inadequate and frequently nonexistent. In some universities a maximum of two hours was set aside for teaching of syphilis, and gonorrhea was not mentioned. Occasionally, if the teachers were interested, gonorrhea might be discussed in the urological department," but there "was no integrated teaching about any of the other sexually transmitted diseases except in two or three medical schools where special programs existed."

The instruction about STD management that physicians do receive in medical school concerns the diseases as they present heterosexually, that is, penile and vaginal clinical presentations. And if the physician's report card for the management of STDs in the heterosexual population is poor, it is even more unsatisfactory in the homosexual population because of the different orifices used by the homosexual male for sexual activity. Consequently, an STD in the homosexual male may be overlooked or misdiagnosed, as was mentioned earlier. For example, unless a physician pursues questions about a patient's specific sexual practices, he might not consider anal gonococcal infection as part of the differential diagnosis to account for the patient's abdominal distress, mucous or blood stools, and mild diarrhea. Instead, he might escalate to colonoscopy, upper and lower GI series, and other unnecessary, costly, and hazardous invasive procedures. This is but one example that serves to emphasize the importance of training physicians to take a sexual practices history, as well as to be aware of the presence of a possible STD and of the differences in disease presentation in persons with other than a heterosexual orientation.*

---

* A study by Stamm et al.[21] has recently been published in which the authors surveyed 127 medical schools in the United States and Canada and showed that 69 (54%) were unaffiliated with any hospital or health department STD clinic for teaching purposes. Further, clinical training for students was absent in 87 (68.5%) of the schools, and 96 (75.6%) offered no training for residents. Stamm et al. showed that in the United States, even when training was available and offered, only 30% of medical students and 45% of residents participated, students receiving an average of six hours of instruction and residents receiving twelve hours. The awareness of inadequate medical education in venereology increases. Currently, The National Conference on Preventing Disease–Promoting Health recommends that by 1990 all medical schools be affiliated with an STD treatment facility and provide at least twenty hours of clinical experience for medical students and residents. If this proposal reaches fruition great strides in the control of STDs should result.

PHYSICIANS' ATTITUDES

The medical attitude toward homosexuality has changed from considering it a sin in the 19th century to classifying it as an illness in the 20th.[22] Not until the 1973 statement by the American Psychiatric Association (APA)[23] was homosexuality accepted as a viable sexual option. As perhaps the leader in this country in shaping medical attitudes toward homosexuality, the APA was the first medical organization to support and endorse openly the rights denied this population and to officially remove the stigma of disease from persons with same-sex preference.

Statements, however, do not control attitudes. A study by Levitt and Klausen,[24] whose results were confirmed by Nyberg and Alston,[25] demonstrated that the majority of white Americans do not approve of homosexual relations. Since physicians as well as nonmedical persons fall into this category, it is reasonable to assume that physicians are as prejudiced about homosexuality as is the population at large.

Two studies do afford an insight into individual physicians' attitudes about treating the homosexual male. The first study,[26] done in 1970, surveyed the attitudes of 937 Oregon physicians about treating homosexual males. Forty-eight percent of physicians reported "some degree of discomfort" when treating homosexual male patients. However, physicians acknowledged fewer negative feelings (5% "always" and 10% "often") than they attributed to "most [other] physicians." (This response reveals an interesting capacity of physicians for self-deception: "I have no negative feelings, but I'm certain my colleagues do.") The breakdown of attitudes by specialty revealed that psychiatrists have the most positive attitudes in treating homosexual males. Ninety-eight percent of the responders in this specialty stated that they "seldom" or "never" were affected by a patient's homosexual preference, followed by 81% of the internists and 70% of the general practitioners. The study also revealed a positive relationship between the physicians' attitudes toward treating the homosexual male and their personal feelings toward sexual problems in general.

A second more detailed study, completed by Golin[27] in 1978 for the American Medical Association, investigated the attitudes of 281 physicians toward treatment of STDs in homosexual males. Of the respondents, 90% of the colon and rectal surgeons, 81% of the public health physicians, 69% of the dermatologists, and 62% of the urologists stated that they are seeing more STDs in the homosexual male population. This fact accounts for the overall awareness of 39% of the respondents that the increases in STDs were attributable to this population.

To a question concerning the taking of a history of sexual practices from patients in whom they suspect an STD, 92% of the general and family practitioners and 81% of the internists stated that they include questions about sexual practices during history taking. Fifty-one percent of the public health physicians and 53% of the urologists stated that they include such questions. Also, 30% of the pediatricians, 30% of the colon and rectal surgeons, and 13.6% of the dermatologists said that they included questions on sexual practices. When asked how they feel about treating homosexual patients, 61% responded "no negative feelings," 33.5% revealed that they are "sometimes uncomfortable," 1.8% stated that they were "often uncomfortable," and 3.7% did not respond to this question.

When asked if their attitudes prompted referral of a homosexual patient to another physician, 93.7% said that they did not prefer that the patient visit another physician. Interestingly, 83.7% of the responding physicians felt that homosexual male patients hesitate to seek medical care because of physician disapproval, 13.8% felt that this statement was untrue, and 2.6% said that they did not know.

When asked, "Do you personally think homosexual male patients would be better off cared for by a homosexual physician," 17.5% said "yes," 79.1% said "no," and 3.3% did not respond.

Concerning training in medical schools for STDs and human sexuality, 84.1% of the physicians stated that they had not received adequate education, 13.8% thought their education was adequate, and 2.1% did not answer.

Both studies indicate that the views of the private physician toward homosexuality and STD management in homosexual males are far more liberal than expected from epidemiologic statistics, which indicate the opposite. In the second of these studies, the most striking finding was that the majority of the responding physicians felt that education about human sexuality and homosexuality had been inadequate during their training. The 84% of the physicians in the second study who felt their training inadequate agree with the 83% of the physician population cited by Pauly who received no formal training whatsoever.

That the majority of the physicians responded positively to sexual practices history taking is probably an indication that they wish to do it but are inexperienced in this matter, or that they ask questions but not necessarily all pertinent questions.

One point is clear from these studies. Physicians are concerned about the lack of training in human sexuality and STDs regardless of their personal prejudices toward individuals whose mores and sexual preferences differ from their own. Many believe that a change in attitude is not what is needed, but rather an ability by physicians and medical students to "tolerate" different sexual preferences even if they do not "accept" them.[28,29] Surely, this is a first step and this approach to attitudinal modification appears to be growing among concerned physicians and educators.

FUNDING FOR STD CONTROL

If physician attitudes seem to be increasingly positive toward the treatment of STDs in the general population and also in the homosexual male population, then other factors besides inadequate medical education must contribute to the inability of the health care system to control the epidemics that currently confront it. Other factors of primary importance are funding and the current health care philosophy that dominates policy.

The federal budget for VD control as administered by the CDC for such programs as consultation visits, screening programs, education and research grants, was $42 million for 1978, up from $35 million in 1977.[10] The amounts of federal funds for VD control have since leveled off and even declined if adjusted for inflation: $39 million in 1979, $47.8 million in 1980, $47.6 million in 1981, $42.75 million in 1982, and a requested $45.6 million in the 1983 budget.[30] These amounts are grossly inadequate, not only in terms of STD statistics, but also in terms of the astounding costs of related health care. We know, for example, that gonorrhea is the most common infectious disease in the country. Annually, $250 million is spent for the treatment of complications of gonococcal pelvic inflammatory disease in women, which accounts for 175,000 hospital admissions.[8] Each year, about $50 million is spent to treat and house the syphilitic insane. If a fraction of the amounts spent on treating complications were channelled into programs providing public education and prevention, it is likely that not only the incidence of STDs but also the overall cost to the country would decline.

And even if current funding is deemed appropriate, is it concentrated where the funds will do the most good? It is well known that the high-risk homosexual male population does not respond to methods of control that are successful within the heterosexual population. The homosexual male prefers to attend a clinic where he will be treated with understanding and a nonjudgmental attitude as well as receive thorough medical attention—criteria all too often lacking in the private sector and public health clinics. In facilities sponsored, operated, and staffed by homosexual men and women, attendance continually increases.[31] Yet community-sponsored clinics that treat homosexual males receive little, if any, local, state, or federal funding. Because these facilities fall outside the standard structure of public health policy, there seems little interest to change present priorities and grant them adequate and necessary funds. While the recent emergence of "new" and more life-threatening STD conditions, in particular the acquired immune deficiency syndrome and its associated diseases and opportunistic infections, deserves all the funding necessary for investigation and ultimate control, it must not divert attention and funding at both the governmental and private levels from control efforts for the traditional STDs.

FUTURE RESPONSIBILITIES

Whether or not separate facilities should be necessary for the homosexual male population for the treatment of STDs is an unanswered question. Surely, these facilities deserve to be an integral part of established VD control programs; their contributions to STD control so far tend to support their inclusion. Separatist programs do seem to be essential today, but one hopes that they may become an anachronism in the future.

Naturally, a great deal of the responsibility for the education of the homosexual male population rests with health care professionals and leaders from within the group. As homosexual men gain information concerning the risks of disease in specific sexual practices, it is to be hoped that they will alter these practices and so produce a decline in STD incidence. Whether or not behavior can be altered remains to be seen, but at least choices will be made by an informed population.

The education of physicians for better STD management and the improvement of policy governing health care funding for STD control and research require concentrated efforts. Only through a tough, realistic, and thorough reevaluation of all aspects of the total STD picture can lasting progress be made. Reorganization on a national scale of existing programs and the institution of viable new approaches at local, state, and federal levels are mandatory if the current situation is to improve at all. The relevance of these needed reevaluations is painfully dramatized by the epidemics of AIDS diseases, whose control currently has insufficient support from the very agencies most concerned. The information contained in this volume is intended to promote increased awareness within the medical profession of the specific problems of STD education, diagnosis, management, and control. By this approach, the knowledge gained through community STD clinics can influence the entire health care system.

REFERENCES

1. Kinsey AC, Pomeroy WB, Martin CE: *Sexual Behavior in the Human Male.* Philadelphia, WB Saunders, 1948.
2. Felman YM, Riccardi NB: Incidence and epidemiology of sexually transmitted diseases. *Curr Ther Res* 26:665–674, 1979.
3. Corey L, Holmes KK: Sexual transmission of hepatitis in homosexual men: Incidence and mechanism. *N Engl J Med* 302:435–438, 1980.
4. Szmuness W, Much MI, Prince AM, et al: On the role of sexual behavior in the spread of hepatitis B infection. *Ann Intern Med* 83:489–495, 1975.
5. Felman YM, Nikitas JA: Sexually transmitted enteric pathogens in New York City. *NY State J Med* 79:1412–1413, 1979.
6. Ferrer R, Felman YM, Nikitas JA: Genital herpesvirus infections. *Sex Transm Dis Newslett* (City of New York) 1:01–04, 1978.
7. World Health Organization: World Health Statistics Report, 1978.
8. Webster B: The medical manpower situation in the United States in relation to the sexually transmitted diseases. *Br J Vener Dis* 52:94–96, 1975.
9. Webster B: Venereal disease control in the United States of America. *Br J Vener Dis* 46:406–411, 1970.
10. Sandholzer TA: STDs—Paradox of the sexual revolution (IMPACT section). *Am Med News,* October 27, 1978.
11. British Cooperative Group: Homosexuality and venereal disease in the United Kingdom. *Br J Vener Dis* 49:329–334, 1973.

12. Drusin LM, Magagna J, Yano K, et al: An epidemiologic study of sexually transmitted disease on a university campus. *Am J Epidemiol* 100:8–19, 1974.
13. Lundin RS, Wright MW, Scatliff JN: Behavioral and social characteristics of the patient with repeated venereal disease and his effect on statistics on venereal diseases. *Br J Vener Dis* 53(2):140–144, 1977.
14. Ronald St. John: Personal communication.
15. Vaisrub S: Homosexuality—A risk factor in infectious disease (Editorial). *JAMA* 238:1402, 1977.
16. Pauly IB, Goldstein SG: Prevalence of significant sexual problems in medical practice. *Med Asp Human Sexuality* 4:48–63, 1970.
17. Masters WH, Johnson VE: *Human Sexual Inadequacy*. Boston, Little, Brown, 1970.
18. Jones E: *Free Associations*. London, Hogarth Press, 1959, p 56.
19. James B, Lord DJ: Human sexuality and medical education. *Lancet* 2:560–563, 1974.
20. Harris JRW: Epidemiologic and social aspects [of syphilis], in Morton RS, Harris JRW (eds): *Recent Advances in Sexually Transmitted Diseases*. New York, Churchill Livingston, 1975, pp 94–95.
21. Stamm WE, Kaetz S, Holmes CK: Clinical training in venereology in the United States and Canada. *JAMA* 248:2020–2024, 1982.
22. Money J: Bisexual, homosexual, and heterosexual: Society, law, and medicine. *J Homosexuality* 2:229–233, 1977.
23. American Psychiatric Association, press release, 15 December 1973.
24. Levitt EE, Klausen AD Jr: Public attitudes toward homosexual behavior. *J Homosexuality* 1:29–43, 1974.
25. Nyberg KL, Alston JP: Analysis of public attitudes toward homosexual behavior. *J Homosexuality* 2:99–107, 1976–1977.
26. Pauly IB, Goldstein SG: Physicians' attitudes in treating male homosexuals. *Med Asp Human Sexuality* 4:26–45, 1970.
27. Golin CB: MDs assess problems in treating gays (IMPACT section). *Am Med News*, October 27, 1978.
28. Cade JD, Jessee WF: Sex education in American medical schools. *J Med Educ* 46:64–68, 1971.
29. Chez RA: Movies of human sexual response as learning aid for medical students. *J Med Educ* 46:977–981, 1971.
30. Joseph Miller, Acting Director, Venereal Disease Control Division, Centers for Disease Control: personal communication, November 10, 1982.
31. Ostrow DG, Shaskey DM: The experience of the Howard Brown Memorial Clinic of Chicago with sexually transmitted diseases. *Sex Transm Dis* 4:53–55, 1977.

Sexual Practices History

DAVID G. OSTROW and ALFRED OBERMAIER

A thorough sexual practices history (SPH) is an essential part of the examination of any patient with a real or potential sexually transmitted or related disease (STD). In fact, the well-informed practitioner is often guided in the choice of physical and laboratory examinations by information gained from the SPH. Yet it is a disturbing feature of the practice of medicine today that less and less emphasis is placed on careful and exact history-taking and that many practitioners deal with their own discomfort when sexual matters are in question by deleting the SPH or making a casual reference to "those matters." This chapter discusses some of the barriers to careful SPH-taking in a clinic or office, offers advice on how to make the SPH process both thorough and nonembarrassing to the examiner and the patient, offers specific approaches for making the SPH an educational process, and provides an outline for actual data gathering.

Table 1 lists the various specific sexual practices performed by homosexual men and the known STDs that are potentially transmissable through each practice. While the table is not exhaustive because "new" STDs continue to appear, it does provide a rational basis for collecting a detailed SPH and for patient education. For example, patients with frequent oral herpes ("cold sores") need to be reminded that they can transmit the infection to a partner's penis or rectum through orogenital or oroanal contact. Conversely, a patient complaining of rectal itching and relating a history of recent anilinction (passive) should have both darkfield and Tzanck smear examination of any rectal lesions present during an anoscopic exam.

The table also illustrates the wide range of sexually related diseases or

DAVID G. OSTROW ● Biological Psychiatry Program, Lakeside Veterans Administration Medical Center, and Departments of Psychiatry and Community Medicine, Northwestern University Medical School, Chicago, Illinois 60611; and Howard Brown Memorial Clinic, Chicago, Illinois 60616. ALFRED OBERMAIER ● Tucson Gay Health Project, Tucson, Arizona 85703.

TABLE 1. Specific Sexual Practices and Associated Disease Problems

Sexual practice (street terms/sample question)	Disease problems/organisms (listed in approximate order of frequency)
Close body contact	Pediculosis pubis Scabies Fungal infections
Masturbation (jacking off, beating off)	Physical abrasions
Douches, lubricants	Allergic reactions Rectal fatty tumors
Amyl and butyl nitrite ("poppers")	Amyl and butyl nitrite burns Contact dermatitis
Fellatio, active ("Do you suck your partner's penis?")	Physical abrasions Oral gonorrhea Herpes progenitalis I and II Nongonococcal pharyngitis (*Chlamydia* and others) Oral condyloma acuminatum Syphilis Hepatitis B Enteric diseases Lymphogranuloma venereum Granuloma inguinale Chancroid
Fellatio, passive ("Does your partner suck your penis?")	Physical abrasions Bites Scrapes Flu Virus Herpes type 1 and 2 Nongonococcal urethritis (*Chlamydia* and others) Gonorrhea *Neisseria meningitidis*
Anal intercourse, active ("Do you put your penis into your partner's rectum?")	Nongonococcal urethritis *Escherichia coli* Gonorrhea Hepatitis A, B, non-A/non-B Herpes Warts—molluscum and condyloma Syphilis Trichomoniasis Epididymitis/prostatitis Fungal infections

TABLE 1 *(Continued)*

Sexual practice (street terms/sample question)	Disease problems/organisms (listed in approximate order of frequency)
Anal intercourse, active *(Continued)*	Lymphogranuloma venereum Granuloma inguinale Chancroid Cytomegalovirus
Anal intercourse, passive ("Does your partner put his penis into your rectum?")	Physical proctitis Rectal gonorrhea Warts—condyloma and molluscum (rare) Nonspecific proctitis (*Chlamydia* and others) Herpes Syphilis Hepatitis B Trichomoniasis *Corynebacterium* Lymphogranuloma venereum Granuloma inguinale Chancroid Cytomegalovirus Candidiasis

Anilinction, active
(scat) ("Do you rim or do scat?")
	Enteric diseases
	  Shigellosis
	  Escherichia coli
	  Hepatitis A, B, non-A/non-B
	  Amebiasis
	  Giardiasis
	  Salmonellosis
	  Helminthic parasites
	Oral warts
	Oral gonorrhea
	Syphilis
	Lymphogranuloma venereum
	Granuloma inguinale
	Chancroid

Anilinction, passive ("Do you get rimmed?")	Rectal herpes Syphilis
Fist/finger insertion, passive ("Have you been fist-fucked?")	Internal scrapes Anal sphincter tears Perforations of the colon Acute abdomen
Fist/finger insertion, active ("Do you fist-fuck?")	Shigellosis *Escherichia coli* Salmonellosis Enteric diseases

(Continued)

TABLE 1 *(Continued)*

Sexual practice (street terms/sample question)	Disease problems/organisms (listed in approximate order of frequency)
Toys/apparatus (cock rings, dildoes, leather, tit clamps, etc.)	Allergic reactions to metal plastic, rubber, or leather Friction dermatitis Physical torsions Varicoceles Peyronie's disease Fungal infections Lost rectal objects Testicular strangulation
S&M, piercing, bondage ("Are you into S&M, piercing, or bondage?")	Lacerations Cutaneous infections Trauma
Group sex	*See* anilinction

pathological conditions that may be present in homosexual men and that are related, at least in part, to specific sexual practices. While this monograph is organized by etiologic agent, we cannot overemphasize that the work-up of homosexual male patients, in fact the work-up of any sexually active patient, is best guided by a thorough SPH based on anatomical sites and their specific role in sexual behavior.

Many readers are probably already asking the question that is most commonly encountered when lecturing on the question of STDs in homosexual males: "How do I know when a patient is homosexually oriented so that I can ask the right questions?" The answer to that question is that you cannot possibly know whether a patient is homosexual or heterosexual, and that simply asking a person about their sexual orientation can often lead to embarrassment and misleading information. It is not the sexual orientation per se, but the specific sexual practices engaged in by homosexual, heterosexual, or bisexual individuals that are important. For example, there are men who are married and consider themselves heterosexual who engage in passive oral or anal intercourse. The physician guided by a simple yes/no response to a question regarding sexual orientation will not examine the oropharynx or anorectum in these individuals. Furthermore, once the subject of sexual orientation has been dealt with in an all-or-none fashion, it is awkward and embarrassing to pry further. Therefore, a correlate to the observation that specific sexual practices are what matter in STDs is the dictum that an SPH must be based on questions about specific anatomical sites and their role in sexual activity if it is to be a useful and important part of the medical examination.

Table 2 presents in outline form a listing of the various sexual activities about which the practitioner should inquire, with sample questions listed under each category of activity. The list is designed to be both thorough and efficient. If an individual denies contact with same-sex partners, then many of the following questions can be omitted. Similarly, if an individual patient answers "yes" to a question concerning passive rectal intercourse, then more detailed questioning concerning frequency, types of lubricants, number of partners, and signs and symptoms of rectal disorders should follow. The list is based upon our experience at the Howard Brown Memorial Clinic (HBMC) in administering a detailed sexual practices questionnaire to over 1000 patients in the course of a study of hepatitis B prevalence and transmission (see Chapter 10). On the basis of that study and the subsequent work relating sexual practices to the risk of acquiring or transmitting specific STDs, the HBMC has been able to establish a relative hierarchy of sexual practices risk factors, and those questions providing the most information regarding risk status are grouped at the beginning of the outline. For example, individuals having sexual contact with multiple anonymous partners are at much greater risk for all STDs than are those having a single monogamous relationship. Therefore, the establishment of the number and type (steady, non-steady identified, or nonsteady anonymous) of sexual partners can serve as an important guide to subsequent questioning.

But where to begin an SPH? Many practitioners feel that they risk embarrassing both themselves and the patient by asking specific questions that imply anything other than monogamous heterosexual activity. This implies, of course, a moral judgment on the part of the physician, patient, or both, a topic discussed in detail in Chapter 1. In this context, it is important to emphasize the need to be nonjudgmental in both the form of one's questioning and the responses, both verbal and nonverbal, to the patient's answers. Questions phrased negatively ("You don't do *that*, do you?") are seen as judgmental and inhibit truthful responses to further questions. Similarly, arched eyebrows or a look of anxiety when a patient begins to discuss homosexual activities quickly communicates the physician's desire to move on to another subject and a presumed disapproval of the patient's life style.

Despite many statements about the need for nonjudgmental attitudes, individual practitioners may still feel uncomfortable when approaching the SPH. This discomfort may be due to moral or ethical feelings or simply to a lack of experience in dealing with sexual topics. Whatever the cause, one is doing a disservice to both one's patients and the profession of healing if the problem of performing a thorough and nonbiased SPH is not confronted directly. Omitting the SPH or postponing it to the end of the interview in the hope that the patient will spontaneously broach the subject and spare the physician the embarrassment of having to probe communicates the desire to avoid the topic to the same degree as the anxious behavior described above. It is imperative that the subject be

TABLE 2. Sexual Practices History Taking Outline[a]

I. Past history of STDs and homosexual activity

This information is useful in determining past risk of sexually transmitted disease and correlates strongly with present seropositivity to hepatitis B. Ask the patient if he has had any of the following, how often, and the date of last infection:

Gonorrhea
—of the mouth/throat
—of the urethra
—of the anus/rectum
Nonspecific urethritis
Nonspecific proctitis
Syphilis (1°, 2°, or 3°? Date and result of last VDRL)
Hepatitis (Was type determined? Date and result of last HBV serology)
Herpes—mouth, penis, scrotum, or anus
Amebiasis, giardiasis, dysentery, or other enteric disorders
Venereal warts
Scabies
Pediculosis

Further, ask the patient about past drug abuse or complications, reactions and allergies to penicillin or other antibiotics, history of trauma to the urogenital or anorectal regions, and present drug use and treatment regimens. The length of time of regular homosexual activity (i.e., sexual contact with another male at least monthly) is helpful in predicting overall exposure to the STDs described above.

II. Current sexual orientation and number of steady/nonsteady partners

This information determines the degree of risk to homosexually and heterosexually transmitted STDs and the frequency of STD examinations required.

"Approximately what percentage of your current sexual partners, that is, in the last four months, were male? Female? Could you say how many were male nonsteady partners (persons with whom you had sex only one or two times in that period)? Male steady partners (three or more times in that period)? Female nonsteady partners? Female steady partners?"

Percentage of sexual activity with men   _____
Number of male nonsteady partners in the last four months   _____
Number of male steady partners in the last four months   _____
   Total number of homosexual partners in the last four months   _____
Number of female nonsteady partners in the last four months   _____
   Total number of heterosexual partners in the last four months   _____
Total number of partners in the last four months   _____

III. Past sexual orientation and relationship history

"Is this [answer to questions under II above] typical of your sexual activity since beginning regular sexual activity?"   _____

TABLE 2 *(Continued)*

"If not, would you describe how the numbers, sex, and types (steady versus nonsteady) of your sexual partners have changed during the past ____ years?"   ____

"Have you been married? Have you had monogamous heterosexual or homosexual relationships or both in the past? What has been the duration of such relationships?"   ____

IVa. Regular sexual partners and specific activities with them

"Let's talk about your ____ (number) regular partners. Are any considered 'lovers'?"   ____

"Do you live with any of them?"   ____

"How often have you had sex with each one during the past four months"   ____

"Now let's talk about specific sexual practices with your steady partners (or lover) [see Section V below]."

IVb. Nonsteady sexual partners ("tricks") and specific practices with them.

"You mentioned ____ (number) nonsteady sexual partners in the last four months. I would like to go through the same set of questions concerning specific practices with this group as we did before for your steady sexual partners."

V. Specific sexual practices (go through with each steady and nonsteady partner as determined in Section IV)

Sexual activity and definition	Sample question
A. Orogenital activity	
Receptive	"Do you engage in fellatio (your partner inserting his penis into your mouth)?"
Insertive	"Do you insert your penis into your partner's mouth?"
Semen swallowed	"Do you swallow your partner's semen?
B. Anogenital activity	
Receptive	"Do you engage in receptive anal intercourse (your partner inserting his penis into your rectum)?"
Insertive	"Do you engage in insertive anal intercourse (you insert your penis into your partner's rectum)"
Ejaculation	"Do you come like this?"
Bleeding	"Do you ever notice rectal bleeding after anal intercourse?"
Douching	"Do you douche before intercourse? If so, what do you use (water, soap, additives)?"
Use of lubricants	"Do you use an anal lubricant? What kind?"
Rectal pain (rectal dysparunia)	"Have you experienced pain with rectal intercourse?"

(Continued)

TABLE 2 *(Continued)*

C. Oroanal activity (anilinction) Receptive ("rimming")	"Do you engage in rimming (your partner inserts his tongue into your anus)?"
Insertive	"Do you rim your partner (insert your tongue into his anus)?"
D. Mutual masturbation	"Do you come to orgasm by masturbating with this partner ('jerking off')? Has the semen entered your eye(s)? Do you use it as a lubricant for other sexual activities?"

VI. Other sexual activities

"Other activities associated with sex may be related to specific health problems. In the past four months, have you been involved in any of the following and, if so, how often?"

Practice	Alternative terms
Manual–anal insertion	Fist-fucking, fist fornication, fisting, hand-balling
Urination onto/into partner	Water sports, golden shower
Defecation, swallowing of feces, or both	Scat
Group sex (three or more persons)	Three-ways, orgies
Dildoes or other objects	
Sadomasochism	S&M, bondage and discipline (B&D),
Type, pain inflicted or received, means,	power and permission, toys
sexual response, fantasies	
Pierced body parts	Tit piercing, cock piercing
Anatomic site(s)	
Erectile aids	Cock rings
How often? How long in place?	

VII. Locations for casual ("recreational") sex with nonsteady partners ("tricks")

"Do you attend bathhouses? If so, about
how frequently?"   _____

"Do you visit homosexual bookstores or movie houses? If so, about how frequently?"   _____

"Do you visit bars with backrooms? If so, about how frequently?"   _____

"Do you visit tearooms, bushes, or other public sites for the purpose of having
sex? If so, about how frequently?"   _____

VIII. Drug use associated with sex

"Drug use, in association with sexual activities and by itself, can be an important factor in your health and in producing certain problems. Therefore, I would like to know how often you use each of the following":

Volatile nitrites ("poppers") (type)   _____

Marijuana ("grass")   _____

Quaaludes, barbiturates, or other sedatives   _____

TABLE 2   *(Continued)*

Preludin, amphetamines, or other stimulants   _____

Frequency of alcohol intake (number of nights per week)   _____

Average number of drinks per occasion   _____

MDA, LSD, DMT, phencyclidine ("angel dust"), or other hallucinogens   _____

IX. Sexual identification and adjustment

An important aspect of sexual practices and the degree of pleasure obtained from them is the way in which actual sexual performance is in harmony with the individual's sexual desires, fantasies, and expectations. While not a primary aspect of an SPH, information regarding your patient's attitudes concerning his sexual performance, gender identification, and satisfaction with his sexual orientation is often elicited during questioning. Failure to inquire about these issues may signal to your patient that you do not wish to deal with psychological issues, but rather wish to focus only on physiological aspects of sexual functioning. This bias will be unfortunate if your patient is experiencing psychological distress, especially if that distress is heightened by inquiries concerning sexual practices that may be the source of that distress. Therefore, it may be appropriate to include in a thorough SPH several questions concerning sexual identification and adjustment and to look for clues to difficulty in this area throughout the interviews.

Sexual orientation adjustment	"How comfortable are you with the pattern of sexual activities that you have described?"
Degree of pleasure derived from sex	"How pleasurable is sex to you?"
Sexual adequacy	"Are you satisfied with the frequency or intensity of your sexual activities? Do you have any concerns about the size, shape, or functioning of your genitals?"
Sexual attractiveness	"Do you feel that you are attractive to potential sexual partners?"

a For male patients indicating homosexual activity.

broached in as direct a manner as possible, a manner that deemphasizes the "special" nature of sexual behavior rather than highlighting it. We have found that putting the SPH into the general context of a social history greatly lessens both our own and our patients' anxiety about discussing sexual topics. In this context, questions about specific sexual behavior lose many of the connotations that make them difficult to deal with in the first place and can be seen in a light more directly related to their actual motivation—the uncovering of important clinically related information, rather than prying into "private" aspects of patients' lives. Specific questions can take the form of general inquiries into modes of behavior that may be related to clinical states: "To understand and treat problems that you may have, I need to know something about aspects of your life [-style] that may increase your chances of having certain diseases or health problems. These include travel to foreign countries; casual and regular sexual partners and the specific activities with each; any special diets and nonprescription medications; and the use of alcohol, caffeine, cigarettes, and other drugs."

Using an introductory comment of this type concerning the need for an in-depth understanding of your patients' behavior makes it relatively simple to begin obtaining the detailed SPH. Table 2 is not intended as a verbatim questionnaire but rather as the basis for the appropriate lines of further inquiry, with appropriate variations. The sample questions are provided simply as helpful hints; the physician's own personal style and vocabulary, as well as the patient's relative degree of comfort with sexual terminology, should determine the actual phraseology employed.

A final note of caution: If, after examining the following outline, you feel unable to ask the types of questions necessary to obtain a detailed SPH without undue embarrassment or moral indignation, then *don't*. Better to tell patients that you are uncomfortable with issues of sexuality, and homosexuality in particular, and refer them to a colleague or gay community clinic than to subject homosexual patients to the types of attitudes and embarrassment that have contributed to the epidemic of STDs in the first place.

Setting Up the Physician's Office for the Diagnosis and Treatment of Sexually Transmitted Diseases

DANIEL C. WILLIAM, JAMES A. NIKITAS, and DAVID G. OSTROW

With a small investment in time and funds, any primary care provider can equip the office and train office personnel to perform a large number of important dignostic and therapeutic interventions in the management of sexually transmitted diseases (STDs), as listed in Table 1. These investments will pay handsomely in the ability to diagnose accurately and thereby offer more precise treatment.

LIGHT SOURCES

By far the most important basic requirement for the diagnosis and treatment of any STD is a well-lit examining room. A brightly lit room with balanced fluorescent lights (or a natural daylight source) facilitates visual examination of

DANIEL C. WILLIAM ● Columbia University College of Physicians and Surgeons, New York, New York 10032; and St. Luke's–Roosevelt Hospital Center, New York, New York 10019.   JAMES A. NIKITAS ● Department of Dermatology, New York Medical College, Metropolitan Hospital Center, Valhalla, New York 10595.   DAVID G. OSTROW ● Biological Psychiatry Program, Lakeside Veterans Administration Medical Center, and Departments of Psychiatry and Community Medicine, Northwestern University Medical School, Chicago, Illinois 60611; and Howard Brown Memorial Clinic, Chicago, Illinois 60616.

TABLE 1.   STD Evaluation Outline

1. Frequency: Every three to six months.
2. Sexual practices and STD exposure history (See Chapter 2).
3. Physical examination: Vital signs, weight, skin, genitals, lymph nodes, oropharynx, anoscopy.
4. Laboratory testing: VDRL or RPR syphilis test, oral and rectal cultures for GC, stool for ova and parasites, hepatitis B serology (unless already known to be immune), baseline CBC with differential, viral serologies, and repeat CBC if indicated. Darkfield examination of any skin lesions, Gram's stain examination of urethral discharge.
5. Treatment: As indicated. See Appendix and individual chapters for regimens.
6. Follow-up: Test of cure for all infections following treatment and before patient resumes sexual activity.
7. Patient education: Discuss risks of sexual practices, treatment regimens, and precautions and need for sexual abstinence until effectiveness of treatment confirmed.

skin lesions, faint rashes, and the difficult-to-see nits and pediculosis commonly encountered in many patients with STDs. An important adjunct to a well-lit room is a high-intensity light source that can be easily manipulated. The authors prefer one of the commercially available headlights equipped with a focusing light source. These lights are available with both regular incandescent light sources and the new, more brilliant, halogen light sources. By using the focusing lens, a narrow light beam is produced that enables the practitioner to examine carefully oral cavities, intrarectal lesions by anoscopy, and faint skin lesions. Visual acuity can be further augmented by the use of a hand-held magnifying glass.

SUPPLIES

The homosexual male patient who presents with any rectal complaint should be examined with a small anoscope. Clear plastic disposable anoscopes are preferable, as they are light, easy to manipulate, and easily disposed of. The use of reusable stainless steel anoscopes is not recommended since fecal contamination can readily transmit a multitude of enteric diseases, including hepatitis A and B, amebiasis, giardiasis, and shigellosis, unless the anoscopes are meticulously cleansed and sterilized. These time-consuming procedures are unnecessary if the readily available, inexpensive disposable anoscopes are used.

Any of the commercially available sterile lubricants can be used to facilitate anoscope insertion. Remember, however, to obtain gonorrhea cultures before performing anoscopy, since most of the sterile lubricating jellies contain bacteriosidal or bacteriostatic agents, which may inhibit the growth of the gonococcus.

A large supply of clean glass slides and coverslips should be kept within arm's length of the examining table. Not uncommonly, while performing anoscopies, exudates may be seen that can be picked up on a swab and smeared onto a slide without having to interrupt the anoscopic exam. The glass slides can also be used when examining skin rashes to differentiate erythematous blanching lesions from true macular lesions.

Both sterile and nonsterile cotton-tipped applicators and applicator sticks should be within arm's length of the examining table as well. Cotton-tipped applicators are useful in drying or cleansing intrarectal condylomata or other lesions, and for obtaining smear specimens from weeping dermatologic lesions, urethral discharges, and exudative proctitis. The plain wooden applicators are used primarily for application of podophyllum or other caustic materials to condylomata accuminata. Sterile cotton-tipped applicators are also necessary to obtain gonorrhea and bacteriologic cultures of stool and skin.

Other miscellaneous supplies for each examination room include wooden tongue depressors, a large supply of vinyl or plastic disposable gloves, and gauze pads. A small plastic squeeze bottle containing normal saline has many simple and important uses. Saline is used to wet and thereby lubricate the cotton-tipped applicator when obtaining rectal cultures, and it is especially useful for the tight-sphinctered anxious patient or in the patient with painful proctitis, for whom any rectal manipulation is extremely uncomfortable. Saline-impregnated gauze pads are useful for cleansing and abrading lesions prior to darkfield examination. Fine scissors and a skin biopsy punch are required if biopsies for Kaposi's sarcoma are to be performed in the practitioner's office.

GRAM-STAINING FACILITY

The basic laboratory should include a good light microscope with low, "high dry," and oil immersion objectives. A gram-staining kit is mandatory for use in conjunction with the microscope. A simple gram-staining kit can be assembled by purchasing four plastic squeeze bottles and filling them with gentian violet, Gram's iodine, acetone–alcohol, and safranin. A small alcohol wick burner is a simple, inexpensive flame source for offices not equipped with a gas jet and bunsen burner. The alcohol burner is used to fix slides prior to gram staining. Gram-stained smears are useful for differentiating gonococcal urethritis from nongonococcal urethritis and for the presumptive diagnosis of symptomatic rectal gonorrhea where an exudate is visualized by anoscopy. Additionally, weeping skin lesions can be gram-stained in order to differentiate between candidiasis and impetigo.

The gram-staining process does not have to be performed in a sink. An excellent sink substitute consists of a small deep-set pan such as can be purchased in any department or variety store. An inexpensive cake rack is placed over the pan and provides an excellent support for the glass slides while staining them. The rapid gram-staining technique takes only seconds to perform for any given slide. A large plastic squeeze bottle filled with tap water suffices for washing off the stains after each step of the gram-staining process. The wet gram-stained slides are then dried with an absorbent paper, available in pads. An inexpensive pair of forceps is useful to keep the fingers clean during the staning process. All gram-stained smears are examined under oil immersion. The oil can be contained in a small test tube and set in a test tube rack, ready for application to the slide by means of a wooden applicator stick.

A small bottle of 10% potassium hydroxide is useful when examining skin scrapings. A standard laboratory centrifuge is also necessary to separate sera when performing any serologic tests. The same centrifuge is used for spinning urine to obtain sediment for microscopic examination.

GONORRHEA DIAGNOSIS

Each of the more common STDs requires a small amount of specialty equipment to facilitate its diagnosis. For gonorrhea, in addition to obtaining gram-stained smears, a suitable culturing system can be employed to perform bacteriologic testing readily in the physician's office. A variety of different culturing systems are available; the choice depends upon the volume of specimens obtained. The JEMBEC® Plate system offers the most advantages and is the least expensive for offices with large volumes of specimens. The heart of the system is a JEMBEC Plate, which is basically a small square plastic plate with a built-in well in which a CO_2-generating tablet is inserted at the time of obtaining the culture. Because of the relatively large surface area of the plate, each plate can be subdivided into two or three divisions, and multisite cultures from one patient can be performed on one plate. The plates need to be warmed prior to culturing. Once the plate receives the material for culture, it is covered and inserted into a plastic zip lock bag and incubated in a standard bacteriologic-grade incubator at 37°C. For smaller-volume practices, the JEMBEC Plate containing the material for culture can be transported to a commerical laboratory for processing.

Persons wishing to read their own plates must examine them at twenty-four hours and forty-eight hours of incubation. Fresh oxidase reagent is flooded onto the small typical mucoid translucent colonies of the gonococcus. A *presumptive* diagnosis of gonorrhea can be made upon the appearance of the characteristic dark-purple color change of oxidase reagent. All oxidase-positive colonies should be smeared onto a glass slide and gram-stained to confirm the gram-negative diplococcal morphology. Caution must be used in interpreting oxidase-positive colonies, especially from pharyngeal or rectal cultures, since *Neisseria menin-*

gitidis can often appear similar to the gonococcus. Sugar fermentation reactions are necessary for a positive differentiation of *Neisseria gonorrhoeae* from *Neisseria meningitidis*. In those male patients without a spontaneous urethral discharge, both cultures and urethral smears must be obtained, using a special thin calcium-alginate swab called a Calgiswab®. This swab is essential for men with small meatal openings, since the standard cotton-tipped applicator is simply too large for adequate intraurethral sampling. The calcium alginate swab is also used for obtaining all urethral cultures for tests of cure, since an intraurethral specimen is mandatory in the absence of frank penile discharge. Thin plastic loops are also useful for intraurethral sampling.

SYPHILIS DIAGNOSIS

The diagnosis of syphilis is made by clinical signs and symptoms as well as laboratory confirmation. Serologic confirmation of syphilis relies on the nontreponemal serologic tests as well as the highly specific treponemal tests. A variety of commercially available kits allow private physicians to perform one of several nontreponemal screening tests in the office setting. These tests are especially useful in patients without prior history of syphilis who present with typical signs and symptoms of either primary or secondary disease. They are also indicated in contacts to known cases of infectious syphilis. The rapid plasma reagin (RPR) diagnostic kit requires little formal training to be used accurately. The simplest RPR kit consists of a hand-held card that is manually rotated for several minutes. Other kits utilize an electric rotator platform to mix the sera precisely with the test reagent. All specimens with a postive RPR screening test should be sent to the laboratory for a titered Venereal Disease Research Laboratory test. Darkfield testing can also be performed with relative ease in the office setting. The equipment necessary for darkfield testing includes the darkfield condenser and a funneled objective with an iris diaphragm for the microscope.

Suspected syphilis lesions should be carefully cleansed with normal saline and should be free of any cellular debris prior to darkfield examination. To obtain sera from the lesion, a simple suction apparatus can be assembled using a 10-cc syringe connected by rubber tubing to a 5-cc syringe with the plunger removed. By applying the plungerless syringe to the lesion, and applying negative pressure to the second syringe and rubber tubing over the course of perhaps one minute, enough sera is obtained from the lesion to be examined by darkfield microscopy. Examiners are cautioned to be certain that the patient has not been taking either systemic or local antimicrobials, which may yield false-negative results. Disposable plastic gloves should be worn during this and any other procedure involving sera, blood, or secretions.

DIAGNOSIS OF CHLAMYDIAL AND VIRAL STDs

Definitive diagnosis of chlamydial and viral infections is not within the capabilities of the physician's private office, for these organisms require special culture media or cell culture procedures, such as complement-fixation immunofluorescence. Office diagnosis of chlamydial and viral infections must thus depend on the clinical impression, and for some diseases, on the direct microscopic examination of the stained smear or biopsy. Definitive diagnosis depends upon a central laboratory equipped and staffed to perform such work on specimens from the patient submitted by the physician. We describe here the procedures for preliminary diagnosis and preparation of samples for submission to a specialized laboratory for definitive diagnosis.

Chlamydial Infections (Nongonococcal Urethritis and Lymphogranuloma Venereum)

As the name implies, nongonococcal urethritis (NGU) is an inflammation of the urethra from which *Neisseria gonorrhoeae* has been excluded as the etiologic agent (Chapter 6). Although the etiology of this infection is not completely known, certain strains of *Chlamydia trachomatis* are often associated with NGU. Definitive diagnosis depends upon isolation of the organism in cell culture. The discharge is collected on an endourethral swab, which is then placed in an antimicrobial transport medium and sent within two hours to the central laboratory. If this is impossible the swab can be stored at $-70°C$.

In actual practice, however, diagnosis of NGU is made by the exclusion of the gonococcus, *Trichomonas,* and *Candida.* The gram-stained slide will show four or more polymorphonuclear leukocytes per oil immersion field ($\times 1000$), few commensal bacteria, and an occasional epithelial cell.

A complement fixation serologic test for the detection of chlamydial antibodies is particularly useful in the diagnosis of lymphogranuloma venereum (LGV). LGV is caused by serotypes L1, L2, and L3 of *C. trachomatis.* The diagnosis of LGV is suggested by the clinical picture, particularly the lymphadenopathy and a positive serologic test. The most widely used serologic test is the LGV-complement-fixation (CF) test. Single-point titers greater than 1 : 64 are highly supportive of LGV; any titer above 1 : 16 is considered significant evidence of exposure to any serotype of *Chlamydia.*

If culture is deemed necessary, the aspirate of a fluctuant bubo is the best specimen. When urethritis is present, the mucous membrane should be vigorously swabbed. The swab or aspirate is transported to the laboratory in a medium containing broad-spectrum antibacterials that will not inhibit the growth of *Chlamydia.* Aminoglycosides and fungicides may be used. If the specimens cannot be processed immediately (within two hours) they must be refrigerated, and if not processed within twenty-four hours they must be frozen at -60 to $-70°C$. On the way to the laboratory such specimens should be packed in dry ice. Sera for serologic tests are stored in the freezer until sent to a specialized diagnostic laboratory.

Genital Herpes

Genital herpes is caused by herpes simplex virus types 1 and 2. The diagnosis is usually arrived at on clinical grounds, but laboratory tests are available for both office and laboratory identification of the organism. The Tzanck smear, which demonstrates morphological changes in infected cells of the lesions, can easily be performed in the physician's office. Culture of the virus and serologic methods require a well-equipped and -staffed laboratory.

The Tzanck smear is prepared by scraping the base of an unruptured vesicle, fixing the specimen on the slide with methanol, and staining with Wright's or Giemsa stain for three minutes. After washing with water and drying, the smear is examined for large, multinucleated, giant cells.

Specimens for definitive diagnosis are obtained with a swab from an open herpetic skin (or other) lesion. The specimen need not be frozen as it will survive transportation when chilled in a medium containing charcoal and agarose. However, if prolonged storage of HSV is necessary, it must be kept at $-60°C$. Serologic tests (generally the complement-fixation test) are performed on paired sera taken at least two weeks apart. A fourfold rise in antibody titer will provide evidence of a primary HSV infection, but is of limited usefulness in the diagnosis of recurrent or latent infection.

Molluscum Contagiosum

Molluscum contagiosum is a benign, often asymptomatic viral infection of the skin and mucous membranes. It is primarily found in children, in whom it usually presents as umbilicated, smooth-surfaced, spherical papules on the face, trunk, and extremities. In sexually active adults, the lesions are usually found on the genitala and adjacent areas. Clinically, molluscum contagiosum is usually diagnosed by the presence of pearly, umbilicated papules from which a plug of caseous material may be extruded. Microscopic examination of Giemsa-stained extruded material will show large characteristic cytoplasmic inclusion bodies.

Cytomegalovirus Infection

Cytomegalovirus (CMV) infection, or cytomegalic inclusion disease, may be acquired congenitally, at the time of delivery, or later in life. In the adult, CMV infection may cause a febrile illness resembling infectious mononucleosis.

The virus has been detected in oral, anal, and urogenital secretions (saliva, feces, semen, urine, milk), and blood has been used to transmit the disease to susceptible individuals. In sexually active adults, transmission is often by the sexual route.

CMV is morphologically indistinguishable from the other herpes viruses (herpes simplex, varicella–zoster, and Epstein–Barr virus) and like them has the ability to remain latent or persistent in the host following infection. Viral excretion can occur for months and years. However, CMV differs antigenically from the other viruses of the groups and can thus be serologically identified. The CMV virus is also species-specific, and human isolates will grow only in human cell cultures.

The definitive method for the diagnosis of CMV infection is direct isolation of virus in human fibroblastic tissue culture from urine, blood, upper respiratory tract, saliva, semen, or biopsy specimens. In the office, however, the demonstration of large nuclear inclusions in the epithelial cells obtained from centrifuged urine specimens may be useful in establishing the diagnosis in a limited number of cases. The cells, affixed to a slide, may be stained with Giemsa, hematoxylin–eosin, or Papanicolaou stain. Unfortunately, although this technique is easy to perform, it is quite insensitive and is of limited value when compared with viral culture and isolation by a specialized diagnostic laboratory.

Serologic techniques are also employed to confirm the diagnosis of CMV infection. A fourfold or greater rise in antibody titer between acute and convalescent serum samples confirms the diagnosis of CMV infection. Complement fixation is the most practical and easily performed test, although other serologic tests are available. Acute and convalescent sera must be sent to the laboratory in the frozen state.

Condylomata Acuminata (Venereal Warts)

Condylomata acuminata, or genital warts, are sexually transmitted lesions caused by a papilloma virus. The diagnosis of condylomata acuminata is made clinically by the appearance of the lesions, which are usually multiple and polymorphic and which may coalesce into large masses. Venereal warts must be differentiated from other growths and lesions. Among these are the pearly penile papules, condylomata lata, carcinoma, benign neoplasms, and donovanosis. Biopsy (requiring a surgical pathology laboratory) may often be advised or necessary, especially with the more extensive or rapidly growing lesions.

TREATMENT OF CONDYLOMATA ACUMINATA

The treatment of condylomata acuminata requires relatively simple office equipment. A small supply of 25% tincture of podophyllum in benzoin is the primary treatment for venereal warts. The podophyllum is best stored in heavy, small, wide-mouthed amber jars to prevent accidental spills. Other chemotherapeutic agents such as bichloracetic acid and trichloracetic acid are useful adjuncts. A wall-mounted hyfrecator can be used to electrodesiccate selected condylomata. A suitable local anesthetic, such as 2% lidocaine, and a suitable small-gauge needle and syringe are needed to anesthetize these lesions locally. Prior to any destructive surgery, lesions should be cleansed with a suitable antiseptic, such as Betadine® solution. Larger warts can sometimes be surgically excised in the office if the physician is comfortable performing minor surgery. A small supply of surgical tools, including scalpels and disposable scalpel blades, hemostats, forceps, and tissue clamps, can be kept in a surgical sterilizing solution. Cryosurgery is also popular, but requires expensive equipment and may be less effective than surgical or electrodesiccation procedures (Chapter 11).

MEDICATIONS

A variety of medications should be stocked to treat the more common STDs. Benzathine penicillin G (Bicillin L-A®) is available in sterile cartridge needles (Tubex®) in either the 1.2 million-unit or 2.4 million-unit dosages. Benzathine penicillin G is appropriately used for the treatment of early syphilis infections. Aqueous procaine penicillin G (APPG) (Wycillin®, Crysticillin®, Duracillin®) is used for the treatment of uncomplicated gonorrhea. APPG is available in 10-cc vials of 600,000 units per cubic centimeter. Five-cubic-centimeter syringes with 1.5-in. 20-gauge needles are necessary for the deep intramuscular injection of APPG. Urethral and rectal gonorrhea can be treated with oral ampicillin, or with amoxicillin, which should also be kept in supply. A supply of probenecid as 500 mg tablets is necessary to augment APPG, ampicillin, or amoxicillin treatment regimens. Spectinomycin hydrochloride (Trobicin®) is available in a 2-g individual dosage form for administration to patients who are gonorrhea treatment failures. Immune serum globulin (gamma globulin) should be stocked for the treatment of contacts of patients with hepatitis A. Tetracycline hydrochloride in 250-mg and 500-mg capsules is necessary for the treatment of nongonococcal urethritis and may be stocked as well. Physicians seeing large numbers of homosexually active patients may wish to keep limited supplies of the hepatitis B vaccine (Heptavax B®) in stock. However, the need to perform serologic testing prior to vaccination and the limited shelf-life and high expense of the vaccine made ordering of vials as needed preferable in most instances.

Emergency Medications and Supplies

Physicians using injectable medications must be prepared to manage severe allergic reactions following the administration of antibiotics. Emergency medications—including epinephrine, aminophyllin, hydrocortisone, injectable diazepam, injectable phenobarbital, intravenous setups, intravenous saline, and adequate needles and syringes—must always be immediately available. Other emergency equipment—including tourniquets, airways, oxygen, and ambubags—should be kept with the emergency supplies. All office staff should have some basic training in recognizing and managing acute medical emergencies. Routine periodic inventories of the emergency medical equipment are necessary to ensure their immediate availability.

PRECAUTIONS IN THE HANDLING OF PATIENTS AND SPECIMENS

Because of the endemic nature of hepatitis B, CMV, herpes, and other viral infections among patients seeking diagnosis and treatment for STDs, as well as the potential infectivity of blood samples for acquired immunodeficiency syndrome (AIDS) (see Chapters 16 and 17), blood handling precautions should always be taken. These include the use of a new set of disposable gloves with each patient and careful handling of blood, sera, biopsy, urine, feces, or other clinical samples. In addition, the Centers for Disease Control have recently proposed the following guidelines in the providing of care to AIDS or pre-AIDS patients[1]:

1. Extraordinary care must be taken to avoid accidental wounds from sharp instruments contaminated with potentially infectious material and to avoid contact of open skin lesions with material from AIDS patients.
2. Gloves should be worn when handling blood specimens, blood-soiled items, body fluids, excretions, and secretions, as well as surfaces, materials, and objects exposed to them.
3. Gowns should be worn when clothing may be soiled with body fluids, blood, secretions, or excretions.
4. Hands should be washed after removing gowns and gloves and before leaving the rooms of known or suspected AIDS patients. Hands should also be washed thoroughly and immediately if they become contaminated with blood.
5. Blood and other specimens should be labeled prominently with a special warning, such as "Blood Precautions" or "AIDS Precautions." If the outside of the specimen container is visibly contaminated with blood, it should be cleaned with a disinfectant [such as a 1 : 10 dilution of 5.25% sodium hypochlorite (household bleach) with water]. All blood specimens should be placed in a second container, such as an impervious bag, for transport. The container or bag should be examined carefully for leaks or cracks.

6. Blood spills should be cleaned up promptly with a disinfectant solution, such as sodium hypochlorite (see above).
7. Articles soiled with blood should be placed in an impervious bag prominently labeled "AIDS Precautions" or "Blood Precautions" before being sent for reprocessing or disposal. Alternatively, such contaminated items may be placed in plastic bags of a particular color designated solely for disposal of infectious wastes by the hospital. Disposable items should be incinerated or disposed of in accord with the hospital's policies for disposal of infectious wastes. Reusable items should be reprocessed in accord with hospital policies for hepatitis-B-virus-contaminated items. Lensed instruments should be sterilized after use on AIDS patients.
8. Needles should not be bent after use, but should be promptly placed in a puncture-resistant container used solely for such disposal. Needles should not be reinserted into their original sheaths before being discarded into the container, since this is a common cause of needle injury.
9. Disposable syringes and needles are preferred. Only needle-locking syringes or one-piece needle–syringe units should be used to aspirate fluids from patients, so that collected fluid can be safely discharged through the needle, if desired. If reusable syringes are employed, they should be decontaminated before reprocessing.
10. A private room is indicated for patients who are too ill to use good hygiene, such as those with profuse diarrhea, fecal incontinence, or altered behavior secondary to central nervous system infections.

The following precautions are advised for persons performing laboratory tests or studies of clinical specimens or other potentially infectious materials (such as inoculated tissue cultures, embryonated eggs, or animal tissues from known or suspected AIDS cases:

1. Mechanical pipetting devices should be used for the manipulation of all liquids in the laboratory. Mouth pipetting is dangerous and should not be allowed.
2. Needles and syringes should be handled as stipulated above.
3. Laboratory coats, gowns, or uniforms should be worn while working with potentially infectious materials and should be discarded appropriately before leaving the laboratory.
4. Gloves should be worn to avoid skin contact with blood, specimens containing blood, blood-soiled items, body fluids, excretions, and secretions, as well as surfaces, materials, and objects exposed to them.
5. All procedures and manipulations of potentially infectious material should be performed carefully to minimize the creation of droplets and aerosols.

6. Biological safety cabinets (Class I or II) and other primary containment devices (e.g., centrifuge safety cups) are advised whenever procedures are conducted that have a high potential for creating aerosols or infectious droplets. These include centrifuging, blending, sonicating, vigorous mixing, and harvesting infected tissues from animals or embryonated eggs. Fluorescence activated cell sorters generate droplets that could potentially result in infectious aerosols. Translucent plastic shielding between the droplet-collecting area and the equipment operator should be used to reduce the presently uncertain magnitude of this risk. Primary containment devices are also used in handling materials that might contain concentrated infectious agents or organisms in greater quantities than expected in clinical specimens.

7. Laboratory work surfaces should be decontaminated with a disinfectant, such as sodium hypochlorite solution, following any spill of potentially infectious material and at the completion of work activities.

8. All potentially contaminated materials used in laboratory tests should be decontaminated, preferably by autoclaving, before disposal or reprocessing.

9. All personnel should wash their hands following completion of laboratory activities and removal of protective clothing and before leaving the laboratory.

REFERENCE

1. Centers for Disease Control: Precaution in the handling of clinical and laboratory AIDS materials. *MMWR* 43:577–579, 1982.

II

Bacterial Sexually Transmitted Diseases

Syphilis

YEHUDI M. FELMAN

HISTORY

> *What varied fortunes*
> *And what germinations*
> *Have produced a fierce and rare disease*
> *Never before seen for centuries.*
>   Gerolomo Fracastoro (Fracastorius),
>   *Syphilis Sive Morbus Gallicus* (1530)

Thus Fracastorius begins his famous poem, which gave us the name *syphilis* for this major venereal disease. Close to five centuries later, the question of whence the disease came is still being debated.

Prior to 1493 syphilis was an unknown clinical entity. It may or may not have existed in some mild form in Europe or may have been confused with other dermatologic conditions. It is known that the disease erupted in virulent form and in epidemiologic proportions in 1494 in Italy and quickly became pandemic. By the year 1499 all of Europe was involved in the pandemic, and soon after the disease appeared in China.

The origin of the disease has never been resolved. Two theories have been promulgated:

1. Syphilis was brought to Europe from the New World by the returning crew of Columbus (post-Columbian theory).
2. Syphilis existed in Europe from time immemorial, but smoldering in a much milder form (pre-Columbian theory).

YEHUDI M. FELMAN ● Departments of Dermatology, Preventive Medicine, and Community Health, State University of New York, Downstate Medical School, Brooklyn, New York 11203.

The evidence for either point of view does not allow for a definitive conclusion.

This evidence comes from three sources:

1. Original contemporary documents*—few in number and often open to question.
2. Anthropological findings—prehistoric to medieval bones that show osseous lesions that are interpreted as characteristically syphilitic (Williams). More evidence of this kind was found in the Americas, especially among the remains of Aztec and Inca aborigines, than in Europe. Most authorities, though by no means all, favor the American origin of syphilis on the basis of these findings.
3. Historical facts—these appear to favor the post-Columbian theory, if the facts are pertinent. In 1493, the year Columbus's crew returned to Spain infected with syphilis, Charles VIII of France invaded Naples and some of the returned crew joined his army, which, of course, had its complement of female camp followers. Spain's army, with whatever syphilis had spread among its soldiers, went to the aid of Naples. There was little fighting and presumably much lovemaking, and the "love sickness" assumed pandemic proportions with the scattering of the troops and their female companions.

Nevertheless, nearly five centuries after Fracastorius asked whence came the disease, there is still no definite answer to the question.

The transmission of syphilis through sexual intercourse was recognized within a few decades of its appearance, as witnessed by its earliest name, the "love sickness." Not long after the mode of transmission was discovered, congenital syphilis was recognized (Fleming, 1594), and this was followed by the understanding of some of the late manifestations [e.g., aortic aneurysm attributable to syphilis (Ambroise Paré)].

During the 17th and 18th centuries the development of our knowledge of syphilis was rapid, save for a considerable setback due to the unfortunate error of John Hunter. By inoculating himself with gonococcal pus from a patient who suffered from both gonorrhea and syphilis, Hunter contracted both diseases. He was convinced that gonorrhea and syphilis were two manifestations of the same disease. He also convinced others, and it was not until 1838 that the two diseases were finally established as two different clinical entities by Ricard.

The 20th century saw six major advances in the understanding, diagnosis, treatment, and prevention of syphilis. We list them in chronological order:

---

* There exist Renaissance documents as early as 1440 referring to a disease similar to syphilis; a typically syphilitic crural ulcer was depicted in a 1461 painting.

1905	Fritz Schaudinn demonstrates *Treponema (Spirochaeta) pallidum*.
1906	August von Wassermann develops the Wassermann test.
1909	Paul Ehrlich introduces arsphenamine (salvarsan, "606").
1936	Thomas Parran drops the euphemisms used in referring to syphilis and brings it out into the open.
1943	J. F. Mahoney uses penicillin in the treatment of syphilis.
1949	R. A. Nelson, Jr., and M. M. Mayer introduce the first of a series of treponemal tests, the *Treponema pallidum* immobilization test.

EPIDEMIOLOGY

After a dramatic drop in the incidence of syphilis owing to the widespread use of penicillin therapy in the late 1940s and early 1950s, the reported number of cases of primary and secondary syphilis began to rise and in the 1960s plateaued, remaining at approximately the same level during the late 1960s and early 1970s. During 1976 and 1977, there was again a dramatic decline in the incidence of syphilis in the United States, followed by a rise in 1978–1981.

These rough data (Figure 1), however, tell only part of the story. When they are broken down to separate the incidence of syphilis in homosexual individuals from that seen in heterosexual individuals, an altogether different picture is seen. The number of patients with infectious syphilis who named same-sex contacts has risen from 25.3% in 1970 to 48.7% in 1980 (Table 1). Indeed, in metropolitan areas with large homosexual male communities, such as New York City, the incidence exceeds 55%. Since infectious syphilis is practically unknown in lesbians, it is homosexual men who presently are responsible for about half of all reported infectious syphilis in the United States. When the natural reluctance of homosexual men to name their sexual contacts is taken into account, especially if their contacts are still "in the closet," the ratio of homosexual to heterosexual patients with syphilis is probably even higher.

Most venereologists are aware that sexually transmitted diseases (STDs) of all types are more common in homosexual men than in heterosexuals of either sex. Since the homosexual male population is estimated to represent not more than perhaps 5% of the total population of the country, it is intolerable that 50% of total infectious syphilis is found within this group. Picture the reaction if some other minority group were victimized by such an awesome prevalence of a disease that can cause all the serious complications known to be part of the picture of tertiary syphilis: blindness, insanity, paralysis, and death from cardiovascular complications. Indeed, the success of the National Venereal Disease Control Program in controlling syphilis in the heterosexual community poses the question of why the program has failed to control syphilis in the homosexual male community.

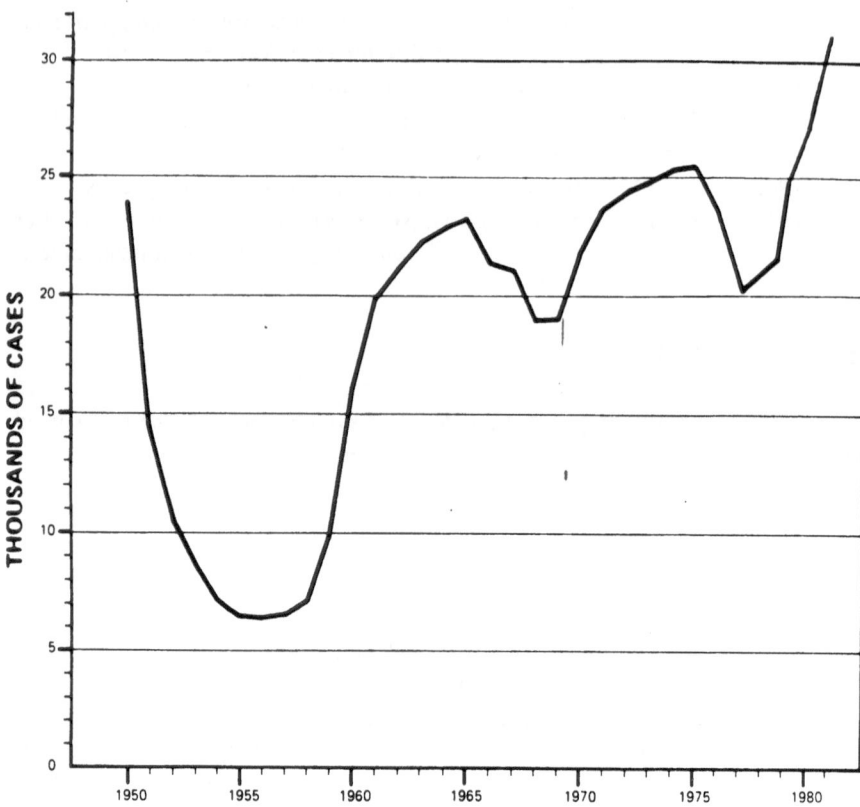

FIGURE 1. Reported civilian primary and secondary syphilis cases by year in the United States, calendar years 1950–1981. Updated from ref. 9.

CLINICAL ASPECTS

Syphilis is caused by a spirochete called *Treponema pallidum*. The genus *Treponema* contains other pathogenic species, including the causative organisms of yaws and pinta, which are not sexually transmitted and are usually found in tropical or semitropical climates. *T. pallidum* is a thin organism, from 6 to 14 μm in length, usually containing 6 to 14 spirals when visualized by darkfield microscopy, which is the definitive diagnostic procedure for syphilis. The pathogenic strain of the organism has never been cultured outside a human or animal host. Attempts to grow it in tissue culture or on egg and duck embryos have been completely unsuccessful. *T. pallidum* is susceptible to physical and chemical agents—e.g., heat, soap and water, storage at refrigerator temperature, and simple drying—all of which bring about its destruction. Consequently, syphilis

TABLE 1. Patients Identifying Contacts by Sexual Orientation[a]

Fiscal year	Heterosexual orientation (percent)	Homosexual orientation (percent)	Bisexual orientation (percent)	Total of homosexual and bisexual (percent)
1970	11,133 (74.7)	2,430 (16.3)	1,345 (9.0)	3,775 (25.3)
1971	12,566 (72.3)	3,244 (18.7)	1,558 (9.0)	4,802 (27.7)
1972	13,286 (70.7)	3,861 (20.5)	1,653 (8.8)	5,514 (29.3)
1973	14,269 (66.8)	5,113 (23.9)	1,993 (9.3)	7,106 (33.2)
1974	13,575 (61.8)	6,271 (28.6)	2,114 (9.6)	8,385 (38.2)
1975	13,512 (56.2)	7,948 (33.1)	2,587 (10.8)	10,535 (43.9)
1976	12,825 (53.7)	8,472 (35.4)	2,598 (10.9)	11,070 (46.3)
1977	10,933 (53.3)	7,492 (36.5)	2,087 (10.2)	9,579 (46.7)
1978	10,560 (51.2)	7,937 (38.5)	2,128 (10.3)	10.065 (48.8)
1979[b]	11,676 (47.9)	10,398 (42.6)	2,328 (9.5)	12,726 (52.1)
1980[b]	12,609 (51.3)	9,819 (40.0)	2,148 (8.7)	11,967 (48.7)
1981[b]	14,222 (55.3)	9,522 (37.0)	1,982 (7.7)	11,504 (44.7)

[a] National figures.
[b] Calendar year.

is almost exclusively sexually transmitted, unlike other STDs, which can sometimes be transmitted by close contact. Syphilis is transmitted through direct skin-to-skin contact, or skin-to-mucous-membrane contact, or mucous-membrane-to-skin contact from an infective lesion on an infected patient to an uninfected individual. The incubation period may be ten to ninety days, with an average of three weeks. Spirochetes pass through abraded skin as well as intact mucous membranes and cause an ulcer to appear at the site of infection. This ulcer, the characteristic lesion of primary syphilis, is known as the chancre.

Primary Syphilis

No one has ever demonstrated convincingly any increased susceptibility of homosexual men to infection with $T.$ $pallidum.$ Consequently, homosexual men cannot be considered biologically or immunologically susceptible to syphilis. The tremendously increased incidence of syphilis in homosexual men must therefore be attributed to sociological and epidemiologic factors and not to constitutional factors.

Clinical Features

Chancres appear either singly or in numbers. They generally possess a firm and indurated margin and are usually completely painless. They are associated with at least unilateral regional lymphadenopathy, especially when the primary lesion is on the penis. In homosexual men, anal, rectal, and oral chancres are quite common and are frequently misdiagnosed. Misdiagnosis, especially of anorectal chancres, has led to serious consequences, including surgical excision of these lesions. The clinical diagnosis in these patients was usually fistula, fissure, or hemorrhoids.[1] Even more extensive surgery has been performed when the clinical misdiagnosis was carcinoma of the rectum. Syphilitic chancres of the rectum are not as asymptomatic as penile chancres.[2] They often cause such symptoms as diarrhea, bloody diarrhea, constipation, dyschezia, pain in the rectum, tenesmus, and bleeding. Unfortunately, these symptoms often lead to the mistaken diagnosis, especially if the examining physician does not take a sexual practices history or take into account the patient's possible homosexuality. On the penis, chancres can be seen anywhere, including the coronal sulcus, shaft, prepuce, glans penis, frenulum, urethral meatus, or intraurethrally. Extragenital chancres may be found on the lip, tonsils, tongue, fingers, eyelids, or nipples. Intraoral lesions are usually accompanied by unilateral lymphadenopathy involving the submental and anterior cervical glands. Rectal chancres are sometimes accompanied by femoral nodes. Occasionally, no nodes are palpable.

Darkfield Examination

The diagnosis of primary syphilis is confirmed by darkfield examination, a technique that requires some experience and that is ordinarily available only in venereal disease (VD) clinics or in the offices of physicians who see a good deal of infectious syphilis. When collecting specimens for examination the examining physician should wear gloves to protect himself from accidental infection. The surface of the suspected lesion should be cleaned carefully with saline, allowed to dry, and then gently abraded. Pressure should be maintained upon the lesion until only clear serum exudes. A drop of serum is picked up directly on the surface of the glass slide and a coverslip is placed over it. Examination is completed under a darkfield microscope. *T. pallidum* can be identified by its typical corkscrew appearance and its wiggly motility.

Chancres are often darkfield-negative, however, because of factors beyond the physician's control. The patient may have used an antibiotic ointment on the lesion or may have received inadequate treatment, such as a short course of oral antibiotics or an injection of an inadequate dose of penicillin. These interventions, though not curative of syphilis, result in a negative darkfield examination. Consequently, if the patient presents with a typical lesion on clinical examination, as well as regional lymphadenopathy and a compatible history of sexual exposure, treatment should not be delayed because of a negative or unavailable darkfield examination. Rather, it is imperative to treat the patient promptly. The alternative is to delay treatment until the patient develops secondary syphilis. The problem with this alternative is that the patient is infectious and will spread the disease if sexually active. Unfortunately, the temptation to continue sexual activity during this period is often too great for the patient to resist. Consequently, the patient should be treated unless the clinician is certain that the patient can be relied upon not to engage in sexual activity during the waiting period.

The differential diagnosis of primary syphilis includes any ulcerative lesion of the genital or extragenital area, other STDs, and non-STDs that can cause such lesions. Table 2 presents criteria that can be used to help differentiate primary syphilis from some of the other diseases that produce similar lesions. The differential diagnosis includes chancroid, granuloma inguinale, lymphogranuloma venereum, herpes progenitalis, carcinoma, lichen planus, drug eruptions, traumatic lesions, and gonorrhea when the chancre is intraurethral. The differential diagnosis of anal chancres includes fistulae, hemorrhoids, sinuses, and fissures, as well as carcinoma. With oral chancres, the differential diagnosis also includes aphthous stomatitis and oral lichen planus.

Secondary Syphilis

A few weeks after the appearance of the chancre the disease enters the secondary stage, manifested by disappearance of the primary lesion and the onset of a number of widely varied signs and symptoms. These usually include generalized or localized eruptions appearing on various areas of the body, particularly the palms and soles. These eruptions, including those on mucous membranes, are the major presenting features of secondary syphilis and are caused by hematogenous dissemination of the organism from the regional lymph nodes. Every single lesion that is seen on physical examination actually contains spirochetes. The skin lesions may be macular, papular, papulosquamous, or pustular, but rarely ever vesicular or bullous. Most often they are macular or papular.

The most outstanding lesions are the whitish, warty excrescences, seen in intertriginous areas, particularly the perianal site, which are called condylomata lata. These lesions teem with spirochetes on darkfield examination, and must be distinguished from condylomata acuminata, also known as venereal warts. Mucous patches are the characteristic lesions of the mouth, throat, and cervix. Upon physical examination, they seem to look like leukoplakia of sudden onset and occur in young patients who are often nonsmokers. Darkfield examinations of specimens from the mouth are unrealiable, as *T. pallidum* cannot be differentiated from nonpathogenic treponemes. Noncicatricial alopecia, especially of the scalp, eyelashes, and eyebrows, may also be a manifestation of secondary syphilis.

Secondary syphilis is a systemic disease and not simply one of the skin and mucous membranes. Systemic signs and symptoms include generalized lymph-

TABLE 2. Differential Diagnosis of Primary Syphilis

Syphilis	Chancroid	Granuloma inguinale	Lymphogranuloma venereum	Herpes progenitalis	Carcinoma	Scabies
Lesion usually single, firm, indurated with raised border. Painless, clean unless secondarily contaminated. Frequently enlarged bilateral lymphadenopathy, hard, painless. Darkfield: Positive for *T. pallidum*. STS: Positive.	Lesions usually multiple. Soft ulcerations. Grayish "dirty" base. Edges undermined. Painful unilateral adenopathy. Darkfield: Negative for *T. pallidum*. *Hemophilus ducreyi* in smears and culture. STS: Nonreactive.	Soft, painless, raised, raw beef-colored. Smooth granulating lesions. No adenopathy. Darkfield: Negative for *T. pallidum*. STS: Nonreactive. *Donovania granulomatis* (Donovan bodies) in tissue smears.	Initial lesion is a small evanescent ulcer. Unilateral painful inguinal adenopathy. *T. pallidum*-, *H. ducreyi*-, and *D. granulomatis*-negative. Complement-fixation test: *Chlamydia trachomatis* in titer of 1 : 32 or higher is diagnostic.	Grouped, painful, vesicular lesions. Usual history of recurrent lesions in the same site. Tzanck smear demonstrates multinucleated cells in herpetic infections.	Lesion usually present a long time. Usually fungating or infiltrating ulcerative lesion. Diagnosis established by biopsy.	Pruritic vesicles with burrow formation. Mite in the burrow is diagnostic. Microtests and STS: Negative.

Trauma	Lichen planus	Drug eruptions	Aphthosis	Reiter's syndrome	Mycosis	Intraurethral chancre
History of injury. Microtests and biopsy: Negative. STS: Negative.	Lesions are annular or the typical polygonal, flat-topped, violaceous papule. May be pruritic single or multiple. STS: Nonreactive.	Dermatitis with history of drug ingestion. STS: Nonreactive.	Round to polycyclic, painful, mucous membrane erosions. Frequently associated with pseudomembranous oral inflammation and ocular lesions.	A triad of nonspecific urethritis, mucopurulent conjunctivitis, and polyarticular arthritis. Lesions, if present, similar to those of erosive circinate balanitis. Clinical diagnosis and biopsy.	Some lesions may resemble chancriform genital lesions. Diagnosis confirmed by KOH preps, culture, and biopsy. STS: Nonreactive.	Lesions not visualized. Nongonococcal discharge if GC not associated. Induration within the urethra near the meatal orifice. Darkfield: Positive. STS: Positive.

adenopathy, hepatosplenomegaly, headache, hepatitis,[3] erosive gastritis,[4] nerve deafness,[5] nephrotic syndrome,[6] iritis,[7] and fever, as well as involvement of the skeletal and central nervous system.[8] These and other symptoms suggesting systemic disease often lead to misdiagnosis of secondary syphilis as intracranial neoplasm, malignant lymphoma, connective tissue disease, or many other conditions. Indeed, syphillis was once known as the "great imitator" because of its propensity to mimic the signs and symptoms of many other diseases. The differential diagnosis of secondary syphilis in its skin and mucous membrane manifestations includes many dermatoses. Among the most important are pityriasis rosea, psoriasis, lichen planus, tinea versicolor, drug eruptions, scabies, and viral exanthems (Table 3).

Fortunately, laboratory diagnosis of syphilis is quite reliable. Any routine serologic tests for syphilis (STS) are positive in the secondary stage of this disease, usually in high titer. The most commonly used nonspecific tests for syphilis are the Venereal Disease Research Laboratory (VDRL) and the rapid plasma reagin test. Both of these tests are positive in a titer of at least 1 : 16 in patients with secondary syphilis, and are often positive in titer as high as 1 : 256. Consequently, treponemal testing either in secondary or primary syphilis is not ordinarily necessary, as diagnosis can be reliably made by other means. Most important, however, the clinician should order a quantitative VDRL to have a baseline for managing the patient.

The VDRL, a nonspecific or nontreponemal test, determines the presence in the serum of an IgG antibody known as reagin. This antibody can be found in a host of other unrelated diseases as well as secondary syphilis. It is first detected in the serum approximately four to six weeks after infection and one to three weeks after the chancre appears. The antibody titer gradually rises as the patient develops clinical lesions of secondary syphilis. If the patient is not treated, the titer gradually falls over a period of several years to a level of 1 : 4 or lower. Sometimes in late cases and in some types of neurosyphilis, the serology actually becomes nonreactive. However, the STS is most important in identifying patients with secondary syphilis. The discovery by Wassermann of reagin was one of the major breakthroughs in the control of this disease. If a test of this type were available for gonorrhea, nongonococcal urethritis, or herpes, it would be of great value in diagnosis and control of these diseases.

Many diseases have been reported to be associated with the chronic biological false positive (BFP) reaction for syphilis. These include lupus erythematosus, other connective tissue diseases, infectious diseases such as malaria and Hansen's disease, and infectious mononucleosis. (Table 4). However, none of these diseases ordinarily presents with an STS of a titer of 1 : 16 or above.

The patient with typical lesions of secondary syphilis, especially on the palms and soles, and a strongly positive STS should be diagnosed as having secondary syphilis and should be treated *immediately*. This axiom applies particularly to homosexual men (and to women), who often are first seen during

TABLE 3. Differential Diagnosis of Secondary Syphilis

Pityriasis rosea	Psoriasis	Lichen planus	Tinea versicolor	Drug eruptions
Erythematous, maculopapulosquamous lesions along lines of skin cleavage. Eruption often preceded by a single lesion for one or more weeks (herald patch). Distal parts of extremities, head, neck, and mucous membranes usually spared. Darkfield: Negative. STS: Nonreactive.	Erythematous, maculopapulosquamous lesion on scalp, elbows, knees, chest, back, and buttocks. Nails may be involved. Removal of scales will produce pinpoint bleeding. Darkfield: Negative. STS: Nonreactive.	Violaceous, papular, pruritic lesions, most commonly on wrists, ankles and sacral areas. Darkfield: Negative. STS: Nonreactive.	Brown, superficial scaly lesions. May be erythematous. Scrapings show mycotic spores and hyphae.	Widely varied skin eruptions. Macular or bullous, localized or generalized. Careful history most important (drug ingestion). Darkfield: Negative. STS: Nonreactive.

"ID" eruption	Scabies	Acute exanthemata (viral, etc.)	Infectious mononucleosis	
Lesions diversified. Dermatophyte or bacterial infection usually demonstrated in other parts of body. Darkfield: Negative. STS: Negative.	Excoriated papules and pustules, mainly in intertriginous areas. Pruritus—severe. Darkfield: Negative. STS: Nonreactive.	Generally associated with fever and constitutional symptoms. Epidemic, generalized moribilliform, occasionally petechial eruptions. Darkfield: Negative. STS: Negative (unless BFP).	Lymphadenopathy and throat manifestations closely resemble those seen in secondary syphilis. BFP STS may be present. Darkfield of lesions when present: Negative. Atypical lymphocytes and positive heterophile agglutination test are diagnostic.	

TABLE 4. Conditions Reported to Produce Chronic
Biological False-Positive Reactions in Reagin Tests[a]

Addison's disease	Lupus erythematosus
Aging (per se)	Lymphatic leukemia
Atopic dermatitis	Lymphosarcoma
Autoimmune disorder	Malaria (usually acute BFP)
Brucellosis	Metastatic carcinoma
Cirrhosis of liver	Multiple myeloma
Cryoglobulinemia	Narcotic addiction
Dermatomyositis	Pemphigus vulgaris
Diabetes mellitus	Periarteritis nodosa
Dysproteinemia	Pernicious anemia
Epilepsy	Pinta (biological true reaction)
Erythema nodosum	Rheumatic fever
Glomerulonephritis	Rheumatoid arthritis
Hashimoto's thyroiditis	Sarcoidosis
Hemolytic anemia	Scleroderma
Histoplasmosis	Subacute bacterial endocarditis
Idiopathic thrombocytopenic purpura	Tuberculosis (also acute BFP)
Leprosy	Yaws (biological true reaction)

[a] Reactive STS of more than six month's duration.

the secondary stage and who often have chancres that are misdiagnosed or that appear at easily missed sites.

Late and Latent Syphilis

The major objective of the national control program for syphilis is not the prevention of primary and secondary syphilis, which are at the present relatively benign diseases, but the prevention of tertiary syphilis, which develops in 40% of all untreated individuals with primary and secondary syphilis.[9] It is not within the scope of this chapter to describe tertiary syphilis in detail. Suffice it to state that there are three major forms of this disease—neurological, cardiovascular, and benign tertiary syphilis. Neurological syphilis can lead to insanity, blindness, deafness, and other major neurological deficits. Cardiovascular syphilis leads to severe disease of the aorta, blood vessels, and heart valves, and eventually death from heart failure. These manifestations occur ten to twenty years (and sometimes even later) after the patient had secondary syphilis. They are not due to further invasion by the spirochetes but are due to a hypersensitivity reaction to the presence of a few treponemes that remain in the body after the body's normal immunologic defenses have destroyed most of the treponemes. More than 50% of patients with late latent syphilis never develop clinical signs of tertiary syphilis.

Latency is defined as that stage of syphilis in which the patient has no clinical signs or symptoms of the disease, STSs are reactive, and spinal fluid is normal. Therefore, the period of time after secondary syphilis and before the onset of tertiary syphilis is known as the latent stage. By this definition, the period of time between resolution of the chancre and the appearance of the secondary eruption is also considered latency. During the year following infection with secondary syphilis, the patient is said to have early latent syphilis and is considered to be still infectious because of relapsing secondary lesions. Thus, patients with primary, secondary, and early latent syphilis are all grouped under the general heading of infectious syphilis. During the period from one year subsequent to the initial infection until the development of some signs or symptoms of tertiary disease, the patient is said to have late latent syphilis and is not considered infectious. The only indication of the disease in patients with latent syphilis is the positive STS. Since there is no way, other than with a history of a previous chancre or typical eruption, of differentiating the patient with late latent syphilis and a positive STS from a patient with a chronic BFP, a specific treponemal test often must be performed. At the present time, the most commonly available specific treponemal test is the FTA-ABS (fluorescent treponemal antibody absorption) test. This test is reliable in most cases in differentiating between a chronic BFP and a patient with late latent syphilis. However, occasional patients with systemic lupus erythematosus have false-positive FTA-ABS results. In addition, as treponemal tests remain positive for many years, even in treated individuals, a serofast individual may have a positive reagin test and a positive treponemal test without falling into the category of latent syphilis. More recently, another treponemal test called the microhemagglutination–*Treponema pallidum* test has been developed and is available in many laboratories, especially municipal health department laboratories. Treponemal tests, of course, do not the secondary stage and who often have chancres that are misdiagnosed or that appear at easily missed sites.

The examining physician realizes that STDs, particularly in homosexual men, do not always occur one at a time. Every patient who has syphilis should be screened for gonorrhea as well. Therefore, all orifices normally used for sexual activity should be cultured. STDs should always be looked for on physical examination. *The highest positive yield of screening for STDs is from screening in a group that already has one STD.*

TREATMENT

The treatment for primary, secondary, and early latent syphilis recommended by the Bureau of Venereal Disease Control of the New York City Health Department is 4.8 million units benzathine penicillin G intramuscularly, given in separate weekly injections of 2.4 million units each. This dosage is based on laboratory observation that the spirochete is most sensitive to a prolonged low blood level of penicillin, unlike the gonococcus, which responds best to a short-acting high level of penicillin. (It is important to emphasize that the Bureau's

TABLE 5. Recommended Treatment Regimens for Syphilis

	Penicillins[a]	Alternate forms of treatment when penicillin is contraindicated[b]	
Early syphilis Primary Secondary Early latent	Benzathine penicillin G 2.4 million units IM injection weekly for 2 successive weeks. Total dosage: 4.8 million units	Tetracycline[c] 0.5 g PO qid for 20 days. Total dosage: 40 g.	Erythromycin succinate, stearate, or base 0.5 g PO qid for 20 days. Total dosage: 10 g.
Late syphilis Late latent Late benign	Benzathine penicillin G 2.4 million units IM weekly for 3 successive weeks. Total dosage: 7.2 million units.	Tetracycline 0.5 g PO qid for 30 days. Total dosage: 60 g.	Erythromycin succinate, stearate, or base 0.5 g PO qid for 30 days. Total dosage: 60 g.
Neurosyphilis, cardiovascular syphilis	Aqueous procaine penicillin G 2.4 million units IM every 2 days for at least 6 treatments. Total dosage: 14.4 million units or more.	Tetracycline 0.5 g PO qid for 30 days. Total dosage: 60 g.	Erythromycin succinate, stearate, or base 0.5 g PO qid for 30 days. Total dosage: 60 g.
Syphilis Epidemiologic Incubating	Benzathine penicillin G 2.4 million units IM in a single injection. It is important to treat patients who have been exposed to infectious syphilis within the preceding 3 months even though the presence of the disease has not been documented.	Tetracycline[c] 0.5 g PO qid for 15 days. Total dosage: 30 g.	Erythromycin succinate, stearate, or base 0.5 g PO qid for 15 days. Total dosage: 30 g.
Syphilis Retreatment	Patients should be retreated if 1. Treatment was suboptimal. 2. Treatment was unknown. 3. Treatment was with drugs other than those recommended.	4. Clinical signs and symptoms of syphilis persist or recur. 5. There is a sustained fourfold increase in the titer of a reagin test. 6. An initially high-titer reagin test fails to decrease fourfold within a year.	

[a] An emergency kit for treatment of allergic reactions should be readily available whenever penicillin is administered.
[b] Allergy to penicillin, ampicillin, or probenecid or previous anaphylactic reaction.
[c] To be given 1 h before or 2 h after meals. Absorption is poor when oral forms are taken with food.

recommended treatment for gonorrhea, 4.8 million units of aqueous procaine penicillin G preceded by 1 g probenecid, aborts incubating syphilis, while the recommended treatment for syphilis is not curative for gonorrhea.)

Patients who are allergic to penicillin should be given 40 g tetracycline, 0.5 g orally four times a day for twenty days, or 40 g erythromycin, 0.5 g orally four times a day for twenty days. Gastrointestinal distress from erythromycin is often overcome by using the pediatric liquid form of erythromycin in the same dosage. *Oral penicillins are not reliable in the treatment of syphilis and should not be used.*

Every patient treated for early syphilis should be warned that within six to twelve hours after treatment there may be a mild reaction with fever, headache, malaise, and worsening of the symptoms. Known as the Jarisch–Herxheimer reaction, it usually lasts several hours and does not recur. The reaction is due to massive destruction of the spirochetes following the first injection of penicillin. By definition it should not occur a second time. If it does, the patient is probably allergic to penicillin.

The patient should be told not to have sex until after treatment is completed. However, it is perfectly permissible to begin sexual activity within one week after the last injection of benzathine penicillin. Patients with late latent syphilis, neurological syphilis, and cardiovascular syphillis are also treated with penicillin, but in different dosages over an extended period of time (Table 5).

FOLLOW-UP

Patients with primary syphilis who are treated with benzathine penicillin G should revert to a negative STS within one year after completion of therapy. Patients who started treatment when they had secondary syphilis should revert to negative within two years of completion of therapy. However, patients treated with erythromycin and tetracycline rarely revert completely to negative, though generally their titers drop considerably and may revert to either a negative or low titer by two years. If a patient who has been treated with benzathine penicillin G does not revert to negative within these specified time periods, treatment was probably inadequate and the patient should be retreated.

It is important to differentiate reinfection syphilis from inadequately treated syphilis. The standard means used to diagnose reinfection syphilis is the presence of a fourfold increase in titer of the STS since the last examination. Examinations are normally performed every three months after treatment until the serology becomes completely negative. Subsequently, syphilis serology should be performed once yearly.

A fourfold increase in titer is suggestive of reinfection. Serology retesting is of great importance in homosexual men who are prone to reinfection syphilis and who often have a positive serology from a previously treated episode of this disease. If a patient is diagnosed as having been reinfected, he must be promptly retreated with the recommended dosage for infectious syphilis.

CONTROL

A national syphilis control program is administered by the CDC through their Bureau of State Services. Epidemiologists, known as public health advisors, are assigned as field investigators to most state and municipal VD control programs in the United States. The program has been in existence for the last thirty years and is based upon several principles. The most imporant of these is that the incubation period of infectious syphilis is twenty-one days. Thus, the sexual partners of a patient with syphilis will not become infectious for three weeks, and the investigator has that period during which to find the sexual contacts of an infected patient before they become infected and transmit the infection to others. Patients with infectious syphilis who are reported to local health departments by private physicians are interviewed promptly by an investigator from the health department, if permission to interview is granted by the examining physician. All patients who are diagnosed as having infectious syphilis in municipal VD clinics are interviewed for contacts as a matter of course. All states require by law that physicians report all cases of infectious syphilis to their local health department so that these interviews can be performed. The purposes of the interview are: to educate the patient concerning the signs and symptoms of syphilis and how to recognize the disease in himself and in his sexual partner, and to locate sexual contacts who may have been infected by the patient, as well as sexual partners of the contacts, before further individuals become infected.

On occasion, a patient with infectious syphilis may have had no additional contacts since becoming infected, but this possibility is unusual. The average homosexual male may be expected to name three or four contacts, and sometimes more than ten. The mobility of the population underscores the necessity that local health departments in various geographical areas of the country be prepared to exchange contact tracing information immediately to insure prompt examination and treatment of infected contacts. This information exchange is made possible through the auspices of the Interstate Communications Control Service, which is available throughout the United States.

Patients with primary syphilis are questioned about sexual contacts during the preceding three months; those with secondary syphilis are asked about the preceding six months; those with early latent syphilis about the preceding eighteen months. However, the chances of successful contact tracing become less likely the longer the time that has elapsed since sexual encounter occurred.

Over the past ten years in the United States, the percentage of individuals who name same-sex contacts upon investigation has been gradually increasing to about 45% of interviewed patients with infectious syphilis.[10] In New York

City the percentage approaches 60. Obviously, the epidemiology of syphilis among homosexual men is quite different from that among heterosexual men, for several reasons. Homosexually active men frequently have far more sexual partners in a given time period than do sexually active heterosexual men.[11] In many incidences, some of these partners are either anonymous or poorly known to the patient. Establishments such as bathhouses, where anonymous sexual activity is the rule, are strong seeding areas for acquiring infectious syphilis. Indeed, many studies have shown that these locations are productive areas for syphilis screening.[12,13] Unfortunately, the managements of bathhouses do not always cooperate with the local health department in allowing routine screening of patrons. VD screening is seen by some managements as bad for business and patrons themselves are often uncooperative, fearing disclosure and lack of confidentiality, despite assurances to the contrary. Indeed, in a recent paper, Wolf and Judson claim that bathhouse screening did not lower the prevalence of infection.[14]

The homosexual male community in the United States has responded to the challenge of high rates of infection by establishing in most large cities facilities where men can be screened, diagnosed, and sometimes treated for syphilis, gonorrhea, and other STDs, in a totally sympathetic environment. In these clinics, physicians and other workers are usually homosexual men and women. The management of these facilities is under the auspices of the homosexual community, while laboratory and epidemiologic support is usually provided by the local health department. Facilities like the Howard Brown Memorial Clinic in Chicago and the Gay Men's Health Project in New York City contribute enormously to controlling syphilis among homosexual men by assuring the patient that there is a place where he can be screened and often treated with complete sympathy and confidence.

Unfortunately, the anonymity of many of the sexual contacts of homosexual men tends to impede contact tracing to a great degree. How can the health department trace the contacts of an individual with infectious syphilis if the patient himself does not know who they are? To a large extent, this is the reason why traditional approaches toward syphilis control, though relatively successful in the past decade in the heterosexual community, are not as successful in the homosexual community. Furthermore, many individuals are understandably afraid to name their sexual contacts for fear that their homosexuality as well as their VD will be disclosed.

PRIORITIES FOR THE FUTURE

The National Venereal Disease Control Program could be improved in many ways. Perhaps one of the most outstanding improvements would be to recruit more openly homosexual men for positions as public health advisors and contact investigators. Homosexual physicians should also be recruited to work in VD clinics and in health departments' central bureaus or divisions of VD control. To accomplish this goal, advertisements have to be placed in newspapers, magazines, and other media read by homosexual men. Strenuous attempts must be made to communicate with bathhouse owners, either by homosexual men working in the VD control program or by other interested and sympathetic individuals, to obtain their cooperation in this effort.

The lack of sensible priorities in national and state VD control programs is perhaps best illustrated by the most expensive tool presently used to control syphilis in the United States—the mandated premarital syphilis serology. This particular procedure costs the American public about $80 million yearly and is of little or no value in syphilis control.[15] In 1976, for example, only 456 patients with infectious syphilis were actually located and treated as a result of this screening procedure, at a cost of almost a quarter of a million dollars per case! The entire National Venereal Disease Control Program in 1976 was budgeted at $25 million. If the premarital syphilis screening serology is of negligible value in the heterosexual community, it is obviously of still less value in the homosexual male population, as homosexual marriage is presently illegal in all 50 states. Premarital syphilis serology should not be required by law. Instead, the public should be educated to realize that syphilis screening should be done primarily in high-risk groups, as with homosexual men. Sexually active men should be encouraged to be screened at least once yearly for their own protection. Dollars spent on this type of screening will be far more productive in terms of disease control than is the premarital syphilis serology.

Patient Education and Counseling

STD education and counseling efforts in the homosexual community should be adequately funded. Unfortunately, the National Venereal Disease Control Program allots relatively little of its budget *directly* to STD education. STD education is included in the contact interviews that are conducted by public health advisors with infected patients. Although it is of value, it is hard to see how this approach will reach individuals who are not patients or friends of patients. Massive educational campaigns must be begun by the homosexual community to inform men of the enormous health hazards of syphilis and the potentially crippling effects caused in late stages. Efforts have already been mounted independently by various organizations. Further, a special national STD education budget must be created that will allow dissemination of STD educational materials to homosexual men and other high-risk groups. STD clinics and facilities such as bars, bathhouses, and any other places where homosexual men congregate should be included in these efforts. The homosexual community must be kept informed of the hazards of syphilis and other STDs and of how these diseases can be prevented, diagnosed, and treated. Films, as well as other audiovisual aids, should also be used as part of a more aggressive educational approach.

Sympathetic VD clinic personnel in municipal clinics are of the greatest importance. Obviously, a homosexual individual presenting at a clinic for the first time will not return if he is made to feel self-conscious or ashamed of his sexual preference. A sympathetic approach is even more important in the private physician's office. Private physicians should be taught in medical school and as part of continuing medical education (CME) how to examine the homosexual male for STDs.[16] Training other health professionals as well as physicians in the community in STDs should be a major feature of CME programs. STDs are the foremost health problem in homosexual men today.

Fortunately, sympathetic physicians have already begun to educate their colleagues. Several papers have recently been published, including some in widely read medical journals, emphasizing the correct approach to examination of the homosexual male patient for STDs. Some of the highlights of this approach are these: Physicians have to be made aware that homosexual men do not look or act differently from heterosexual men and that all the stereotypes are a myth. Physicians have to demonstrate from the outset a nonjudgmental, sympathetic attitude, since, otherwise, the homosexual patient is often deterred from adequate examination and treatment.

It is to be hoped that informational booklets, as well as other materials describing the signs and symptoms of primary and secondary syphilis in simple and easy to understand language, will become available for the homosexual male. Men will thus become aware of the signs and symptoms of this disease while it still is in the primary stage, and seek treatment at that time. The patient's knowledge of the signs and symptoms may even enable him to suggest to a physician unaware of anal and intrarectal chancres that rectal examination be performed.

A homosexual man who consults a physician because he suspects an STD ordinarily has to make an open admission of sexual orientation. Unfortunately, all too often, health professionals can barely conceal their aversion. As a result, many patients neglect to seek examination, fearing discrimination or anxiety about their and their contacts' sexual orientation. These fears can also keep the homosexual man from being completely forthright with his physician. In addition, the examining physician can often cause alienation by assuming that his patient is heterosexual and failing to test or examine for rectal chancre or pharyngeal gonorrhea. This assumption, of course, is not necessarily due to hostility, but simply to ignorance.

The key element in motivating the homosexual male to seek health care services related to STDs is for him to know that he will receive appropriate care. Use the word *gay* when you talk to the patient, not the word *homosexual*.

Homosexual sounds stiff and formal to many patients. *Gay* connotes awareness, understanding, and acceptance. To avoid the out-and-out question "Are you gay?" it is helpful simply to ask the patient what orifices he wishes to have cultured. If the patient tells you that he wishes to have his anus and mouth cultured, it is not difficult to guess his sexual practices. If a medical professional really feels uncomfortable caring for a homosexual patient, it is both ethical and sound practice to refer the patient to another physician who does feel comfortable, or to a counseling agency or an organization designed to offer advice on sexually related diseases and other matters to the homosexual male population.[16]

RECENT RESEARCH

The most important development on the horizon in syphilis research, aimed at eliminating and eradicating this disease, is the work that has been done on the development of a syphilis vaccine. This work holds great promise precisely because infectious syphilis, if untreated, does confer lifetime immunity against another attack of infectious syphilis. In other words, if a patient has secondary syphilis and *goes untreated,* he may develop tertiary syphilis, but he will never again get secondary syphilis. Once the patient has been treated with penicillin or other curative agents, however, the patient can acquire infectious syphilis again and again. After each time a patient is successfully retreated, he can become reinfected. Nonetheless, the lifetime immunity that would ordinarily occur against infectious syphilis if the patient had not been treated offers the possibility of developing a vaccine that will confer the same lifetime immunity against infection. The most promising work in this area has been done by Metzger[17] in Poland and Miller[18] at the University of California. Metzger and co-workers presented evidence showing that weekly injections of 2.4×10^8 *T. pallidum* protected rabbits against dermal challenge. Subsequently, Miller produced immunity by injecting rabbits with 10^7 irradiated *T. pallidum* twice weekly for thirty-seven weeks. Though presently impractical for human use, immunization against syphilis is indeed possible.

REFERENCES

1. Drusin LM, Homan WP, Dineen P: The role of surgery in primary syphilis of the anus. *Ann Surg* 184:65–67, 1976.
2. Cluckman JB, Kleinman MS, May AG: Primary syphilis of the rectum. *NY State J Med* 74:2210–2211, 1974.
3. Feher J, Somogyi T, Timmer M, et al: Early syphilitic hepatitis. *Lancet* 2:896–899, 1975.
4. Butz WC, Watts JC, Rosales-Quintana S, et al: Erosive gastritis as a manifestation of secondary syphilis. *Am J Clin Pathol* 63:895–900, 1975.

5. Wilcox RR, Goodwin PG: Nerve deafness in early syphilis. *Br J Vener Dis* 47:401–406, 1971.
6. Hellier MD, Webster ADB, Eisinger AJM: Nephrotic syndrome: A complication of secondary syphilis. *Br Med J* 4:404–405, 1971.
7. Stokes JH, Beerman H, Ingraham NR: *Modern Clinical Syphilology*, ed 3. Philadelphia, WB Saunders, 1945, pp 604–605.
8. Tight RR, Warner JF: Skeletal involvement in secondary syphilis detected by bone scanning. *JAMA* 235:2326, 1976.
9. Clark GE, Danbolt N: The Oslo study of the natural course of untreated syphilis. *Med Clin North Am* 48(3):613–623, 1964.
10. Center for Disease Control: CDC-HSM Form 9.54. Atlanta, HEW-PHS-CDC, VD Control Division, Evaluation and Statistical Services Section, 1979.
11. Bell AP, Weinberg MS: *Homosexualities. A Study of Diversity Among Men and Women.* New York, Simon and Schuster, 1978, pp 85–102.
12. Merino HI, Bennett D, Judson FN, et al: Screening for gonorrhea and syphilis in the gay bathhouses. A comparative study of programs in Denver, Colorado, and Los Angeles, California. Presented at the 105th Annual Meeting of the American Public Health Association, Washington, DC, Oct 30–Nov 3, 1977.
13. Judson FN, Miller KG, Schaffnit GN: Screening for gonorrhea and syphilis in the gay baths—Denver, Colorado. *Am J Public Health* 67:740–742, 1977.
14. Wolf FC, Judson FN: Intensive screening of gonorrhea, syphilis, and hepatitis B in gay bathhouse does not lower the prevalence of infection. *Sex Transm Dis* 7:49–52, 1980.
15. Felman YM: Should premarital syphilis serologies continue to be mandated by law? *JAMA* 240:459–460, 1978.
16. Felman YM, Morrison JM: Examining the homosexual male for sexually transmitted diseases. *JAMA* 238:2046–2047, 1977.
17. Metzger M, Smogor W: Artificial immunization of rabbits against syphilis. Effect of increasing doses of treponemes given by the intramuscular route. *Br J Vener Dis* 45:308–312, 1969.
18. Miller JN: Immunity in experimental syphilis. V. The immunogenicity of *Treponema pallidum* attenuated by gamma irradiation. *J Immunol* 99:1012–1016, 1967.

5

Gonococcal Infections

DAVID G. OSTROW

Gonorrhea is the world's most common sexually transmitted infectious disease. Approximately 1 million cases of gonorrhea are reported each year in the United States.[1] Figure 1 shows the overall trends in gonorrhea infections in the United States as reported to the Centers for Disease Control (CDC). Unreported cases are estimated to be as high as 3 million per year. Several comprehensive reviews concerning gonococcal infection have recently been published,[2,3] and the reader is referred to these sources for general information regarding the subject.

Specific aspects of gonococcal infection in the homosexual male relate to sexual practices in this group, particularly orogenital (fellatio) and anogenital (anal intercourse) sexual activity, which can result in oral, anal, and urethral infection. A homosexual male who participates in the full range of sexual activities has three possible sites for infection, rather than the single (urethral) site for the heterosexual male who practices only penile–vaginal intercourse. The overall high incidence of gonococcal infection in the homosexual male, as well as the possibility for multiple sites of infection occurring simultaneously, makes the risk of infection substantially greater than in his heterosexual counterpart. The problem is compounded since both anal and pharyngeal infections are frequently asymptomatic (see page 60).

ETIOLOGY

The causative organism of gonorrhea, *Neisseria gonorrhoeae,* is one of six members of the genus *Neisseria,* which also includes *N. meningitidis,* all of

DAVID G. OSTROW ● Biological Psychiatry Program, Lakeside Veterans Administration Medical Center, and Departments of Psychiatry and Community Medicine, Northwestern University Medical School, Chicago, Illinois 60611; and Howard Brown Memorial Clinic, Chicago, Illinois 60616.

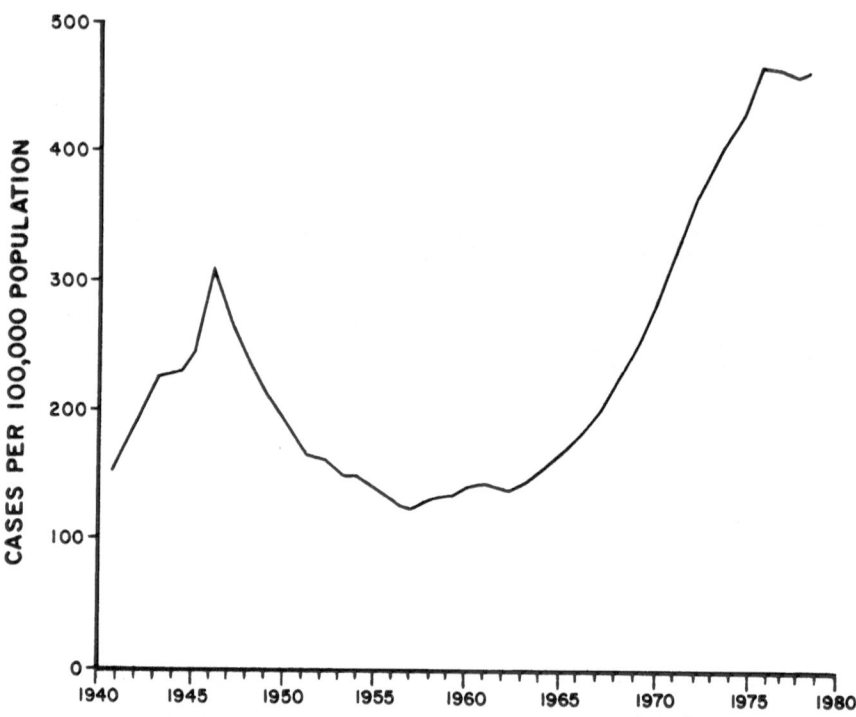

FIGURE 1. Reported civilian gonorrhea case rates by year in the United States, calendar years 1941–1978. From ref. 1.

which are gram-negative diplococci. Identification of *N. gonorrhoeae* is either by gram stain of exudates or by colony morphology and fermentation characteristics of suitably cultured specimens. Gram stain may provide immediate identification, but this must be considered a presumptive diagnosis as other species of *Neisseria*, particularly those commonly found in the oral and anal cavities, have a similar gram-stained appearance. In a recent study of homosexual males attending the Howard Brown Memorial Clinic (HBMC), over 40% of pharyngeal cultures yielded *N. meningitidis*, in contrast to 7% for heterosexual males tested at a university student health clinic.[4]

Transmission of *N. gonorrhoeae* in adults occurs almost exclusively by sexual contact. Fomite transmission is theoretically possible, but the fastidious nature of the organism makes survival outside the host for more than several hours relatively rare. Several recent studies have failed to recover viable organisms from toilets used by patients attending venereal disease (VD) clinics,[5,6] but occasional anecdotal reports of gonococcal infection acquired from contaminated surfaces have appeared. Anal infection secondary to dildo or digital insertion in a group sex or bathhouse situation is possible, but such cases are rare and not of epidemiologic significance. Transmission of the organism from urethral and rectal sites to all three possible sites in the sexual partner has been well documented through both epidemiologic and experimental investigations.[7,8] While pharyngeal gonorrhea may well be transmitted to partners through fellatio or oroanal (anilinction) sexual practices, these routes of infection have not been documented. An important consideration in the epidemiology of gonorrhea in homosexual men is the high rate of cotransmission of other sexually transmitted diseases (STDs), such as genital herpes, syphilis, hepatitis, and warts (condylomata acuminata). Not at all infrequently, homosexual patients who initially present at a VD clinic with rectal pain and discharge have pus containing numerous gram-negative diplococci, typical anal herpes lesions, and a positive Venereal Disease Research Laboratory test on follow-up examination two to three weeks later.

The recent discovery of penicillin-resistant forms of *N. gonorrhoeae,*[9] as well as the identification of unusual nutritional or morphological characteristics of asymptomatic urethral isolates,[10] suggests that a variety of subtypes of *N. gonorrhoeae* exist, with variable clinical manifestations of infection that depend upon the particular subtype and site of infection.

CLINICAL ASPECTS OF UNCOMPLICATED INFECTIONS

Gonococcal Urethritis

Uncomplicated gonococcal urethritis is usually symptomatic in homosexual men.[11] Asymptomatic infection of the urethra has been described,[10,12] but less than 2% of the urethral isolates at the HBMC have been from asymptomatic individuals. Incubation time is usually one to three days but may be as long as seven days. Symptoms include urethral discomfort, dysuria, and purulent discharge. The discharge usually ranges in color from white to yellow to green and is often copious, although the nature and quantity of discharge may be affected by the patient's prior (and usually inadequate) self-medication with antibiotics. Occasionally the discharge will be clear and/or scanty, even in the absence of prior medication.

The differential diagnosis of urethral discharge includes other causes of urethritis, such as *Chlamydia, Trichomonas,* herpes simplex, and "nonspecific urethritis." Occasionally, a urinary tract infection, most commonly prostatitis or epididymitis, presents as a scant urethral discharge. The features of the discharge in terms of quantity and gram stain appearance as well as incubation period, history of exposure, and previous urinary tract infection often permit the differentiation of gonococcal infection from these other types of urethritis at the time of initial examination. Patients presenting with wads of toilet tissue or Kleenex matted to their penis or underwear by a copious purulent discharge will invariably turn out to have gonococcal urethritis.

Gonococcal Proctitis

Gonococcal proctitis may be symptomatic, asymptomatic, or intermittently symptomatic.[13,14] The most frequent symptoms (seen in less than 40% of patients with rectal gonorrhea) include rectal discomfort, tenesmus, a pus or mucous discharge, and scant blood in stool (hemafecia). Clinical signs are rectal discharge and mucopurulent material of varying amount, which is frequently positive on gram stain for gram-negative intracellular diplococci. The rectal mucosa is usually normal in appearance, but patchy mucosal lesions sometimes are seen that may resemble ulcerative colitis on proctologic examination but that rarely extend beyond the rectum. The differential diagnosis includes other infectious conditions, such as amebic or herpetic proctitis, shigellosis, inflammatory bowel disease, "nonspecific proctitis," and traumatic or allergic proctitis. Specific diagnostic procedures used to determine the etiology of proctitis are described on page 62.

Gonococcal Pharyngitis

The patient with uncomplicated gonococcal pharyngitis is usually asymptomatic, but florid infections, including sore throat, dysphagia, and tender swollen anterior cervical lymph nodes, may be seen.[15–17] When present, clinical signs include pharyngeal erythema with and without exudate. Differential diagnosis of acute pharyngitis must include streptococcal pharyngitis, mononucleosis, and other viral infections. At least one study suggested that pharyngeal gonorrhea had a relatively high rate of systemic dissemination,[18] but this complication has rarely been observed in the clinical population at the HBMC. This may be due to the relative rarity in homosexual men[4] of those strains known to be a frequent cause of disseminated gonorrhea. Alternatively, patients with systemic infection may preferentially be seen in facilities, such as hospital emergency rooms, known to be equipped for the handling of severe illness, or may have developed pharyngeal infection secondary to the disseminated gonorrhea.

CLINICAL ASPECTS OF COMPLICATED INFECTION

Disseminated Gonococcal Infection

The major complication of gonococcal infection is disseminated gonococcal infection (DGI).[19,20] Though DGI is more common in women than in men, it may occur as a consequence of pharyngeal infection.[17,18,20] Estimates place the incidence of DGI in men at approximately 0.5% of all gonococcal infections. The presumed pathogenesis of the disease is that gonococci enter the bloodstream from the initial site of infection and are then disseminated to the skin, joints (common), heart valves, and meninges (rare). Symptoms include fever, general malaise, and arthralgias. Clinical signs include skin lesions, which are typically hemorrhagic pustules on the extremities. Joint lesions are also common, and erosion of cartilage and atrophy of adjacent bony structures are easily recognized on X ray and confirmed by culture of aspirated synovial fluid. In the early stage of the disease, tenosynovitis of multiple joints is usually present; later, during the course of the illness, septic arthritis of one or more joints is common. The differential diagnosis must include Reiter's syndrome, rheumatic fever, gout, and meningococcemia. Diagnosis of DGI is usually made by laboratory identification of *N. gonorrhoeae* in material aspirated from one or more involved joints.

Other Complications

Infrequent complications of gonorrhea infection are gonococcal epididymitis and prostatitis. While the overall incidence of both of these complications is low, several series have been reported and their incidence may be higher in men with frequent urethral gonorrhea or with coexisting prostatitis.[21,22] Urethral strictures, once a frequent complication of untreated urethral gonorrhea or treatment with preantibiotic silver nitrate instillation, are now rare except in geriatric patients. Rectal strictures associated with recurrent anorectal gonorrhea have not been reported, but this complication is possible and should be considered in patients presenting with anorectal complaints.

DIAGNOSIS

The diagnosis of gonococcal infection remains relatively straightforward, specific, and highly accurate if physical examination is thorough and laboratory techniques are precise. The mainstays of diagnosis are trisite culture and examination of gram stain smears. Provine and Gardner have described a rapid gram stain technique, involving sequential ten-second rinses with crystal violet, Gram's iodine, 95% ethanol, and safranin, which yields excellent results.[23] Handling and interpretation of specimens are described in most basic texts of clinical microbiology as well as in the review by Morton.[2] Most important are the use of selective growth media to inhibit overgrowth by nonpathogenic commensal organisms and rapid transfer of plates to a CO_2-enriched atmosphere at 37°C.

Symptomatic Urethral Gonorrhea

Diagnosis of symptomatic urethral gonorrhea is made by gram-stained smear of fresh urethral exudate, while confirmation depends upon fermentation testing of cultured organisms. Contamination of urethral specimens with *Neisseria* species other then *N. gonorrhoeae* is relatively rare. To detect early or asymptomatic urethral gonorrhea, deep urethral specimens are obtained by passing a fine calcium-alginate swab (Inolex®; Calgiswab®) or urethral loop approximately 2 to 4 cm into the urethral canal, gently scraping the urethra in all four quadrants, and culturing the obtained material into a suitable medium. Pain and trauma are minimal when a small-caliber swab is used for this procedure, but many patients are reluctant to undergo urethral cultures in the absence of symptoms. The small yield of yield of asymptomatic gonococcal infection in homosexual men (approximately 1% of the population at an STD clinic such as the HBMC) has led to questioning of the routine use of this procedure.[24] Many STD clinics seeing large numbers of homosexual men therefore do not include urethral cultures of asymptomatic patients as part of a routine STD check-up.

Gonococcal Proctitis

Gonococcal proctitis is more difficult to diagnose and requires visual examination of the anal canal to obtain adequate specimens for gram stain smear and culture. However, any physician with sexually active patients should have the necessary equipment for anoscopic examination. Figure 2 diagrams the method used at the HBMC for anoscopic examination and for obtaining samples for testing. We have found the use of an 8-cm plastic disposable anoscope most suitable as it eliminates the problems of sterility and cross-contamination. The physician should ready all material needed for obtaining gram stain smears and cultures beforehand. Many authorities warn against applying lubricant to the tip of the anoscope. However, a small amount of a water-based lubricant applied to the obturator makes the procedure more tolerable to the patient and does not interfere with subsequent testing. Once the anoscope has been fully inserted, the obturator is removed and the instrument slowly withdrawn while visual examination for friable and ulcerative lesions is performed under suitable illumination. Headset illumination provides the most easily directed light source since it leaves one hand free to obtain samples for cultures. Any lesions are carefully swabbed for both gram stain and culture. Generally, as the anoscope is withdrawn, a variable amount of pus will collect distal to the collapsed mucosa. This "pearl" of pus is easily picked up by cotton-tipped swab and provides material for both smear and culture.

Table 1 illustrates the results of this procedure in a series of symptomatic

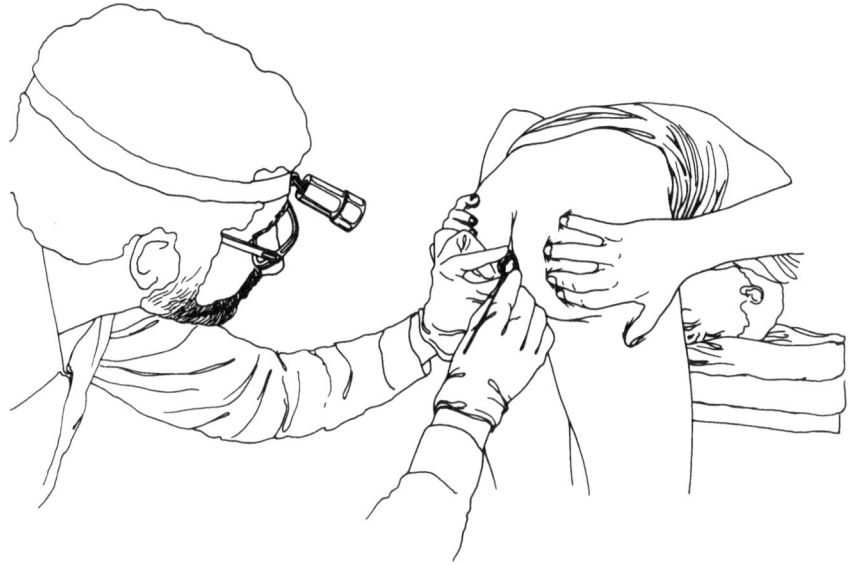

FIGURE 2. Anoscopic examination procedure in an STD clinic setting.

homosexual men examined at the HBMC. Most notable is the high yield of presumptive diagnoses of gonococcal proctitis obtained by careful examinations of gram stain smears of rectal exudates obtained via anoscopy in symptomatic patients. In contrast to the results for gram stain examination of material obtained either blindly or from asymptomatic patients, these results support the use of

TABLE 1. Rectal Gram Stain Results in Diagnosing Gonorrhea Infections[a]

| Culture result | Gram stain result | |
	Positive (I or II)	Negative (III or IV)
Positive	36	10
Negative	3[b]	24

[a] Gram stain readings were performed according to the criteria of Jacobs and Kraus.[11] All samples were obtained by anoscopy on patients with anorectal symptoms.

[b] Rapid cessation of symptoms followed treatment with 4.8 million units aqueous procaine penicillin G IM, preceded by 1 g probenecid PO, in all three patients.

gram stain examinations of material obtained by anoscopy from men with rectal symptoms. These results are similar to those obtained by McMillan and Young[25] in men attending two STD clinics in Scotland. These investigators reported a somewhat higher percentage of false-negative gram stain smears, but admitted that the few false-positive readings may have actually represented loss of viable gonococci prior to transfer to culture medium. Other sources of "false-positive" gram stain readings may be the presence of other rectal organisms that resemble *Neisseria* and are phagocytized, or inadequate culture methodology in the identification of "atypical" or slow-growing colonies. In any case, our experience in finding a high rate of correlation between gram stain results and response to adequate treatment with penicillin or ampicillin in patients with proctitis suggests that this technique be more widely used.

Pharyngeal Gonorrhea

Diagnosis of pharyngeal gonorrhea is made by culture of any exudate present at oropharyngeal examination. Gram stain examination of oral exudates is not useful because other *Neisseria* species are normally present in the throat. In addition, definitive identification of oral cultures requires fermentation tests because all *Neisseria* species appear identical to *N. gonorrhoeae* in terms of colony morphology and oxidase positivity. The yield of asymptomatic oral gonorrhea infections in homosexual men is quite high, ranging from 3% to 5% in bathhouse screening (Table 4) to 10% to 15% at STD clinics.

Various techniques have been developed for the culturing and subsequent identification of *N. gonorrhoeae*, but most clinics now use modified Thayer–Martin medium or New York City medium. In addition to traditional petri dishes, several manufacturers now produce "mini-plates" (e.g., the JEMBEC® Plate). These include a tablet that, when added to the plate, produces a CO_2-enriched environment, allowing immediate transfer of the sample to a standard 37°C incubator. Culture specimens must be placed in a CO_2-enriched environment and incubated immediately since the yield of positive cultures falls off rapidly if they remain under room-temperature conditions. Results of urethral cultures can usually be obtained within twenty-four to forty-eight hours, but because of the need for fermentation testing of oral and anal cultures, confirmation of these results requires more time. To overcome this difficulty, investigators are working to develop more rapid means of detecting gonococcal infection, including the use of specific immunofluorescent reagents, DNA transformation techniques, and serologic tests. While some of these tests show promise, none is yet reliable in diagnosing acute infection. Their possible usefulness in field locations, especially in such high-risk environments as bathhouses, requires further investigation.

TREATMENT

Table 2 summarizes the most recent recommendations by the CDC for the treatment of uncomplicated gonorrhea and DGI.[26] While these schedules include four different antibiotics as first choice for the treatment of uncomplicated gonorrhea, aqueous procaine penicillin G (APPG) remains the drug of choice and, except in the special situations discussed in the next section, remains the most effective, fastest, and least expensive therapy. Recent shortages of APPG supplies have led to the investigation of alternative treatment regimens, the results of which are also discussed.

TABLE 2. Centers for Disease Control Recommended Antibiotics Treatment Regimens for Gonococcal Infections

I. Uncomplicated infections in adults
   A. *Preferred treatment:* 4.8 million units aqueous procaine penicillin G IM, divided and injected into two sites at first visit, preceded by 1 g probenecid PO to block renal secretion of penicillin.
   B. *If the organism is resistant or the patient is allergic to penicillin:* 0.5 g tetracycline hydrochloride PO qid for 5 days (total dosage 10 g).[a] Other tetracyclines (e.g., doxycycline) may be substituted at equivalent dosage, but no single-dose tetracycline therapy is effective.
   C. *Or, if the patient cannot tolerate tetracyclines:* 3.5 g ampicillin PO or 3.0 g amoxicillin PO. Precede either drug with 1 g probenecid PO. Controlled studies evaluating the effectiveness of the latter alternative regimen have not been published, but anecdotal reports testifying to the efficacy of amoxicillin in the treatment of anal gonorrhea have appeared.
   D. *If the organism is resistant to penicillin, tetracyclines, or ampicillin or amoxicillin:* 2 g to 4 g spectinomycin hydrochloride IM. This treatment has a high failure rate in oropharyngeal gonococcal infection.

II. Complicated or disseminated infections in adults (arthritis–dermatitis syndrome)
   A. 3.5 g ampicillin *or* 3 g amoxicillin PO, either one preceded by 1 g probenecid PO. Then 0.5 g of the drug of choice orally qid 7 days.
   B. *Or* 0.5 g tetracycline hydrochloride PO qid for 7 days.[a]
   C. *Or* 2 g spectinomycin hydrochloride IM bid for 3 days. *Treatment of choice for penicillinase-producing gonococcal infections.*
   D. *Or* 0.5 g erythromycin PO qid for 7 days.
   E. *Or* 10 million units aqueous crystalline penicillin G IV per day until improvement occurs. Then 0.5 g ampicillin PO qid to a total of 7 days' treatment.

[a] Food, especially dairy products, interferes with the absorption of all tetracyclines. Oral tetracycline should be taken on an empty stomach (at least 1 h before and 2 h after meal). Further, if the patient is taking iron preparations, these should be separated from the tetracycline by at least 1 h. The patient should be instructed to avoid prolonged exposure to sunlight while taking tetracyclines. The use of alcohol during tetracycline therapy is not contraindicated but should be minimized.

Special Problems in the Initial Treatment of Gonorrhea

Several difficulties arise from the frequency of oral and rectal gonorrhea in the homosexual male population and the lack of adequate studies of the efficacy of various managements for infections in these locations. Generally, oral gonococcal infections are more difficult to treat than urethral infections,[27] with relatively high rates of treatment failure with any parenteral single-dose regime and with all oral regimens. Whenever possible, 4.8 million units APPG, divided and injected at two sites and preceded by 1 g oral probenecid, should be administered at the first visit. If the patient is allergic to penicillin or the organisms are resistent to penicillin therapy, administer 0.5 g tetracycline hydrochloride orally four times a day for five days. While many regimens propose a loading dose of 1.5 g tetracycline hydrochloride, the efficacy of therapy is as high as when the loading dose is omitted. The frequency of gastrointestinal side effects is also significantly reduced.[28]

Published data on the therapeutic efficacy of the various treatment regimens in anorectal gonorrhea are scarce. In some studies[13,29] the failure rates in men ranged from 0% to 29%, with perhaps the most consistently low treatment failure rates in patients treated with 4 g spectinomycin hydrochloride intramuscularly (0% to 14%). Table 3 lists the treatment failure results obtained in a recent CDC study of anorectal gonorrhea.[30] These data illustrate that spectinomycin hydrochloride was the most effective drug for treatment of anorectal gonorrhea. Markedly increased failure rates are noted for single-dose ampicillin and four- to seven-day tetracycline regimens for anorectal gonorrhea, especially as compared to their efficacy for management of urethral gonococcal infections. Recent studies suggest that a two-dose regimen of 3.5 g oral ampicillin plus 1.0 g probenecid given eight to twelve hours apart results in an acceptably low (1% to 2%) failure rate in the treatment of anorectal gonorrhea.[31,32] The high failure rate for spectinomycin in the treatment of oral gonorrhea plus the observation that men with rectal gonorrhea are at high risk for oral infections makes penicillin APPG plus

TABLE 3. Therapy Failures in Men by Infection Site and Treatment Regimen[a]

Regimen	Rectum			Urethra		
	Tested	Failed	Percent	Tested	Failed	Percent
Penicillin, IM	40	2	5.0	2324	101	4.3
Ampicillin, single dose PO	34	7	20.6	1363	100	7.3
Tetracycline, multiple dose PO	38	9	23.7	921	21	2.3
Spectinomycin, IM	17	0	0	1155	59	5.1

[a] From ref 30.

probenecid the preferred treatment for anorectal gonorrhea. If APPG continues to be in short supply, the two-dose ampicillin plus probenecid regimen may become a standard alternative. This latter regimen is now standard at the HBMC for patients with urethral gonorrhea and a history or symptoms suggestive of possible concurrent rectal infection.

The cause of the relatively high failure rates for oral antibiotic therapy of anorectal gonorrhea is unknown, but it may be related to the easily traumatized nature of the rectal mucosa (as hypothesized for the sexual transmission of hepatitis B via this route), drug penetration factors, or unreported reinfections. Accordingly, it is imperative that careful follow-up with test-of-cure by post-treatment cultures at seven to fourteen days be done in all patients with anorectal and oral gonorrhea infection. Posttherapy anorectal cultures should be obtained via direct visualization of the anal canal; otherwise there is a 40% chance of a false-negative culture result. Patients must be strongly advised to abstain from sexual contact of any kind during the time between treatment and follow-up, both to protect sexual contacts from infection and to prevent reinfection. Persons allergic to penicillin or suspected of having penicillin-resistant anorectal infection should be treated with 2 g to 4 g spectinoymcin intramuscularly.

Treatment Failures

The patient who presents with continuing or recrudescent symptoms of gonorrhea one to two weeks after initial treatment represents a difficult therapeutic problem. Attempts should be made to distinguish reinfections from treatment failures, as based on the patient's history. The longer the period between the initial treatment and the patient's presentation, however, the more arbitrary and potentially misleading the distinction. If a definite history of reexposure to gonorrhea is elicited, the original treatment regimen should be prescribed. Contact tracing and treatment of sexual partners must be attempted, especially if the patient's contact was a person with asymptomatic anorectal or pharyngeal gonorrhea. Individuals with these forms of the disease serve as the greatest potential reservoir for gonococcal infection in the homosexual male population, but are among the least likely to seek medical intervention. The reinfected sexual partner should be prompted to discuss the situation with his asymptomatic contacts (with or without help from clinic workers). This approach is more likely to induce contacts to seek diagnosis and treatment than reliance on traditional state board of health epidemiology contact tracing or form letters.

Treatment failures or relapses may be due to a variety of factors other than antibiotic-resistant organisms. These include patient noncompliance in the case of multiple-dose oral antibiotic regimens, poor tissue penetration of antibiotics in the case of gonococcal prostatitis, and breakdown of the prescribed antibiotic by endogenous penicillinase-producing organisms in the bowel. While these organisms may be the cause of some anorectal gonorrhea treatment failures, penicillinase-producing gonococci have been isolated from increasing numbers of patients in the United States[33] and are now the predominant organisms in several Far East countries.[34] Any apparent treatment failure following adequate APPG treatment should be suspected as being due to a β-lactamase-producing strain, and a culture or subculture isolate should be sent to the CDC or state laboratory for tests of antibiotic resistance and β-lactamase production. The treatment of choice for these infections appears to be spectinomycin,[33,35] but data are inconclusive on whether 2 g or 4 g of spectinomycin intramuscularly are required for treatment. Multiple resistance factors are frequently found in penicillinase-producing organisms, and a high proportion of organisms have been found to be resistant to tetracycline and a smaller amount to spectinomycin. The high failure rate for the treatment of oropharyngeal gonorrhea with spectinomycin (up to 50% in one study[18]) makes the routine use of this antibiotic unwise. Rather, actual determination of the in vitro antibiotic concentrations necessary for growth inhibition ["minimum inhibitory concentration" (MIC)] of a particular isolate and treatment with a high dosage of a selectively chosen effective antibiotic are the preferred treatment options. Thus far, no organisms have been found that are resistant to all known antibiotics. To ensure that treatment-resistant organisms do not become established, the appropriate antibiotic should be administered in a dosage that attains a blood concentration level three to five times the in vitro MIC. These steps should be sufficient to treat most of the "resistant" organisms presently found and should help to ensure that alternative antibiotics, such as spectinomycin, sulfa-trimethoprin, and new cephalosporins, retain their effectiveness. Successful treatment of a case of penicillin-resistant gonococcal polyarthritis (stemming from pharyngeal infection acquired in the Phillipines) with 2 g oral tetracycline daily for three weeks followed by 2 g oral erythromycin daily for an additional 10 days[36] has been reported, but this novel regimen has not been further tested.

Postgonococcal Urethritis

A common complication following the treatment of urethral gonorrhea is the emergence of postgonococcal urethritis (PGU). PGU presents similarly to nongonococcal urethritis with scant mucoid discharge that is negative on gram stain examination for gram-negative intracellular diplococci and may be caused by the same organisms (see Chapter 6). The prevalence of this condition (about 1% to 2% of STD patients) is probably due to coexistent infection with penicillin-insensitive organisms. PGU may also be caused by commensal urethral organisms that become invasive in the wake of gonococcal damage to the urethral mucosa. Tetracycline, 2 g daily for five to seven days, is the treatment of choice.[37]

Tetracycline therapy has been considered as the drug of choice for gonococcal urethritis to minimize the risk of PGU. However, the relatively low rate of PGU that follows adequate treatment of initial infection with APPG, and the risk of inadequate gonorrhea treatment when a multiple oral antibiotic dose regimen is employed, argue strongly against such a change.

Although recent developments have complicated the treatment of gonococcal infection, an initial dose of 4.8 million units of APPG intramuscularly, divided and injected in two sites and preceded by 1 g oral probenecid, remains the treatment of choice in almost all gonococcal infections. The problems produced by multiple-site infections, treatment failures, and the rising frequency of penicillin-resistant organisms do not argue for any change in the suggested regimen, but rather for more stringent retesting for cure and antibiotic sensitivity testing in all apparent cases of treatment failure.

EPIDEMIOLOGY OF GONOCOCCAL INFECTION IN HOMOSEXUAL MEN

The reasons for the exceedingly high rate of gonococcal infection in the homosexual male population include nonspecific factors (multiple sexual partners and anonymity of sexual partners) as well as specific factors (the high rates of asymptomatic infection and treatment failure for anorectal infection). Large-scale screening programs for gonorrhea in homosexual men in several major cities in the United States have yielded important information concerning the incidence and epidemiologic characteristics of this infection.

Table 4 summarizes the results of trisite (oral, rectal, and urethral cultures and gram stain) gonorrhea testing in the homosexual male community of Chicago. The lower number in each range is for confirmed *N. gonorrhoeae* isolates and the higher number is combined positive and suspicious isolates. Owing to the practice of the Chicago Department of Health Laboratories of reporting as "suspicious" those rectal and oral isolates that are not confirmed by sugar fermentation tests, the latter number undoubtedly includes a certain number of *N. meningitidis* isolates. The three types of testing programs are as follows:

1. *HBMC patients*. This population includes mainly symptomatic patients who have had recent sexual contact with an infectious individual. The range of sexual activities, the number of steady and nonsteady partners, and the types of specific complaints are as broad as the homosexual male population of Chicago. The average age of patients with gonococcal infection is approximately 27 years within a range of patients aged 15 to 80.

2. *"VD Van"/Winter Carnival outreach programs*. These programs are held routinely and are operated in collaboration with the Chicago Department

TABLE 4. Summary of Gonorrhea Testing Results by Anatomic Site and Screening Program

Testing location; testing period; total no. of patients	Oral culture positives Percent tests performed Percent total patients	Rectal culture positives Percent tests performed Percent total patients	Urethral culture positives Percent tests performed Percent total patients
HBMC July 1975– December 1978 15,465 patients	3.3%–5.5% 2.9%–4.8%	10.1%–11.4% 9.2%–10.4%	[a] 13.6% Overall: 21.1% patients positive
"VD Van"/Winter Carnival 1976–1978 1537 patients	1.7%–2.4% 1.7%–2.4%	4.5%–5.1% 2.3%–2.6%	4.5%–4.9% 0.6%–0.7% Overall: 4.5% patients positive
Bathhouse testing February 1978– January 1979 1030 patients	1.5%–5.2% 1.5%–5.1%	7.6%–9.2% 6.5%–7.9%	8.2%–8.9% 1.2%–1.3% Overall: 8.8% patients positive

[a] As gram stain was performed on symptomatic patients and cultures were performed on asymptomatic and gram-negative patients with discharge, percent tests performed "positive" is not given.

of Health Venereal Disease Control Program. Testing is performed periodically throughout the year, either in a mobile "VD Van" that is stationed in front of various bars and other business establishments or at a major citywide social event, the Winter Carnival. Individuals attending these functions are assumed to be largely asymptomatic and to be a random selection of sexually active persons, engaging in polygamous sexual relationships with a mean number of nonsteady sexual contacts of about four per month. The aim is to identify those asymptomatic carriers of gonorrhea or syphilis who might otherwise not come to a VD clinic, as well as to raise the level of awareness of the community to the need for routine STD screening.

3. *Bathhouse testing program.* This program is operated on weekend evenings at the major bathhouses in Chicago in an attempt to identify asymptomatic individuals. Individuals tested in this program are representative of the most sexually active homosexual male population, with an average number of nonsteady partners of three to four persons per visit. While both outreach programs are assumed to represent random cross-sections of asymptomatic individuals, a certain percentage of participants at these "off-clinic" sites are individuals with early or mild

symptoms, who take advantage of the convenience of being tested and thus skew the data by an indeterminate amount.

Not surprisingly, the urethral positivity rate (combined culture and gram stain results of 13.6% of patients) was highest in patients attending at the HBMC. However, the 3% to 5% oral gonorrhea and 9% to 10% anorectal gonorrhea rates for clinic patients are surprising when one considers that only a fraction of these patients had oral or rectal symptoms indicative of gonococcal infection. These results are similar to those observed by McMillan and Young[25] in homosexual males tested at public STD clinics in Scotland, with the exception that a somewhat smaller proportion of pharyngeal gonorrhea infections were observed than at the HBMC.

Both oral and anal gonorrhea positivity fell to approximately 2.5% when testing was done at the "VD Van" or Winter Carnival outreach programs. Urethral gonorrhea was less than 1%, which probably approximates the incidence of asymptomatic gonorrhea. Overall, 4.5% of persons presenting at mobile testing sites at or near social activity centers had gonococcal infection in one or more anatomic sites. Results for testing at bathhouses are for one year only and are intermediate between the clinic and mobile testing center rates. Most striking was the high rate of anorectal gonorrhea infections in this group (6% to 8%), which accounted for the majority of infections found in the bathhouse patrons. The low rate of urethral infections in this group (1.2%) argues against a large proportion of symptomatic individuals being included among those tested at these programs.

Epidemiologically, the asymptomatic carrier of anorectal gonorrhea causes the most concern. The data indicate that the carrier rate for anorectal gonorrhea ranges from 2.5% to 8%, with the incidence of infection paralleling the degree of sexual activity. HBMC data are surprisingly similar to those of Judson et al.,[38,39] who tested patrons at the Denver and Los Angeles bathhouses (6.6% rate). Based on this rate and the average of four to five sexual contacts per visit to the baths, Judson estimated that bathhouse patrons ran a one in three chance of having contact with gonococcal infection. Considering that the anal gonococcal carrier is a proven efficient vector for transmission of gonorrhea to sexual contacts, and the findings that individuals practicing anal receptive intercourse have the highest number of nonsteady sexual contacts,[40] the contribution of asymptomatic rectal carriers to the overall incidence of gonorrhea must be significant.

Obviously, efforts to identify carriers of asymptomatic anorectal gonorrhea have high priority within overall gonorrhea control programs. However, the difficulties in utilizing gram stain exams for diagnosis of anorectal gonorrhea and the three- to five-day delay in gonorrhea culture screening make identification programs difficult if not impossible. Experimentation with the use of anal gram stains for the identification of gonorrhea carriers has been carried out at the

HBMC, but this technique appears to be useful only in symptomatic individuals.[41] Further attempts have been made to determine if certain mild or chronic symptoms might be present in a major proportion of anorectal gonorrhea carriers.[40] Results of these studies are negative. If the rate of anorectal gonorrhea carriage and thus the rate of transmission of gonococcal infection in the homosexual male population are to be reduced, then ways to treat persons who are at highest risk selectively must be developed. This author has suggested that bathhouse screening programs be expanded to include prophylactic treatment of gonorrhea.[41] Certainly, persons who practice anal receptive intercourse with multiple partners need to be examined at frequent intervals and suspected gonococcal infection treated prior to further sexual activity. The development of rapid "on-site" diagnostic procedures for anorectal gonorrhea should be a major priority of STD control programs. The use of such procedures in selective screening and prophylactic treatment programs would afford the best chance of interrupting the cycle of gonorrhea transmission within the homosexual male community.

PROPHYLAXIS

Mechanical methods of prophylaxis are unlikely to gain any significant degree of acceptance in the gay community. Attempts to educate persons having multiple sexual contacts in the use of condoms have been uniformly disappointing, except for several recent campaigns in Sweden and Denver that used advertising, posters, and the distribution of free condoms. Many of the patients at the HBMC claim that rectal douching following anal intercourse helps reduce the chance of catching anorectal gonorrhea, but there have been no published controlled studies of the efficacy of this practice. In addition, the use of antibiotic or chemical douching agents would be expected to carry a significant risk of allergic or chemical proctitis, and rectal douching has been implicated as a risk factor in the sexual transmission of hepatitis B.[42] Patients at the HBMC are advised to wash their genitals and to urinate as soon as possible after insertive anal intercourse as a possible method of reducing the chances of acquiring urethral infection. Again, no controlled studies of the efficacy of this practice exist. However, in bathhouses or other group sex situations, these practices would at least lessen the likelihood of fecal–oral transmission of hepatitis B, giardiasis, amebiasis, and other enteric disorders.

Antibiotic prophylaxis to reduce the risk of urethral gonorrhea during time-limited exposure periods (i.e., shore leave) has been demonstrated to be effective.[43] However, the widespread use of penicillin prophylaxis in the Far East and Africa by prostitutes is implicated as a major cause of the emergence of penicillin-resistant organisms in those areas. Their use has led to skepticism concerning the use of antibiotic prophylaxis in endemic situations. However, a recent study by Holmes and associates[44] suggests that 200 mg doxycycline taken after sexual contact can dramatically reduce the rate of gonococcal infection without any significant morbidity in terms of antibiotic resistance or allergic reactions. In this study, the relative rate of gonococcal infection at each anatomic site for two groups of homosexual men with multiple sexual partners (the patients who received antibiotic prophylaxis and those who received placebos) was calculated. Protection was highest against urethral and anorectal gonorrhea infection, with little protection afforded against pharyngeal infection. Overall, there was a fivefold reduction in the incidence of gonococcal infection in the group who received the doxycycline prophylaxis. The benefit of prophylactic administration to the homosexual male community may be even greater, as the rate of transmission of infection to secondary contacts would presumably also be significantly decreased by the use of doxycycline prophylaxis. This study needs to be expanded to include a larger cohort of men, with testing of sexual contacts to document the efficacy of this form of antibiotic prophylaxis and to monitor the long-term risk of emergence of antibiotic-resistant strains. The major advantage of utilizing community STD clinics for studies of postexposure prophylaxis in specific target groups at high risk is that the dose of antibiotic and return testing for asymptomatic infection can be more rigidly controlled than in other settings. A well-controlled long-term study that demonstrated a significant impact on the overall rate of gonococcal infection in the homosexual male community through antibiotic prophylaxis in high-risk groups would be a major breakthrough. However, extreme caution needs to be used in the extrapolation of the results of any such study to the uncontrolled use of antibiotic prophylaxis, lest we repeat the Far East experience.

CONTROL

In the area of STD control in the homosexual male population, great problems arise because of widespread personal prejudices and public attitudes toward both STDs and homosexuality. Nevertheless, sophisticated and innovative education and control programs aimed directly at this population have been shown to be highly effective in limiting the spread of STDs.[45] Much has been said about the need for education of the public about STD control; education of the health care provider to the particular difficulties and anxieties of the homosexual patient seeking consultation for a real or imagined sexually related condition is also of prime importance. The reader is referred to the introductory chapters of this book as well as to several recent articles on the problems of homosexual male patients interacting with the health care system.[46,47]

Any control program tailored for the homosexual male population should stress the need for periodic STD testing, institute community participation in the form of screening programs directed toward the high-risk individual, and provide confidential contact tracing and treatment of sexual partners within a professional setting. The first of these elements, the education of the homosexual community to the importance of periodic STD testing, is a fundamental aim of community-oriented health care facilities such as the HBMC. This is accomplished by the distribution of circulars and posters in bars and bathhouses and the placement of regular ads in homophile newspapers. Entrance and exit personnel remind each client of the importance of regular and periodic testing to halt the spread of gonorrhea and other STDs. However, it is primarily by providing a convenient and comfortable setting for inexpensive, confidential, and thorough STD testing that periodic STD testing is best encouraged.

Outreach can be accmplished in a number of ways. In Chicago, Los Angeles, and elsewhere, a collaborative group composed of Department of Health workers and community clinic staff conduct on-site gonorrhea testing and syphilis serotesting at the major bathhouses, an especially high-risk area. In Chicago, this group also sponsors the "VD Van," already discussed. Finally, on-site mini-clinic and educational resource centers operated at large community-wide social events or "health fairs" are especially effective in introducing the concept of asymptomatic STD testing to persons who might otherwise be unaware of the importance of this procedure. In communities lacking a homosexual STD clinic, similar projects co-sponsored by the local Department of Health and community advisors or business establishments can also help to target diagnostic services, with persons detected as having an STD referred to appropriate clinics or private practitioners for treatment.

Contact referral and epidemiologic treatment of sexual contacts, the major elements of federally funded VD control programs, have an important role in the gay community, provided that certain modifications and safeguards are employed.[45] Gaining the confidence and trust of the patients coming for diagnosis and treatment is the major step in determining ability to identify and treat sexual contacts. Once the patient knows that he or she will be respected and treated in a confidential and dignified manner, there is usually no problem in having that patient self-refer his or her sexual contacts for diagnosis and epidemiologic treatment. Clinic staff is available to aid in that task, but will never communicate with a patient's sexual contacts without the request and permission of that patient.

One of the major drawbacks to contact tracing in the homosexual male community is the existence of anonymous sexual contacts. It has been suggested that mass treatment of persons frequenting such places as bathhouses be undertaken to decrease the infective pool of persons not otherwise accessible to diagnostic and treatment programs. The problems with these prophylactic measures were discussed in the previous section. Provided that selective prophylactic treatment is shown to be effective, and adequate measures are taken to reduce the risk of adverse drug reactions and the emergence of antibiotic-resistant strains, such programs may ultimately be useful in the homosexual male community. Meanwhile, the most effective way of decreasing the pool of asymptomatic gonococcal carriers within the homosexual male community is through education programs and on-site testing programs as previously described.

RESEARCH

For a variety of reasons, research into new means of preventing the spread of gonorrhea has been extremely slow. Recent developments, spurred on by changing public attitudes and a new awareness among government agencies charged with VD control, suggest an increased interest and activity. Several important questions raised by the experience of community clinics working with the homosexual male population must be answered before more effective control measures can be implemented. Two major lines of investigation at present focus on the development of rapid tests for gonococcal infection and on *N. gonorrhoeae* vaccine. Since the body's immune reaction to gonococcal infection is rather weak and nonspecific, serologic testing is difficult and does not discriminate between acute and chronic or past infection. Furthermore, the high incidence of meningococcal colonization in homosexual males[4] will require serologic or immunofluorescent tests capable of distinguishing between the antigenically related *N. gonorrhoeae* and *N. meningitidis*.

Similarly, the immune response produced in experimental animals to injections of whole gonococci does not appear to confer immunity against subsequent infection by a different strain of *N. gonorrhoeae*. Several groups are experimenting with vaccines prepared from the external pili purified from the gonococcus, which appear to stimulate the more effective and broader range of immunity when tested in chimpanzees. Other gonococcal antigens currently being investigated as potential vaccine constituents include lipopolysaccharide antigens, serum opacity factors, and the so-called "POMP" and "MOMP" peptides. As the *N. gonorrhoeae* auxotypes in homosexual men appear to differ from auxotypes of strains commonly found in heterosexual patients, particular attention must be paid to the selection of specific antigens and gonoccocal strains for inclusion in any proposed vaccine.

As an understanding of the sexual practices of individuals at high risk of acquiring repeated gonococcal infections increases, numerous mechanisms to interrupt the natural cycle of reinfection have been suggested. The use of chemical methods to destroy the gonococci at the time of sexual contact rather than through systemic antibiotics—a chemical shield that could replace the condom as the most effective means of gonorrhea prophylaxis while avoiding problems of compliance and toxicity—might revolutionize gonorrhea prophylaxis and control. Similarly, the usefulness and safety of rectal douching or chemical mouthwash for the prevention of rectal or pharyngeal infection need to be systematically investigated. Other research areas should determine what biological or sociological variables confer seeming "immunity" to gonococcal infection and what is the nature of that immunity. Recent studies have suggested that the anal and pharyngeal canals of many homosexual males harbor an unusual population of nonpathogenic and meningococci, raising the question of whether cohabitation with such organisms reduces the chance of acquiring gonococcal infection. Are there substances produced by nonpathogenic organisms that are toxic to pathogenic organisms? Several groups of investigators have identified gonococci with unusual nutritional requirements or lipid sensitivities from homosexual patients with recurrent or anal infections. Can control measures be developed that take advantage of these properties, thus selectively attacking more virulent and contagious strains of gonorrhea? Research in these areas is most promising and urgently needed. At the same time, the widespread community clinics that are designed specifically to meet the needs of homosexual males provide ideal locations for clinical research programs aimed at the reduction of gonococcal infection.

REFERENCES

1. Center for Disease Control: Gonorrhea: Reported Morbidity and Mortality in the United States. *MMWR* 27(Suppl):27–29, 1979.
2. Morton RS: *Gonorrhoea*. London, Saunders, 1977.
3. Skinner FA, Walker PD, Smith H: *Gonorrhoea: Epidemiology and Pathogenesis*. London, Academic Press, 1977.
4. Janda WM, Bohnoff M, Lerner SA, et al: Epidemiology of pathogenic *Neisseria* in homosexual men. *J Homosexuality* 5(3):289–290, 1980.
5. Gilbaugh JH, Fuchs PC: The gonococcus and the toilet seat. *N Engl J Med* 301:91–93, 1979.
6. Rein MF: Nonsexual acquisition of genital gonococcal infection (Letter to Editors). *N Engl J Med* 301:1347, 1979.
7. Harnisch JP, Wiesner PJ, Holmes KK: Clinical epidemiology of VD: The role of the homosexual. *Cutis* 9:221–224, 1972.
8. British Cooperative Clinical Groups: Homosexuality and venereal disease in the United Kingdom. *Br J Vener Dis* 49:329–334, 1973.
9. Seigel MS, Thompson SE, Perine PL: Penicillinase-producing *Neisseria gonorrhoeae*. *Sex Transm Dis* 4:32–33, 1977.
10. Crawford G, Knapp JS, Hale J, et al: Asymptomatic gonorrhea in men: Caused by gonococci with unique nutritional requirements. *Science* 196:1352–1353, 1977.
11. Jacobs NF, Kraus SJ: Gonococcal and nongonococcal urethritis in men. *Ann Intern Med* 82:7–12, 1975.
12. Handsfield HH, Lipman TO, Harnisch JP, et al: Asymptomatic gonorrhea in men. Diagnosis, natural course, prevalence and significance. *N Engl J Med* 209:117–123, 1974.
13. Klein EF, Fisher LS, Chow AW, et al: Anorectal gonococcal infection. *Ann Intern Med* 86:340–346, 1977.
14. Kilpatrick ZM: Gonorrheal proctitis. *N Engl J Med* 287:967–969, 1972.

15. Felman YM: Pharyngeal gonorrhea. *Sex Transm Dis Newslett* (City of New York) 2:1–4, 1979.
16. Hallquist L, Lindgren S: Gonorrhea of the throat at a venereological clinic. Incidence and the results of treatment. *Br J Vener Dis* 51:395–397, 1975.
17. Wiesner PJ: Gonococcal pharyngeal infection. *Clin Obstet Gynecol* 18:121–129, 1975.
18. Wiesner PJ, Tronca E, Bonin P, et al: Clinical spectrum of pharyngeal gonococcal infection. *N Engl J Med* 288:181–185, 1972.
19. Kraus SJ: Complications of gonococcal infection. *Med Clin N Am* 56:1115–1125, 1972.
20. Holmes KK, Counts GW, Beaty HN: Disseminated gonococcal infection. *Ann Intern Med* 74:979–993, 1971.
21. Harnisch JP, Alexander ER, Berger RE, et al: Aetiology of acute epididymitis. *Lancet* 1:819–821, 1977.
22. Furness G, Kamat NH, Kaminski Z, et al: Relationship of epididymitis to gonorrhea. *Invest Urol* 11:312–314, 1974.
23. Provine H, Gardner P: The gram-stain smear and its interpretation. *Hosp Pract* 9:85–91, 1974.
24. Sands M: Nonsymptomatic urethral gonorrhea in homosexual men. *Sex Transm Dis* 7:206, 1980.
25. McMillan A, Young H: Gonorrhea in homosexual men: Frequency of infection by culture site. *Sex Transm Dis* 5:146–150, 1978.
26. Centers for Disease Control: Sexually transmitted diseases: Treatment guidelines, 1982. *MMWR* 31(Suppl):37s–40s, 1982.
27. Kraus SJ: Incidence and therapy of gonococcal pharyngitis. *Sex Transm Dis* 6(Suppl):143–147, 1979.
28. Jaffe H: Personal communication.
29. Washington AE: Experience with various antibiotics for treatment of anorectal gonorrhea. *Sex Transm Dis* 6(Suppl):148–151, 1979.
30. Zaidi AA, Reynolds GH, Jones OG, et al: Rectal gonorrhea. Presented by SE Thompson at the symposium on Recent Advances in STDs, Chicago, June 22, 1979. Unpublished study of CDC National Gonorrhea Therapy Monitoring Network.
31. Legedeft DA, Hochman EB: Rectal gonorrhea in men: Diagnosis and treatment. *Ann Intern Med* 92:463–466, 1980.
32. Sands M: Therapy of anorectal gonorrhea in gay men. Presented at Current Aspects of Sexually Transmitted Diseases II, San Francisco, June 19, 1980.
33. Jaffe HW, Biddle JW, Thornsberry C, et al: National Gonorrhea Therapy Monitoring Study: In vitro susceptibility and its correlation with treatment results. *N Engl J Med* 294:5–9, 1976.
34. Ng WWS, Echeverria P, Rockhill R, et al: Antibiotic sensitivities of *Neisseria gonorrhoeae* in the Far East: Comparison of plasmid species in isolates from six countries. *Sex Transm Dis* 9:120–123, 1982.
35. Reynolds GH, Zaidi AA, Thornsberry C, et al: The National Gonorrhea Therapy Monitoring Study. II. Trends and seasonality of antibiotic resistance of *Neisseria gonorrhoeae*. *Sex Transm Dis* 6(Suppl):103–111, 1979.
36. Leftik MI, Miller, JW, Brown JD: Penicillin-resistant gonococcal polyarthritis. *JAMA* 239:134, 1978.
37. Holmes KK, Handsfield HH, Wang SP, et al: Etiology of nongonococcal urethritis. *N Engl J Med* 292: 1199–1205, 1975.
38. Judson FN, Miller KG, Schaffnit GN: Screening for gonorrhea and syphilis in the gay baths— Denver, Colorado. *Am J Pub Health* 67:740–742, 1977.
39. Merino HI, Judson FN, Bennet D, et al: Screening for gonorrhea and syphilis in gay bathhouses in Denver and Los Angeles. *Pub Health Rep* 94:376–379, 1979.
40. Altman N, Ostrow DG: Methods of risk factor identification in gay men. Presented at Current Aspects of Sexually Transmitted Diseases II, San Francisco, June 20, 1980.
41. Ostrow DG, Shaskey D, Steffen G, et al: Epidemiology of gonorrhea infections in gay men. *J Homosexuality* 5:285–288, 1980.

42. Schroeder MT, Thompson SE, Hadler SC, et al: Epidemiology of hepatitis B infection in gay men. *J Homosexuality* 5:307–310, 1980.
43. Harrison WO, Hooper RR, Wiesner PJ, et al: A trial of minocycline given after exposure to prevent gonorrhea. *N Engl J Med* 300:1074–1079, 1979.
44. Holmes HH: Unpublished study, data presented at the symposium on Current Aspects of STDs, Chicago, June 22, 1979.
45. Merino HI, Richards JB: An innovative program of venereal disease casefinding, treatment, and education for a gay male population. *Sex Transm Dis* 4:50–52, 1977.
46. Ostrow DG: Spotting and treating STDs in gay men. *Mod Med* 47:42–47, 1979.
47. Felman YM, Morrison JM: Examining the homosexual male for STDs. *JAMA* 238:2046–2047, 1977.

Nongonococcal Urethritis

YEHUDI M. FELMAN and KING K. HOLMES

ETIOLOGY

The etiology of urethritis in homosexual men differs from its etiology in heterosexual men in at least two major ways. First, it is quite clear that the relative frequencies of gonorrhea and nongonococcal urethritis are different for the two groups. Homosexual men have predominantly gonococcal urethritis (GU), and, in many areas of the United States, heterosexual men have predominantly nongonococcal urethritis (NGU). The relative frequency of GU/NGU is also related to race, but this may be for different reasons. In sexually transmitted disease (STD) clinics, heterosexual black men with urethritis more often have GU than NGU, while the reverse is true for heterosexual white men. This has suggested to some that blacks may be more susceptible to gonorrhea and whites more susceptible to NGU. However, in a United States Navy cohort study[1] done recently on an aircraft carrier, it was found that black men had a higher risk of GU than white men, but they also had a higher risk of NGU. GU is more symptomatic than NGU; it is therefore possible that racial or cultural differences in the response to symptoms account for some of the differences in apparent frequency of GU and NGU in various population groups in the STD clinic setting.

The Centers for Disease Control estimate that approximately 2.5 million cases of NGU occurred in 1981, while 999,500 cases of gonorrhea were reported out of an estimated total of 2.7 million actual cases.[2] In Great Britain, the reported incidence of NGU exceeds that of gonorrhea in men by a factor of nearly two.[3] Demographic data from several studies in the United States indicate that NGU

YEHUDI M. FELMAN ● Departments of Dermatology, Preventive Medicine, and Community Health, State University of New York, Downstate Medical School, Brooklyn, New York 11203.   KING K. HOLMES ● Division of Infectious Diseases, Seattle Public Health Hospital, and Department of Medicine, University of Washington at Seattle, Seattle, Washington 98144.

is more prevalent than gonorrhea among university students and higher socio-economic groups.[4,5] The New York City Health Department has been tabulating NGU since 1951 and has reported nearly a threefold increase over the last decade. Tabulations from the Social Hygiene Clinics in New York City for 1977 have shown that 38% of the cases of urethritis reported among male patients were nongonococcal.

Despite the high rate of NGU, some physicians consider it a "minor" STD without serious complications. From an etiologic viewpoint, this is clearly not the case. NGU can be transmitted to sexual contacts and *Chlamydia* proctitis has been reported in patients engaging in receptive anal intercourse with NGU-infected partners.[6] Prostatitis and epididymitis are known complications of NGU in males, while 5% of venerally acquired Reiter's syndrome is associated with a primary NGU infection.[7]

While various microorganisms have been implicated in NGU, the only proven causal agent is *Chlamydia trachomatis. Chlamydia* is an obligate intra-cellular organism that multiplies by binary fission in the cytoplasm of its host cells, is susceptible to certain antimicrobial agents, contains RNA and DNA, and possesses ribosomes and cell walls resembling gram-negative bacteria. The application of a microimmunofluorescent antibody typing test has demonstrated separate serotypes within *C. trachomatis:* types A, B, Ba, and C mainly associated with trachoma; types D, E, F, G, H, I, J, and K associated with urethral, cervical, and ocular infections; and three clearly defined types—L1, L2, and L3—that cause lymphogranuloma venereum. Evidence to support the etiologic role of *C. trachomatis* in NGU is based on studies in which the organism was isolated from the urethra in from 30% to 50% of men with NGU and infrequently from sexually active men without urethritis. Additional supporting evidence that *C. trachomatis* is the agent in a large number of NGU infections is provided by IgM immunofluorescent antibody data, the isolation of the organism from sexual contacts, and response to therapy.[8]

Another of the organisms that have been implicated is *Ureaplasma urealyticum*, a minute, gram-negative, coccobacillary organism often found within the cytoplasm of epithelial cells. These organisms have distinctive cultural characteristics, colony morphology, and staining reactions that differentiate them from the classical mycoplasmas. Although *U. urealyticum* can be isolated from healthy individuals, it has been recovered more often from men with *Chlamydia*-negative NGU than from either *Chlamydia*-positive NGU or from men with no urethritis.[9]

While approximately 40% of heterosexual men with NGU have *C. trachomatis* infection, only about 10% to 20% of homosexual men with NGU have *C. trachomatis* infection. Similarly, about 20% of heterosexual men with GU have simultaneous *C. trachomatis* infection, whereas mixed urethral infection with these two pathogens is significantly less common in homosexual men (Table

TABLE 1. Recoveries (in Relation to Sexual Preference) of *Chlamydia trachomatis* (C) and *Ureaplasma urealyticum* (U) from the Urethras of Men with Gonorrhea[a]

Group	No. of men with indicated culture results				
	C+ U+[b]	C+ U−	C− U+	C− U−	Total no.
Homosexual	0	0	7	11	18
Bisexual	1	0	2	5	8
Heterosexual	8	14	27	46	95
TOTAL	9	14	36	62	121

[a] From refs. 9 and 10.
[b] C+, *C. trachomatis* culture positive; C−, *C. trachomatis* culture negative; U+, *U. urealyticum* culture positive; U−, *U. urealyticum* culture negative.

1). *C. trachomatis* is a major cause of postgonococcal urethritis after penicillin, ampicillin, or spectinomycin therapy of gonorrhea in heterosexual men, but not in homosexual men. Thus, *C. trachomatis* is not isolated less often from homosexual men with gonorrhea or NGU than from heterosexual men. The etiology of NGU in homosexual men is not at all apparent at this time.

We have no idea today what causes *Chlamydia*-negative, plasma-urea-negative NGU in either heterosexual or homosexual men. The etiology may well be different in men acquiring NGU by rectal intercourse than in men acquiring it by vaginal intercourse. Enteric organisms might be more likely pathogens after rectal intercourse, for example. Whatever the cause, however, it is probably an organism sensitive to the tetracycline and the macrolide antibiotics, since many patients with NGU improve during therapy with either of these antibiotics, even if infection recurs. The C-negative, U-negative type of NGU represents the greatest treatment problem in homosexually active men. Among a predominantly heterosexual population we have found that, following a seven-day course of therapy with a tetracycline congener, the recurrence rate within six weeks was just over 50% among men with C-negative, U-negative NGU. Further data are needed concerning the efficacy of tetracycline or macrolide antibiotics for homosexual men with NGU, but it would not be surprising if failure rates were higher in homosexual men than in heterosexual men because of the predominance of C-negative, U-negative NGU in the former.

DIAGNOSIS

Since facilities for isolating chlamydial and ureaplasmal organisms are usually not available, diagnosis of NGU is made by establishing the presence of a significant degree of urethritis and by excluding gonococcal infection. The diagnostic procedure should include a culture specimen for *Neisseria gonorrhoeae* and microscopic examination of a gram-stained smear of the urethral discharge or the sediment of a centrifuged urine specimen (first 10 ml) collected at least two hours after the last micturition. In asymptomatic patients, first-void overnight urine specimens are preferable. The presence of ten or more polymorphonuclear leukocytes per high-power field on the urethral smear or twenty or more polymorphonuclear cells per high dry field with magnification $\times 400$ in the urinary sediment in at least two of five random fields has been accepted as a criterion for urethral inflammation or pyuria.

A common situation is presented by the patient with symptoms of urethritis, such as dysuria and a painful meatus, but no objective signs of urethral discharge. If the initial urethral smear or urinary sediment examination is negative, the patient should return the next day and examination for discharge as well as the gram stain of endourethral secretions should be repeated. If an increased number of leukocytes is not seen, other possible causes of symptoms, such as urinary tract infections, bacterial or herpetic prostatitis, or functional complaints should be considered. In the latter case, treatment of the symptoms blindly with a broad-spectrum antibiotic can reinforce the psychological cycle of functional dysuria, antimicrobial therapy, relief of symptoms. Referral to a psychotherapist for treatment of the underlying psychological conditions is often necessary in patients with recurrent functional dysuria.

TREATMENT

Since most facilities do not culture for *C. trachomatis* or *U. urealyticum*, treatment for NGU is usually empirical. Tetracycline, minocycline, and doxycycline, which have been demonstrated effective in the treatment of NGU, have also been shown to be active against these two organisms and are considered the drugs of choice. However, there will be a certain percentage of cases that fail to respond to these drugs, probably because *Chlamydia* and *Ureaplasma* are not causing the condition. Other factors to be considered are noncompliance with the prescribed drug regimen, reinfection, and underlying prostatitis.

There is no general consensus as to duration of treatment. Treatment schedules of one to three weeks have been recommended. Some investigators were able to eradicate the infection on a seven-day course of tetracycline therapy at 0.5 g four times a day, while others recommend 0.25 g four times a day for two to three weeks. Minocycline at 100 mg twice a day for one to three weeks has also been recommended. Since 10% of male patients presenting with a urethral discharge that are gram-negative for *Neisseria gonorrhoeae* and who are treated with a tetracycline regimen later turn out to be culture-positive for gonorrhea, the Bureau of Venereal Disease Control of New York City recommends the following approach. To prevent inadequately treated gonorrhea in those cases of gonococcal urethritis with negative initial smears, all diagnosed cases of NGU are treated with 500 mg tetracycline four times a day for the first week followed by 250 mg of tetracycline four times a day for an additional two weeks, for a total dosage of 28 g given over a period of three weeks. If the culture report turns out to be positive for *Neisseria gonorrhoeae,* no further treatment after the first week is necessary. The diagnosis in these cases is changed to gonococcal urethritis.

In patients who do not respond or are allergic to tetracycline (or minocycline, if this drug is used), erythromycin given orally in the same regimen as tetracycline may be substituted. Cure is achieved when the patient is asymptomatic and shows no evidence of urethritis as defined by microscopy of a gram-stained smear or by determination of pyuria.

CONTROL

It is important to treat both the patient and his sexual contacts. Most contacts of homosexual men with NGU are asymptomatic. Examination of contacts may reveal proctitis or cervicitis, but will often be negative. Clinical relapses or so-called treatment failures in a large number of cases are probably due to reinfection from the original sex partner, male or female, who was never treated. The contact is given the same course of therapy, except in the case of the pregnant female, in whom erythromycin is substituted. Both partners should be treated simultaneously to prevent a ping-pong infection. Additionally, the female contact should be evaluated so as to exclude gonorrhea, trichomoniasis, and candidiasis (which may be activated as a result of tetracycline therapy).

Patients should be reexamined weekly for one month. In addition to the clinical examination, the urethra or urine should be evaluated for urethral inflammation. If there is no response to medication either clinically or microscopically, the patient should be reassessed in terms of new sexual contacts and presence of other organisms (thought to be responsible for some cases of urethritis). If one week of therapy was prescribed initially, a longer course of three weeks may prove more efficacious. In treatment-resistant patients, urological consultation should be considered to rule out anatomic abnormalities, prostatitis, or other urogenital diseases.

REFERENCES

1. Harrison WO, Hooper RR, Wiesner PF, et al: A trial of minocycline given after exposure to prevent gonorrhea. *N Engl J Med* 300:1074–1078, 1979.
2. Evaluations and Statistical Services Section, Venereal Disease Control Division, Centers for Disease Control, Atlanta.

3. Willcox RR: How suitable are available pharmaceuticals for the treatment of sexually transmitted diseases? 1. Conditions presenting as genital discharges. *Br J Vener Dis* 53:314–323, 1977.
4. Wiesner PJ: Selected aspects of the epidemiology of nongonococcal urethritis, in Hobson D, Holmes KK (eds): *Nongonococcal Urethritis and Related Infections.* Washington, DC, American Society for Microbiology, 1977, pp 9–14.
5. McCormack WM: Etiology of nongonococcal urethritis—One piece in the puzzle. *N Engl J Med* 292:1238–1239, 1977.
6. Goldneier D, Darougar S: Isolation of *Chlamydia trachomatis* from throat and rectum of homosexual men. *Br J Vener Dis* 53:184–185, 1977.
7. Simmons P, Senior Registrar, St. Bartholomew's Hospital, London, England, personal communication.
8. Bowie WR, Wang SP, Alexander ER, et al: Etiology of nongonococcal urethritis. Evidence for *Chlamydia trachomatis* and *Ureaplasma urealyticum. J Clin Invest* 59:735–742, 1977.
9. Holmes KK: Nongonococcal urethritis: General considerations and specific considerations for homosexual men. *J Homosexuality* 5:295–298, 1980.
10. Bowie WR, Wang SP, Alexander ER: Etiologies of postgonococcal urethritis in homosexual and heterosexual men: Role of *Chlamydia trachomatis* and *Ureaplasma urealyticum. Sex Transm Dis* 5:151–154, 1978.

III

Enterically Transmitted Diseases

Amebiasis

DANIEL C. WILLIAM

Over the past ten years, a group of protozoal diseases have been increasingly recognized as being venereally transmissible. Significant outbreaks of Amebiasis and giardiasis have been reported from both California and New York. Available evidence strongly suggests that these two diseases are major problems within the homosexual male community.

EPIDEMIOLOGY

Although homosexuality is irrelevant to disease transmission, the frequent practices of anilinction and fellatio within the homosexually active male population most likely account for the high incidence of these diseases.

Amebiasis is an infection caused by the protozoan *Entamoeba histolytica*. Although approximately 10% of the world population harbors *E. histolytica*, the prevalence in the United States is thought to be less than 3%.[1] Traditionally, this illness has been associated with poverty and poor sanitation. In tropical countries, up to 40% of the population may be infected.

Individuals are infected after ingesting the cysts of *E. histolytica*, usually through fecally contaminated water or food. Until recently, most new cases in the United States occurred in travelers returning from tropical areas or in the rural southern states. Rare urban outbreaks have occurred only when drinking water has been inadvertently contaminated with raw sewage.

The first hint of the venereal transmission of amebiasis occurred in 1968 when Harry Most, M.D., of New York University reported a small cluster of

DANIEL C. WILLIAM ● Columbia University College of Physicians and Surgeons, New York, New York 10032; and St. Luke's–Roosevelt Hospital Center, New York, New York 10019.

presumptively sexually acquired amebiasis among homosexual men who had never traveled outside New York.[2] In 1972, Ben Kean, M.D., of Cornell Medical Center in New York reported a case of venereal amebiasis in an asymptomatic young homosexual man.[3] Initially suspecting contaminated drinking water, the New York City Department of Health was unable to demonstrate sewage contamination in the Greenwich Village water supply. During this time, the phenomenon of venereally transmitted amebiasis became increasingly well-recognized by a small group of New York City parasitologists. Unfortunately, most of the medical community failed to appreciate the magnitude of this problem. Several studies, reported in 1977–1979, finally underscored the frequency of venereally acquired amebiasis.[4–7] In a retrospective study of hospital records of all adult male patients with proven amebiasis at New York Hospital in the early 1970s, 20 infected men in the study population had never traveled outside of metropolitan New York City. All patients were subsequently found to be homosexual males. In the last year of the study, the majority of all new patients with amebiasis were homosexual males, suggesting that in New York City venereal transmission had become the most important mode of disease acquisition.

A second, prospective study, conducted at the Gay Men's Health Project in New York City in cooperation with the New York City Department of Health, examined stool specimens from 89 male volunteers. Of these, 20% were infected with *E. histolytica*. In 1976 in San Francisco, 89% of all amebiasis occurred in men aged 20 to 39, corresponding to the same population with other sexually acquired diseases. The absence of reported venereal amebiasis elsewhere probably reflects continued ignorance within the medical community as well as insufficient diagnostic laboratory facilities.

By far the most important mechanism of venereal spread is fecal–oral (anilinction). In the Gay Men's Health Project study, all infected men had engaged in anilinction. Men who never practiced anilinction were free of amebiasis. Although confirmation is still pending, fellatio also may be a risk factor, especially if performed on those who previously practiced rectal (insertive) intercourse without intervening genital washing. The transmission of amebiasis from rectum to rectum, bypassing the fecal–oral route, has been confirmed in an outbreak of amebiasis secondary to a contaminated colonic enema machine.[8] The implications of this report are that rectal–rectal transmission may occur via shared contaminated enemas, as well as via fecally soiled genitalia in bathhouse group sex situations.

Cysts of *E. histolytica* are able to survive for nine days in fecal material left at room temperature (Table 1). After ingestion, the cysts pass to the lower small intestines. Here, under the influence of the digestive juices, the cysts disintegrate, liberating the immature amebas which migrate to the large intestine and there multiply into the adult trophozoite organisms. The freely moving amebas can live as commensals within the intestinal feces of an asymptomatic

TABLE 1. Survival of *E. histolytica* Cysts in Feces[a]

Temperature	Days
37°C (98.6°F)	2
22°C (71.6°F)	9
0°C (32°F)	60

[a] Unlike most other venereal diseases, the infectious agents of amebiasis remain viable outside the body for days. Transmission of the disease can, therefore, involve fomites such as contaminated towels, mats, and even genitalia.

carrier. Alternatively, the trophozoite may invade the wall of the intestine, especially in the cecum and rectosigmoid areas of the colon.

The pathogenicity of the infection depends upon a variety of factors, including the dose of the inoculum, host resistance, the diet of the host, and the virulence of the ingested amebic strain. Most amebiasis acquired in the United States is relatively mild compared with the often virulent and occasionally life-threatening infections that can be acquired in the tropics. Possible explanations for the relatively mild temperate zone disease include the high-protein American diet, good overall nutritional status, and the mild virulence of locally encountered strains.

CLINICAL ASPECTS

The clinical symptomatology of an amebic infection is exceedingly variable (Table 2). Amebic dysentery, that is, fulminant diarrheal disease, is rarely encountered today in the United States. More often, most infections are either

TABLE 2. Symptoms of Intestinal Amebiasis[a]

Change in bowel habits; onset of disease usually insidious; diarrhea; soft bowel movements
Abdominal cramps
Bloating
Flatulence
Rarely: weight loss, bloody diarrhea, fever, prostration

[a] Symptoms of amebiasis are often nonspecific and often mimic common gastrointestinal illnesses. A significant percentage of patients present asymptomatically.

asymptomatic or minimally symptomatic. This clinical picture is a mixed blessing since the so-called healthy carrier may unknowingly pass millions of cysts a day and subsequently infect a large number of sexual partners. Most patients with symptomatic amebiasis complain of vague abdominal discomfort, mild diarrhea alternating with constipation, increased flatulence, and bloating. Symptoms characteristically develop insidiously, and many patients fail to appreciate the change in bowel habits for months after the onset of disease. Others report a waxing and waning of symptoms, with frequent periods of normalcy punctuated by occasional episodes of pasty or soft, poorly formed stools. More severe symptoms, which include weight loss, bloody diarrhea, fever, and prostration, are rarely encountered in uncomplicated venereally acquired amebic colitis.

For reasons that are still unclear, the major complications of amebic colitis, including amebic hepatic abscess, pulmonary abscess, and brain abscess, are distinctly rare in venereally transmitted disease in the United States.

DIAGNOSIS

Diagnosis of amebiasis should be entertained in any homosexually active male patient who reports the characteristic insidious onset of lower intestinal symptoms. A high index of suspicion is indicated in patients who frequently engage in oroanal and orogenital sexual practices, especially with multiple sexual partners. Frequently, patients with amebiasis have been in contact with infected sexual partners. Another diagnostic clue is the temporary amelioration of symptoms that may occur with incidental administration of tetracycline or tetracyclinelike antibiotics for the treatment of unrelated venereal infections. On physical examination, most patients with mild or even moderate amebiasis have a completely normal examination.

One of the major problems in the control of amebiasis is the difficulty and expense of diagnosing the disease. Unfortunately, the only reliable diagnostic test is a careful stool examination, which it is not always possible to perform, since few laboratories have adequate proficiency in parasitology (Table 3). Since the natural life cycle of the ameba involves intermittent cyst production, the chance of finding cysts in a single direct smear from an infected individual is about 20%. This chance increases to 50% for three stool examinations, and six or more tests may be required to establish a reliable diagnosis. Fresh purged stool examinations, when available, may circumvent the low sensitivity of a casual stool examination. Patients are given a potent cathartic and fresh diarrheal stools are examined directly for both cysts and motile trophozoites. A purged specimen examination has a much greater sensitivity than its cold casual counterpart.

In symptomatic patients with amebiasis, the problem of diagnosis is further

TABLE 3.   Tests for Enteric Protozoa

Purged, fresh stool examination
Warm stool
Cold stool
Serologic tests are only of value for invasive tissue disease
Direct smear

[a] Ideally, stool specimens should be examined for enteric protozoa within
hours of production. Sensitivity is improved by examining a fresh
specimen as soon as possible. Watery movements must be examined
while warm since viable trophozites disintegrate within hours. The
performance of a direct smear obtained by anoscopy should be limited
to physicians trained in parasitology.

compounded by the presence of the diarrheal stool. In this instance, patients are rarely excreting the stable cyst form, but rather expel the fragile motile trophozoites. Unless these stools are examined immediately while they are still warm, the trophozoites disintegrate to produce a false-negative examination.

The multiple interfering substances commonly ingested by patients also affect the reliability of stool examination results. These substances include antidiarrheals containing bismuth or alkaline salts such as kaolin, the nonabsorbable antacids, and many antibiotics, including tetracycline and sulfonamides. Barium sulfate, mineral and castor oil, and magnesium hydroxide also interfere with test results. A dependable examination of stools for amebiasis cannot therefore be made for a period of at least ten to fourteen days after the last ingestion of an interfering substance.

Patients with stool examinations negative for *E. histolytica* but positive for protozoal cysts (including the nonpathogens) should always have additional examinations performed to rule out amebiasis. Although nonpathogenic protozoa are not associated with clinical disease, they are frequently excellent markers for the presence of fecal contamination. *E. histolytica* travels in the company of its nonpathogenic friends, and in the experience of the Gay Men's Health Project study, fully two-thirds of patients with nonpathogenic cysts on casual stool examination are found to harbor *E. histolytica* when additional stool examinations are performed. In addition, some clinicians now feel that these so-called nonpathogens may cause symptoms and may become pathogenic in immunocompromised patients. These practitioners thus advocate the necessity of treating all intestinal protozoa according to the regimens that follow. Not infrequently, mixed infections with more than one protozoan occur. In a prospective prevalence study of 176 sexually active homosexual men, 9.5% were infected with *E. histolytica* and *Giardia lamblia*. This frequent occurrence of "mixed" infections may be responsible for treatment failures, since all organisms have not been identified (Table 4).

Anoscopy or sigmoidoscopy performed in the absence of colonic cleansing

TABLE 4. Results of Parasitological Examination of Stool
Specimens from Two Biased Populations[a]

Protozoan/protozoa isolated	Gay men's health project study (1977)[b]		New York Hospital study (1976–1977)[c]	
	No.	Percent	No.	Percent
One or more	61	48.4	305	5.2
Entamoeba histolytica	39	31.7	74	1.3
Giardia lamblia	23	18.3	123	2.1
Entameba coli	15	11.9	82	1.4
Endolimax nana	19	15.1	84	1.4
Iodameba butschlii	4	3.2	13	0.2
E. histolytica and G. lamblia	12	9.5	5	0.08
E. histolytica or G. lamblia	50	39.7	192	3.3

[a] From ref. 5.
[b] N = 126 sexually active men.
[c] Inpatients and outpatients. N = 5885.

is a valuable adjunct to the diagnosis of amebiasis. Occasionally, small discrete hemorrhagic ulcerations can be seen on a background of essentially normal rectal mucosa. Barium studies of the colon are primarily of value in ruling out other causes of diarrheal illness. Contrast studies are rarely abnormal in mild to moderate amebic colitis, and, even when abnormal, the radiographic changes lack the specificity necessary to differentiate amebic colitis from idiopathic ulcerative colitis.

Various serologic tests, including hemagglutination and precipitation tests, may be of value in diagnosing patients with invasive disease. Unfortunately, these tests are rarely, if ever, positive in the asymptomatic cyst carrier. Also, once the patient is infected with invasive disease, these tests remain positive long after the infection has been eradicated.

TREATMENT

Treatment of patients with amebiasis remains a difficult and frustrating dilemma.[9] For the asymptomatic cyst carrier three drugs are currently available (Table 5). All have unique limitations and liabilities.

The drug of choice is still considered to be diidohydroxyquin, 650 mg orally three times a day for twenty days.[10] Although usually well-tolerated, this drug has been associated with optic neuropathy and visual loss, especially when given chronically. Unfortunately, diiodohydroxyquin has a single-treatment failure rate of perhaps 30% to 40%. Treatment with this drug is further complicated by its frequent nonavailability.

Alternatives to diiodohydroxyquin include metronidazole (Flagyl®), 750 mg orally three times a day for five to ten days. Metronidazole is a drug poorly tolerated by patients. Side effects include metallic taste, dark urine, alterations in mood, fatigue, and a potentially dangerous interaction with ethanol. The safety of metronidazole is clouded by its carcinogenicity in rats and mice. Furthermore, many instances of treatment failures have occurred using metronidazole alone.

A third drug, diloxanide furoate (Furamide®) is available from the Centers for Disease Control in Atlanta, Georgia, as an investigational drug for the treatment of the asymptomatic cyst carrier. The dose is 500 mg orally three times a day for ten days. The drug is nonabsorbable and the most common side effect is increased flatulence. Furamide's major limitation is its narrow spectrum of activity, which is restricted to *E. histolytica* cysts. In symptomatic patients with trophozoites, diloxanide furoate is rarely effective when used alone. Other drugs that have been tried in combination with diiodohydroxyquin include tetracycline and its analogs, erythromycin, carbazone (an arsenical), and chloroquine. In any multiple-agent regimen, one must weigh the benefits in terms of potential increased amebacidal activity against the increased risk of adverse drug reactions.

For mild to moderate intestinal disease, no single drug (or drug combination) has been clearly shown to be the treatment of choice. Possible combinations include a twenty-day course of diiodyhydroxyquin given concurrently with paromomycin sulfate (Humatin®) as 25 to 30 mg per kilogram of body weight per day in three divided doses for five to ten days. Paromomycin is a nonabsorbable antibiotic with an excellent safety record. Unfortunately, it is expensive. Alter-

TABLE 5.   Treatment of Amebiasis

Asymptomatic cyst carrier
  Diiodohydroxyquin, 650 mg PO tid for 20 days, *or*
  Metronidazole (Flagyl®), 750 mg PO tid for 5 to 10 days, *or*
  Diloxanide furoate (Furamide®), 500 mg PO tid for 10 days
For patients with mild to moderate intestinal disease
  Diiodohydroxyquin, 650 mg PO tid for 20 days, *plus* paromomycin sulfate (Humatin®), 25 to
    30 mg per kilogram of body weight per day in three divided PO doses for 5 to 10 days, *or*
  Diiodohydroxyquin, 650 mg PO tid for 20 days, *plus*
  Metronidazole, 750 mg PO tid for 5 to 10 days
For patients with recurrent or persistent disease, additional drugs in combination with the above
    may include
  Erythromycin
  Tetracycline or its analogs
  Carbazone
  Chloroquine

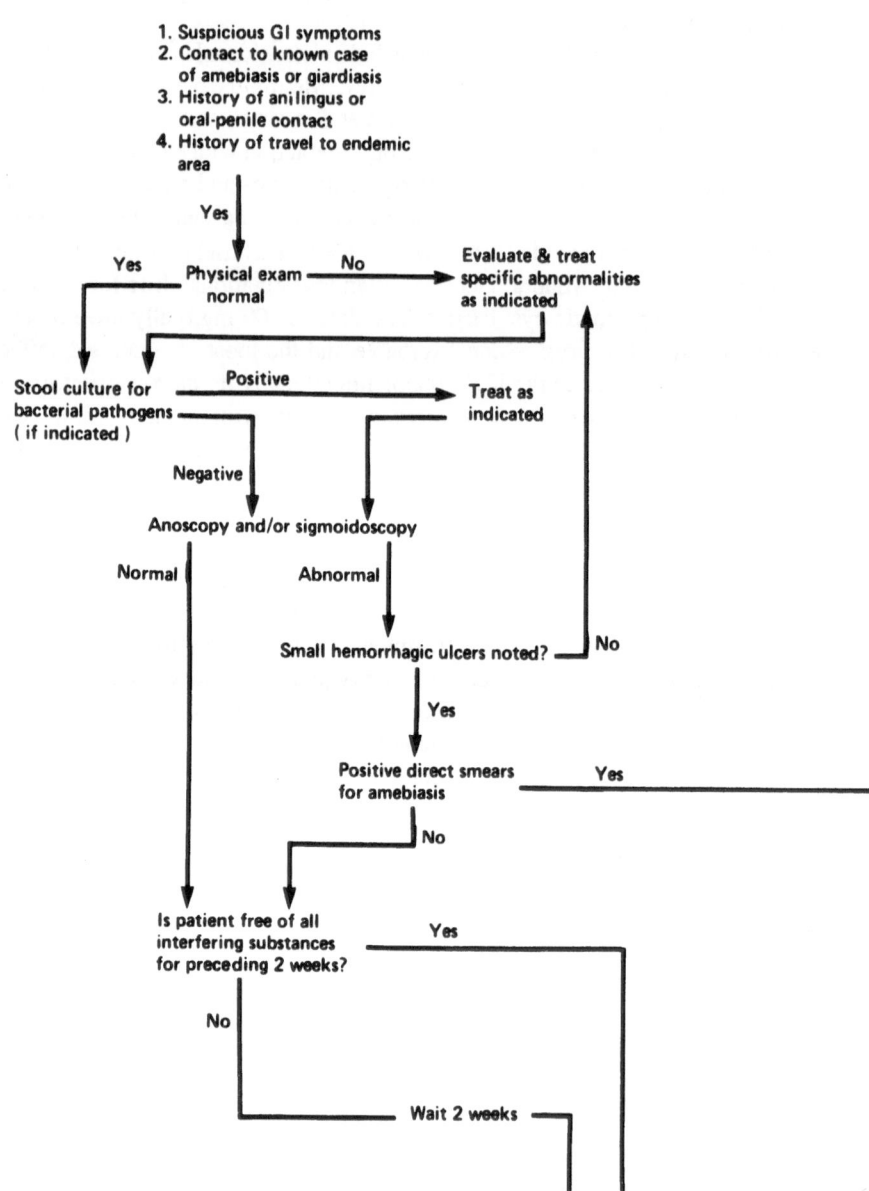

FIGURE 1.   Flowchart for the diagosis and treatment of suspected amebiasis.

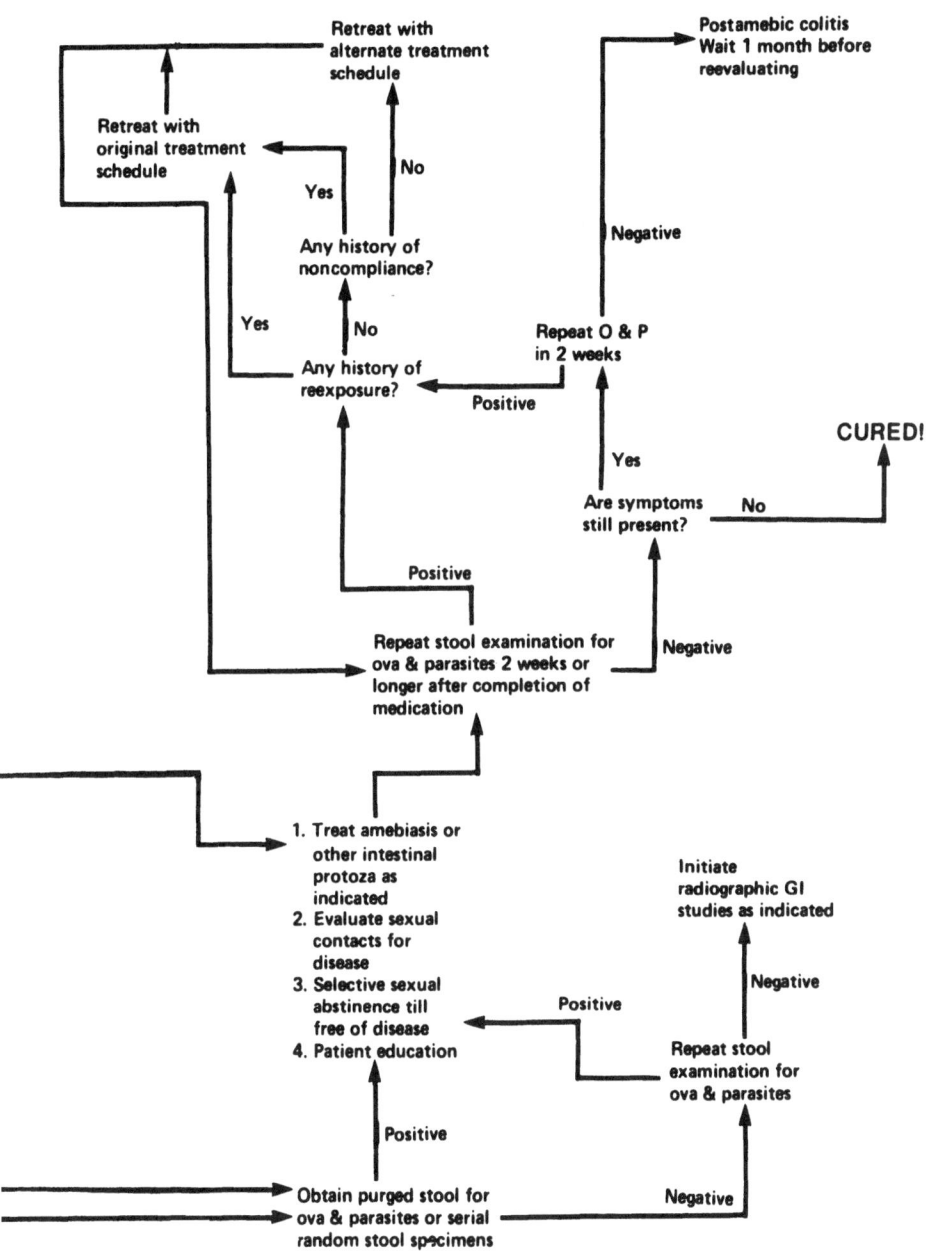

nately, a twenty-day course of diiodohydroxyquin can be given concurrently with a five- to ten-day course of metronidazole. Patients treated with any of these drugs must be serially rechecked at least two weeks after completion of therapy for a test of cure since treatment failure as well as reinfection commonly occurs. The patient's regular sexual partners should also be tested for the presence of protozoa and treated if they are infected. Not infrequently, patients treated for amebiasis become stool-negative but remain symptomatic. This "postamebic colitis" syndrome apparently represents some as yet undefined mucosal abnormality of the previously infected colon. These patients should be reassured that this illness does not represent progressive diseases and in many instances will clear with time.

The steps in the diagnosis and treatment of amebiasis are summarized in Figure 1.

CONTROL

Counseling

Patients infected with venereally acquired amebiasis should be told frankly and honestly about their disease (Table 6). They should know that anilinction ("rimming") is the primary mode of transmission, though occasionally fellatio may be the source of infection. Until their infection is absolutely cured, common sense dictates that the perirectal and rectal areas of infected patients should be off limits for oral sexual practices. Good personal hygiene with thorough handwashing after defecation and urination is mandatory to diminish the likelihood of nonvenereal transmission. Since amebiasis is quite prevalent in the homosexually active male community, and often presents asymptomatically, patients should know the risks associated with anilinction. Finally, patients should know that the probabilities of developing an amebic hepatic abscess in the United States are luckily remote.

TABLE 6. Patient Education[a]

Caution! Aniliction ("rimming") is harmful to your health.
Notify all at risk contacts, including sexual contacts without symptoms.
All treated patients must be retested two weeks or longer following completion of therapy.
Meticulous personal hygiene is mandatory to prevent nonvenereal transmission.
Selective sexual abstinence until follow-up specimens are negative.

[a] Patients should be told frankly about their disease. Sexual practices should be discussed and the importance of following medical advice should be underscored.

Prevention

Little is known about the prevention of venereally acquired amebiasis. Avoidance of oroperineal contact with multiple casual sexual partners will diminish the risks of disease acquisition. Careful attention to personal hygiene, including washing one's penis after anal insertive intercourse may decrease the risk of spread of this infection by fellatio. Carefully washing the anus and perirectal tissues may decrease the spread by anilinction.

Clearly, however, anilinction should be discouraged, especially with casual sexual contacts. I also advise infected patients to quarantine their anus from others until several follow-up stool examinations have been negative. Since the cysts of intestinal protozoa may survive for long periods outside the body, I caution patients about possible fomite contamination following any rectal penetration or manipulation.

Prospects for Control

Amebiasis and the other intestinal parasites are diseases that have historically been controlled by the development of sanitary facilities and food supplies. Today, even in countries with rapidly rising standards of living and modern health systems, these diseases are never controlled until adequate preventive public health measures are instituted. This same reality applies to venereally transmitted infection. Clearly, these infections will never be eradicated or even contained by improved medical access or improved medical care. Prevention alone can control these diseases.

To prove this point, let us follow the outcome of 100 sexually active homosexual men infected with venereally acquired amebiasis. assuming that the best medical care is readily available and no restriction on medical funds is imposed. Since half the men will be asymptomatic, only 50 will have one or more amebic symptoms. Characteristically, there is a huge spectrum of symptoms. Many patients have only mild intestinal dysfunction. Perhaps only 40 of these symptomatic men will seek medical care. Since many of the symptoms are rather nonspecific even under the best of circumstances, probably no more than three-fourths of the consulting physicians will suspect intestinal parasites. Of the 30 men with suspected disease, probably no more than 20 men will actually be diagnosed. Unfortunately the sensitivity of stool examinations is all too low. Unless multiple examinations are performed, many infected cases will always escape detection. Of the 20 men probably diagosed, only between 50% and 75% will be cured following a single course of therapy. Obviously, if only 15 of the original 100 men infected will be cured under the best of circumstances, the actual percentage cured in the real world is significantly less.

The immediate prospects for improved diagnostic testing and treatment regimens are not good. The only sensible control strategy is prevention. All homosexually active men must be informed about these diseases. But information is not enough. The prospect of disease control will only become a reality when sexual behavior is significantly modified to prevent disease transmission.

REFERENCES

1. Brown HW: *Basic Clinical Parasitology*, ed 4. New York, Appleton-Century-Crofts, 1975, pp 18–45.
2. Most H: Manhattan: "A tropical isle?" *Am J Trop Med* 17:333–354, 1968.
3. Kean BH: Venereal amebiasis. *NY State J Med* 76:930–931, 1972.
4. Schmerin MJ, Gelston A, Jones TC: Amebiasis: An increasing problem among homosexuals in New York City. *JAMA* 238:1386–1387, 1977.
5. Will DC, Shookhoff HB, Felman YM, et al: High rates of enteric protozoal infections in selected homosexual men attending a venereal disease clinic. *Sex Transm Dis* 5:155–157, 1978.
6. Kean BH, William DC, Lumanais SK: Epidemic of amebiasis and giardiasis in a biased population. *Br J Vener Dis* 55:375–378, 1979.
7. Mildvan D, Gelb AM, William DC: Venereal transmission of enteric pathogens in male homosexuals: Two case reports. *JAMA* 238:1387–1389, 1977.
8. Amebiasis associated with colonic irrigation—Colrado. *MMWR* 13(30a):101–102, 1981.
9. Kean BH: The treatment of amebiasis: A recurrent agony. *JAMA* 235:501, 1976.
10. Drugs for parasitic infections.*Medical Letter on Drugs and Therapeutics* 21(26):105–106, 1979.

Giardiasis

DANIEL C. WILLIAM

Giardia lamblia, a flagellated protozoan with worldwide distribution, shares with *Entamoeba histolytica* the possibility of venereal transmission by the fecal–oral route.[1,2] Venereally transmitted giardiasis is slightly less frequent in incidence than amebiasis.[3,4] As with amebiasis, infected individuals exhibit a spectrum of symptoms. Many adults with giardiasis are asymptomatic, while others have unrelenting diarrhea and malabsorption. However, metastatic infections to other organs do not occur in patients with giardiasis, as they do in patients with amebiasis.

EPIDEMIOLOGY

The epidemiology of venereally acquired giardiasis is essentially identical to that of amebiasis, with several slight qualifications. *G. lamblia* is the most common enteric protozoal pathogen isolated within the United States today. *Giardia* cysts are exceptionally stable and survive for months outside the host under moist conditions. This survival rate suggests that suitable fomites may play a potentially significant role in disease transmission. The amebiasis risk factors of anilinction, multiple sexual partners, and orogenital contact apply equally to venereally acquired giardiasis. *G. lamblia* is truly endemic in this country, with many contemporary nonvenereal outbreaks being traced to faulty municipal water filtration plants.[5] Unlike that of amebiasis, the nonvenereal transmission of giardiasis is almost always associated with contaminated drinking water.

DANIEL C. WILLIAM • Columbia University College of Physicians and Surgeons, New York, New York 10032; and St. Luke's–Roosevelt Hospital Center, New York, New York 10019.

Characteristically, the venereally infected homosexual male lacks a travel history. At New York Hospital, all male patients with giardiasis between 1971 and 1976 had no history of travel and were found to be homosexual. Most patients also had a prior history of other sexually transmitted diseases. Because of the short period from infection to cyst excretion (nine days in experimental infection), giardiasis may be rapidly spread among sexual contacts of those already infected.

The risk of infection is directly related to the number of cysts ingested. Virtually all individuals become infected following ingestion of 100 or more cysts. Following ingestion, the cysts pass unharmed through the gastric acids and undergo excystation in the duodenum. The flagellated trophozoite inhabits the duodenum and upper jejunum and attaches itself to the mucosal wall via a sucking disc. Rarely, organisms extend into the bile ducts and gall bladder. Because of the sucking disc attachment, trophozoites are uncommonly found in the stool except in the presence of diarrhea and a rapid transit time. The exact mechanism by which attached trophozoites cause clinical disease is still unknown. Both functional and anatomic changes of the duodenum can be seen on small bowel radiographic studies in a percentage of infected persons.

CLINICAL ASPECTS

Symptoms of giardiasis may characteristically begin explosively with foul-smelling, loose, and frequent bowel movements that are absent of blood and pus. The diarrhea is often associated with nausea and crampy abdominal pains. Bloating, flatulence, anorexia, and fatigue may also be present. Some patients may experience a modest weight loss, especially if chronically symptomatic. Although the symptoms of amebiasis and giardiasis often overlap, patients with giardiasis more frequently have epigastric symptoms, while lower abdominal complaints more often characterize the patient with amebiasis. The individual's host response is largely responsible for the magnitude of the symptoms. Patients with abnormalities of gamma globulin (e.g., dysgammaglobulinemias) and achlorhydria typically have increased symptoms.

The incubation period for giardiasis averages about two weeks. Infectivity, however, often precedes the onset of symptoms by several days. Symptomatic giardiasis usually is a self-limited illness lasting several weeks. Only a minority of patients remain ill for protracted periods.

Patients with chronic giardiasis usually have episodic recurrences of symptoms usually separated by periods of normalcy. Not uncommonly, chronic giardiasis induces a relative lactose deficiency and resulting milk intolerance, which may even persist following successful eradication of the infection.

DIAGNOSIS

Most patients with giardiasis have an essentially normal physical examination and, in the absence of malabsorption, routine chemistries and blood counts are normal. The diagnosis of giardiasis is usually dependent upon finding the cysts or trophozoites in fresh stool specimens. Since cyst excretion is often intermittent, several alternate-day specimens may be required to find the organism. When repeated stools are negative in a patient with suspected disease, the duodenal fluid should be sampled for trophozoites. This examination may be accomplished by duodenal intubation and aspiration or by using the "enterotest" device, which is basically a weighted gelatin capsule attached to a nylon string. One end of the string is taped to the patient's face and the capsule is swallowed. After the capsule has passed into the duodenum, the string is withdrawn and the bile-stained mucus from the distal string is examined fresh for trophozoites.

TREATMENT

Treatment of giardiasis is usually highly effective, inexpensive, and well-tolerated by the majority of patients (Table 1). The drug of choice is quinacrine hydrochloride (Atabrine®), 100 mg three times a day after meals for five to ten days. Side effects include headache, nausea, vomiting, and abdominal pains. Rarely, a toxic psychosis, drug fever, or severe skin rash may occur. The yellow skin discoloration seen with chronic quinacrine administration is rarely encountered with the dosage used to treat giardiasis.

Although treatment failures are more common with this drug, metronidazole (Flagyl®) can also be used to treat giardiasis. The dosage is 250 mg three times a day for ten days. As with amebiasis, follow-up stool examination should be obtained to assess efficacy of treatment no sonner than two weeks following completion of therapy. Most treatment failures respond to a second course of therapy. All at-risk sexual contacts should be evaluated for the presence of disease. A third alternative regimen is Furoxone®, 100 mg taken orally four times daily for seven days.[6] Alcohol is contraindicated while taking any of these regimens.

TABLE 1. Treatment of Giardiasis

Quinacrine hydrochloride (Atabrine®), 100 mg PC tid for 5 to 10 days, *or*
Metronidazole (Flagyl®), 250 mg PO tid for 10 days, *or*
Furazolidone (Furoxone®), 100 mg PO qid for 7 days

TABLE 2.   Factors Associated with the Increasing
Incidence of Venereally Acquired Amebiasis and
Giardiasis in the Homosexually Active Male Population

Failure by physician to diagnose and treat infected patients
Large asymptomatic pool never seek medical care
Misdiagnosis, e.g., functional bowel disease
Insensitivity of routine tests
Presence of interfering substances
Practice of anilinction and fellatio
Multiple sex partners
Imported disease secondary to foreign travel
Patterns of immigration
  Southeast Asia
  Caribbean
  Illegal aliens

CONTROL

Patient education in cases of giardiasis is identical to that for amebiasis (see pages 96 to 98).

REFERENCES

1. Myers JD, Kuharic HA, Holmes KK: *Giardia lamblia* infection in homosexual men. *Br J Vener Dis* 55:54–55, 1977.
2. Schmerin MJ, Jones TC, Klein H: Giardiasis: Association with homosexuality. *Ann Intern Med* 88:801–803, 1978.
3. William DC, Shookhoff HB, Felman YM, et al: High rates of enteric protozoal infections in selected homosexual men attending a venereal disease clinic. *Sex Transm Dis* 5:155–157, 1978.
4. Kean BH, William DC, Lumanais SK: Epidemic of amebiasis and giardiasis in a biased population. *Br J Vener Dis* 55:375–378, 1979.
5. Maguire JH: Giardiasis: An update. *Infect Dis Pract* 1(4):1–5, 1978.
6. Drugs for parasitic infections. *Med Lett* 24:8, 1982.

Shigellosis

DANIEL C. WILLIAM

Shigellosis is the most common cause of bacterial dysentery seen in homosexually active men. In fact, a significant proportion of all cases of shigellosis has occurred in homosexual men in recent years. At New York Hospital, a retrospective study found that homosexual men comprised the majority of adult men with shigellosis; in Seattle, 30% of all cases of shigellosis occurred in this population.

ETIOLOGY

The genus *Shigella* is associated with a large spectrum of colonic diarrheal disease. Many infected patients have nonspecific watery diarrhea while others have severe infection with bloody diarrhea, severe cramps, and fever. Only two of the fours groups of *Shigella*—which consist of short gram-negative rods— are common in the United States: group B, which includes *S. flexneri,* and group D, which has a single serotype, *S. sonnei.* The biological characteristics of *Shigella* determine both their epidemiology and pathology. Unlike the non-typhoidal salmonella, *Shigella* have no intermediate host outside of man. Transmission is, therefore, person-to-person and always involves fecal–oral contamination. Since the organism survives poorly outside the gastrointestinal tract of man, both waterborne and foodborne outbreaks are uncommon.

DANIEL C. WILLIAM ● Columbia University College of Physicians and Surgeons, New York, New York 10032; and St. Luke's–Roosevelt Hospital Center, New York, New York 10019.

EPIDEMIOLOGY

Intimate sexual contact provides an excellent opportunity for these organisms to spread. *Shigella* are highly infectious organisms. Less than 200 bacteria are required for the inoculum to cause clinical disease. *Shigella* has the dubious distinction, therefore, of being the most infectious enteric pathogen known.

CLINICAL ASPECTS

The biology of *Shigella* determines the signs and symptoms of clinical infections. Since the organism multiplies rapidly, symptoms of shigellosis appear after a brief incubation period averaging thirty-six to seventy-two hours. This short incubation period provides physicians with an important clinical clue to proper diagnosis. All patients presenting with any symptoms of shigellosis should be questioned carefully about the possibility of any at-risk sexual activity during the three-day period prior to the onset of symptoms.

Since shigellosis rarely disseminates beyond the gastrointestinal tract, the disease is almost always a self-limited infection. The organisms, however, penetrate the epithelium of the large bowel and multiply in the submucosa and lamina propria to cause microabscesses and superficial bleeding. The resultant symptoms include diarrhea, which may be blood-stained or grossly bloody.

Shigellosis usually presents with the acute onset of a fever, often high, and severe crampy abdominal pains, which rapidly progress to severe diarrhea. This dysenteric syndrome is, however, only the tip of the *Shigella* iceberg. Patients with mild disease may only have watery diarrhea of brief duration. Unfortunately, these patients rarely present to physicians and are often responsible for the continued spread of the disease to their sexual contacts. Patients with shigellosis often complain of myalgias involving the lower back and thighs. On physical examination, bowel sounds may be increased and there is often diffuse abdominal tenderness to deep palpation, usually described by the patient as "soreness." Anoscopy may reveal hyperemia, edema, and occasional small bloody mucosal ulcers with a purulent mucoid exudate. Gram-stained smears of rectal swabs reveal pus cells, red blood cells, and macrophages.

DIAGNOSIS

A presumptive diagnosis of shigellosis can be made when typical signs and symptoms are present. A rectal swab should be cultured prior to initiating therapy. Since the organism survives poorly, swabs must be rapidly inoculated into the appropriate media to prevent false-negative results.

The typical course of untreated shigellosis usually lasts approximately one week. Fever usually resolves before the diarrhea. The main complications encountered are dehydration and electrolyte imbalance, both of which are relatively uncommon in otherwise healthy adults. Although the clinical illness lasts only a week, stools may remain positive for as long as one month following resolution of all symptoms. All patients suspected of having shigellosis should, therefore, refrain from all rectal sexual activity until follow-up has been completed.

TREATMENT

Since immunity is species-specific, recurrent infections with shigellosis are both possible and common. The therapy for shigellosis involves supportive measures to assure adequate hydration and specific antimicrobials. A combination medication drug that contains both sulfamethoxazole (800 mg) and trimethoprim (160 mg) (Bactrim DS®; Septra DS®), is effective when taken as a tablet twice a day for five days. Ampicillin, 500 mg every six hours for five days, is also a suitable therapy for most cases. Resistance to antimicrobials may occur, requiring antibiotic sensitivity tests. In those regions where ampicillin-resistant shigellosis has been reported, the sulfa-trimethoprim regimen may be the preferred treatment.

The need for therapy in mild cases has been questioned since the disease is intrinsically self-limited. Unlike antibiotic treatment of salmonellosis, which appears to prolong the carrier state, antimicrobial therapy of shigellosis appears to shorten the carrier state. In San Francisco, where antimicrobial therapy has been widely applied in an attempt to decrease the reservoir of infected carriers, an increased resistance to antimicrobials, especially ampicillin, has been noted (personal communication from William Owen, M.D.). The use of antidiarrheal medications, which may reduce peristalsis, is relatively contraindicated, since they impair the ability of the bowel to eliminate the *Shigella* organisms.

CONTROL

As with any sexually transmitted disease, contacts of all patients should be notified and appropriately treated if infection is present.

10

Viral Hepatitis

DAVID G. OSTROW and TERENCE C. GAYLE

Viral hepatitis ranks fourth in the annual number of reported cases of communicable diseases in the United States.[1] Moreover, there is a likelihood that the morbidity is much higher since only 10% to 20% of diagnosed cases are reported by physicians to public health officials.[2] The total cost of viral hepatitis in the United States is currently estimated to be in excess of $1 billion.[3]

ETIOLOGY

Acute viral hepatitis encompasses at least three separate diseases that are dissimilar immunologically but are clinically similar. The etiologic viral agents for hepatitis A (HA) [hepatitis A virus (HAV)] and hepatitis B (HB) [hepatitis B virus (HBV)] have been identified; the search continues for the agent(s) responsible for a third type, hepatitis non-A/non-B (Hep NA/NB).

The discovery of the Australia antigen and its association with HBV was part of the foundation for subsequent research in viral hepatitis.[4] The development of techniques to detect virus-specific antigens and host antibodies resulted in greater understanding of the epidemiology and pathology of acute viral hepatitis.

Of the three types of viral hepatitis that are currently recognized, it is HB that is most often present in homosexual men. The physician will, however, probably encounter patients exhibiting a variable extent of signs and symptoms suggestive of HA and Hep NA/NB. Because of differences in the modes of

---

DAVID G. OSTROW • Biological Psychiatry Program, Lakeside Veterans Administration Medical Center, and Departments of Psychiatry and Community Medicine, Northwestern University Medical School, Chicago, Illinois 60611; and Howard Brown Memorial Clinic, Chicago, Illinois 60616. TERENCE C. GAYLE • Department of Psychiatry and Behavioral Sciences, University of Washington, Seattle, Washington 98195.

transmission, periods of incubation, immunologic response, duration of illness, and occurrence of sequelae between the various hepatitides, a specific diagnosis should be differentiated as soon as possible after a patient seeks consultation.

CLINICAL ASPECTS

A comparison of several laboratory and clinical diagnostic features of each of the three main types of viral hepatitis is presented in Table 1. While the main focus of this chapter is on HB in homosexual males, the reader is referred to several excellent reviews of the general subject of viral hepatitis.[2,5–9]

Acute Hepatitis

The clinical spectrum of acute hepatitis infection in homosexual men is similar to that seen in any group of well-nourished and otherwise healthy individuals and thus ranges from totally asymptomatic and anicteric (subclinical) patients to severe and fulminant illness that may culminate in death. The results of readily available serologic tests for HB at venereal disease (VD) clinics for homosexual men have increased awareness of the preponderance of asymptomatic infection seen in this population. As many as 40% to 50% of patients with seroconversion are asymptomatic, and a similar proportion of subclinical patients are probably present in other "healthy" populations in the United States. In contrast, the specialized nature of community sexually transmitted disease (STD) clinics and the severely ill patient's need for close clinical observation will selectively exclude some of the more symptomatic patients from presenting in an STD clinic setting. However, as the result of long-term follow-up of sexually transmitted STD clinic patients with acute infection, an increasing number of chronic active HBV cases have been identified over the last seven years at the Howard Brown Memorial Clinic (HBMC), and private practitioners with large homosexual male patient populations have reported several dozen cases during the last several years. The following description of acute viral hepatitis is based on both the authors' experience and the published and unpublished accounts of others.

Acute hepatitis infection in the homosexual male population seen at the HBMC averaged 4% of all patients visiting the clinic between January 1976 and December 1981. Clearly, the majority of patients presented with HB, which had an overall incidence of 3.5% during that period, with HA and Hep NA/NB each seen in less than 0.5% of clinic patients. For the most part, the symptoms of all three types of acute hepatitis infections are similar. Information concerning asymptomatic infection is available only for the patients with HB. Of a total of 1086 who seroconverted to HB_sAg positivity, 50% experienced prodromal symp-

TABLE 1. Laboratory and Clinical Diagnostic Features of the Viral Hepatitides[a]

	Hepatitis A	Hepatitis B	Hepatitis non-A/non-B
Etiologic agent	HAV	HBV	Possibly more than one agent?
Virus type	RNA	DNA	Unknown
Virus size, shape	27 nm, cubic	42 nm, spherical	Unknown
Host range	Man, marmoset	Man, chimpanzee	Man, chimpanzee
Incubation period, average (range)	30 days (15 to 50)	75 days (50 to 180) (may vary with route of transmission)	50 days (15 to 150)
Seasonal incidence	Autumn, winter	All seasons	Unknown
Routes of infection			
1. Orofecal (food, water, shellfish)	Yes	Probably not the dominant mode of transmission	Unknown
2. Close contacts, especially sex partners	Yes	Yes	Yes
3. Parenteral (inoculations, transfusions, dialysis, and needle-stick)	Rare	Yes	Yes
4. Vertical transmission (mother to fetus or neonate)	Unknown	Yes	Unknown
Viremia	Transient: late incubation and early acute phases (7 to 20 days)	Prolonged: late incubation and acute phases (sometimes months or years)	Unknown
Virus in feces	Late incubation period and early acute phases (2 weeks before and 1 week after onset of jaundice)	Unresolved	Unknown
Virus in semen, saliva, urine, nasopharyngeal secretions, mother's milk, and other secretions	No	Yes	Unknown

(Continued)

TABLE 1 *(Continued)*

	Hepatitis A	Hepatitis B	Hepatitis non-A/non-B
Serologic tests			
1. Antigens	HA antigen (only recently available)	HB_sAg, HB_cAg, HB_eAg in serum	None yet
2. Antibodies	Anti-HA	Anti-HB_s, anti-HB_c, anti-HB_e	None yet
3. Other		DNA polymerase and DNA polymerase inhibitory substances	
Carrier state	No	Yes	Unknown
Immunity	Homologous only	Homologous only	Probably homologous but may be more than one agent
Acute viral hepatitis			
Clinical features			
1. LFT ranges			
a. Aminotransferases (SGOT and SGPT) SGOT/SGPT not of diagnostic use	500 to 2500 IU/liter Rise during late incubation and acute phases and return to normal within 6 weeks in uncomplicated cases	Same as for HA Rise during late incubation and acute phases and may take 6 weeks to several months to return to normal in uncomplicated cases	Same as for HB Same as for HB
b. Alkaline phosphatases	Mildly elevated or normal	Mildly elevated or normal	Mildly elevated or normal
c. Total bilirubin (serum)	1 to 20 mg/dl	1 to 20 mg/dl	1 to 20 mg/dl

2. Percent icteric cases	Unknown	Possibly 30 to 50% in adults	Less than for HB
3. Onset of symptoms	Usually abrupt	Usually insidious	Usually insidious
4. Prodromal symptoms	Influenzalike symptoms: fever, anorexia, nausea, vomiting, dark urine, light-colored stools, right upper quadrant tenderness (2- to 7-day period)	Same as for HA with the addition of serum-sickness-like syndrome: arthritis, arthralgia, and urticaria seen in a minority of cases (2- to 30-day period)	
5. Clinical severity	Usually mild	Spectrum from mild to severe debilitating disease	Probably between those of HA and HB
Chronic infection and sequelae	Rare	6 to 10% or more of cases	Unclear: probably less than that for HB
Prophylaxis	Gamma globulin (ISG)	HBIG, HB vaccine (Heptavax B®, Merck Laboratories)	Unclear

[a] Abbreviations: HA, hepatitis A; HAV, hepatitis A virus; HB, hepatitis B; HBIG, hepatitis B immune globulin; HBV, hepatitis B virus; ISG, immune serum globulin; LFT, liver function test; SGOT, serum glutamic oxaloacetic transaminase; SGPT, serum glutamic pyruvic transaminase.

toms, most of which were related to cholestasis (dark urine, light stools, diarrhea) and liver inflammation. Right upper quadrant tenderness, which was present in half of the symptomatic patients, usually preceded the development of jaundice or scleral icterus. Other common symptoms included fatigue, anorexia, and bowel disturbances. Nausea, vomiting, and pruritic eruptions were seen in approximately 5% of symptomatic patients, and only three patients with HB had associated arthralgia or arthritis.

When liver function tests are compared in asymptomatic versus symptomatic patients, the presence of symptoms, and more specifically jaundice, correlates with more severe liver disease based on the degree of elevation of the serum transaminases. Whereas the peak serum glutamic pyruvic transaminase (SGPT) levels averaged 328 IU in asymptomatic patients, 610 IU for symptomatic patients without jaundice, and 1255 IU for jaundiced patients, alkaline phosphatase levels showed a similar moderate elevation for all three groups of patients. Serum glutamic oxaloacetic transaminase (SGOT) elevations generally paralleled SGPT levels, with an overall SGOT/SGPT ratio of 2 : 2.5. Fatigue was the earliest prodromal symptom, followed by gastrointestinal and then cholestatic symptoms prior to the peak elevation of serum transaminases (Figure 1). None of the patients with acute HB evidenced disorders of liver protein synthesis; serum proteins and prothrombin times of these patients were within normal limits.

The most common symptom cluster in patients presenting at the HBMC was that of right upper quadrant tenderness, fatigue, and dark urine, accompanied by jaundice or scleral icterus and mild hepatomegaly. Finally, a small but significant number of patients (approximately 5%) reported depression or altered mood as the major initial symptom. Only a small proportion of symptomatic patients, and none of the asymptomatic patients, complained of inability to perform routine daily tasks. Indeed, most patients continued to work throughout the acute episode. Requests by patients for letters documenting their fitness to continue work far outnumbered sick leave requests. Thus, the clinical picture of acute HBV infection in the homosexual male population (mean age 27 years) presents as a relatively benign course in most patients, with symptoms present in half of the patient population. Presenting symptoms and liver test abnormalities resolved within two months of the initial serum transaminase elevations. In most cases, the discovery of HB_sAg positivity corresponded with the major rise in SGPT and SGOT levels, but a number of patients had variable delays ranging from two to twenty weeks between antigenemia and serum transaminase elevations. Similarly, conversion from antigen to antibody positivity usually coincided with the return of serum transaminase values to normal. However, 15% to 25% of patients evidenced prolonged (greater than six months) antigenemia or elevated transaminase levels or both. For these reasons, we considered as chronic cases or carriers only those individuals with antigenemia of greater than one year's duration.

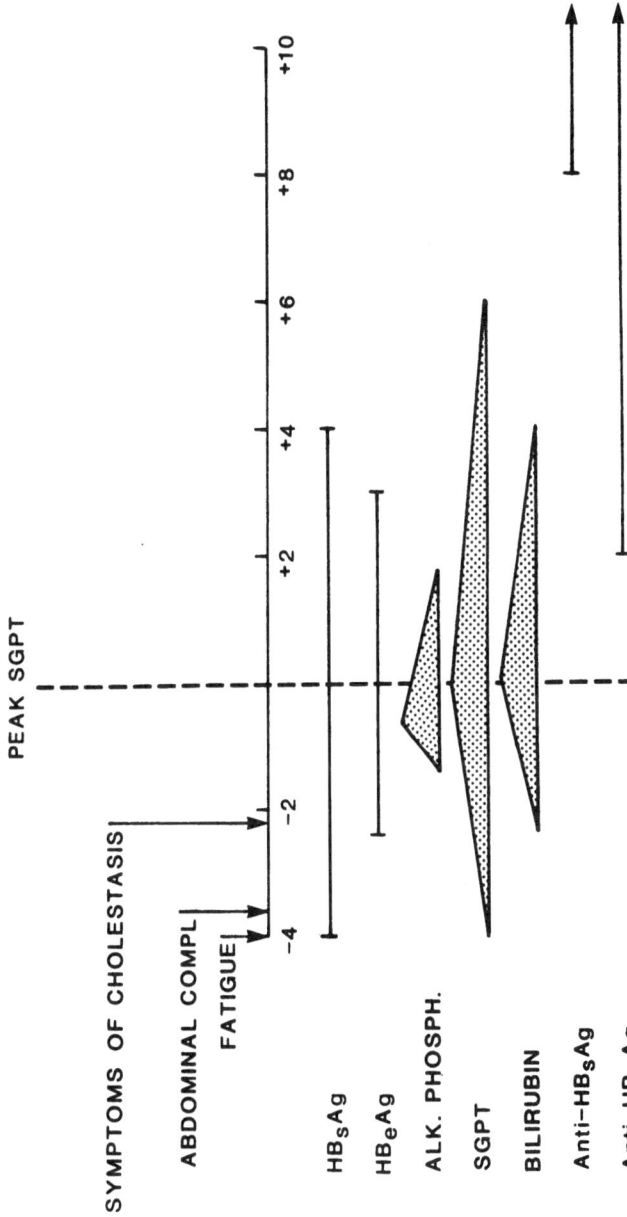

FIGURE 1.   Time course of symptoms and laboratory abnormalities in patients with acute hepatitis B. Time intervals along x axis are in weeks. Adapted from ref. 80 by permission of the publisher and authors.

Work-Up of Patient with Acute Hepatitis

Because of the clinical similarity of all three types of viral hepatitis, serologic testing for HBV is necessary from both management and epidemiologic standpoints. The diagnostic work-up of any patient with suspected viral hepatitis must reasonably exclude toxic etiologies, such as ethanol, drugs, occupational exposures, and gallstones, even though the incidence of these forms of hepatitis is remarkably low in otherwise healthy men. Previous viral hepatitis history, known seropositivity, and the coexistence of other enterically transmitted infections, such as giardiasis and amebiasis, help in narrowing the etiology of the current episode. Counseling of patients and the prophylaxis of close sexual contacts is based on making a definitive etiologic determination (see page 131). The laboratory evaluation of acute hepatitis is summarized in Figure 2.

Hepatitis A

HA was previously known as infectious or epidemic hepatitis. The etiologic agent is an RNA virus that has recently been classified as Enterovirus Type 72 of the picornaviruses.[10] Ingestion of even small amounts of HAV via the fecal–oral route through direct or indirect person-to-person contact is the chief mode of transmission in homosexual men. Parenteral transmission of HAV is possible, but documented cases are rare, presumably due to the short duration of viremia. The "epidemic" picture of HAV infections arose from the higher incidence seen in lower socioeconomic groups, institutions for the mentally retarded, and other situations associated with overcrowding and poor hygiene. Recently there has been renewed interest in an epidemic and virulent form of HA seen in India and perhaps Africa.[11]

Indirect transmission of HAV infection through the ingestion of raw or insufficiently cooked oysters or clams from contaminated waters is also well known but probably of insignificant importance in transmission to homosexual men. While the incidence and age distribution vary widely by world geography, the suggestion that HA in the United States has become a predominantly adult disease is supported by prevalence rates for antibody to HAV and a sharp peak of incidence rates in 19- to 25-year-olds.[12] No differences in susceptibility by sex have been reported.

Clinical Aspects of Hepatitis A

The incubation period of HA ranges from fifteen to fifty days, with an average of thirty days. In temperate climates, HA is seen more frequently during the fall and winter seasons. Transient viremia occurs during the late incubation and acute phases. HAV is likewise present in feces during the second half of

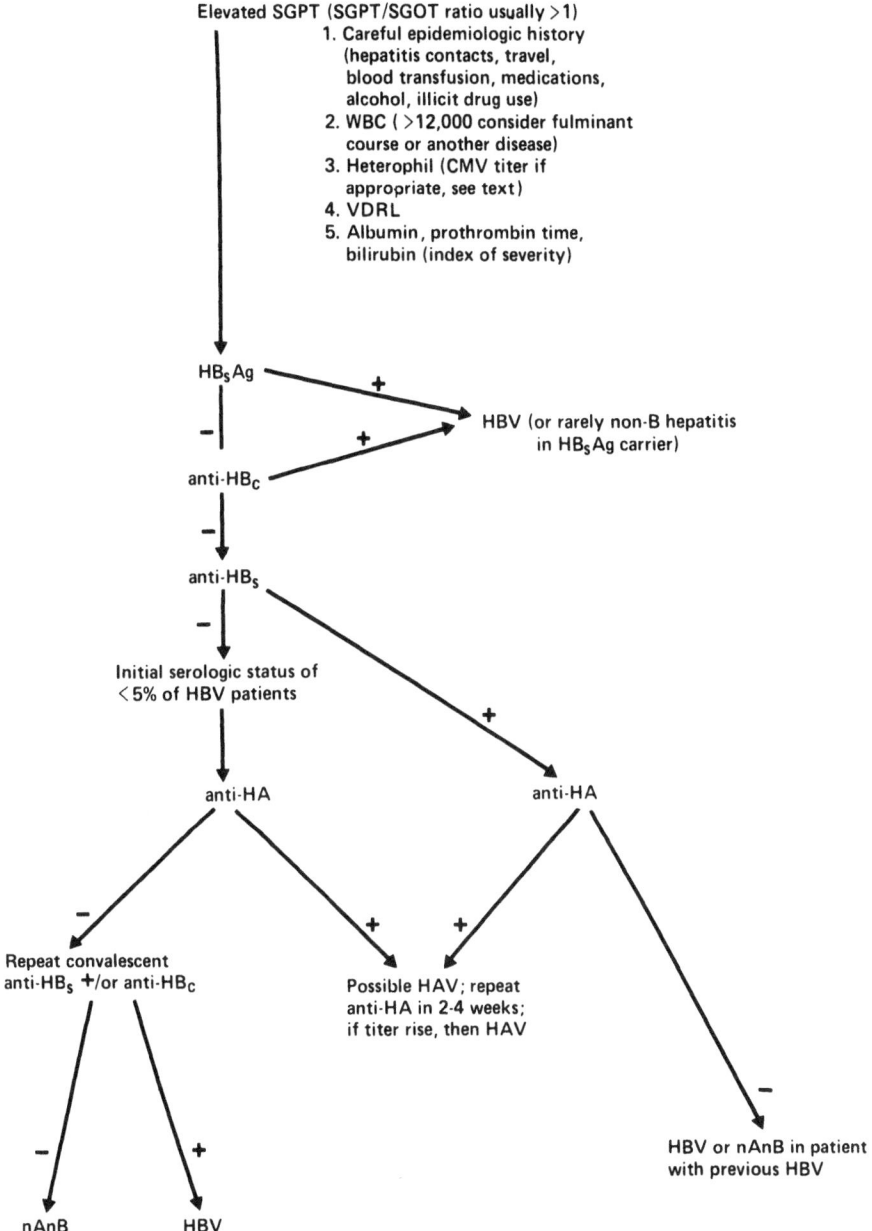

FIGURE 2.   Laboratory evaluation of acute hepatitis. Modified from ref. 7 by permission of
the publisher and authors.

the incubation period and the first eight to ten days after the onset of jaundice.[13] The three-week period of fecal virus shedding corresponds to the period of contagiousness, although determination in an individual patient may be difficult since many cases are subclinical or anicteric. Unlike for HB and Hep NA/NB, no chronic carriers of HAV have been identified. SGPT and SGOT levels begin to rise in the late incubation period, reaching their maximum during the icteric phase. Immunoglobulin M (IgM) anti-HAV can be detected by a commercially available test at the time of onset of jaundice and may remain elevated for variable periods. HAV antigen testing is clinically not useful since viremia is transient and of low titer and since fecal shedding ceases with the onset of symptoms.

Role of Sexual Practices in Transmission of HAV Infection

The role of sexual contact in the transmission of HAV infection has recently been clarified. While an early study in New York City revealed no significant difference in the prevalence of anti-HAV between heterosexual and homosexual populations,[14] it would seem likely that a number of sexual practices common among homosexual males could facilitate fecal–oral transmission of HAV infection. Enteropathogenic infections such as amebiasis, giardiasis, and shigellosis are transmitted by the same route and their incidence is increasing dramatically in this population.[15] The specific risk factors include anilinction and subsequent contact with a penis, finger, hand, or other object that has been inserted into the partner's anus and contaminated with feces. A subsequent study done in Seattle by Corey and Holmes[16] revealed a much greater incidence of HAV infection in homosexual men when compared to heterosexual STD clinic patients. Not surprisingly, frequency of anilinction was the major specific sexual practice risk factor. A recent epidemic outbreak of HAV infection among homosexual males in Denver appears to be of venereal origin.[17]

Hepatitis B

HB was previously known as serum hepatitis because of an earlier mistaken notion that it was transmitted only by inoculation with infected serum. The agent responsible for HBV infection is a DNA virus (also called the Dane particle, after its discoverer). The spherical virus is 42 nm in diameter and consists of a 28-nm inner core surrounded by a 7-nm-thick shell. The inner core contains circular 3200-base-pair-long double-stranded DNA and DNA polymerase. The outer shell contains a complex HBV surface antigen (HB_sAg) with identifiable antigenic subgroups. HB_sAg can be detected in the patient's serum during infection. A second "core" antigen, HB_cAg, is associated with the inner core and is found in the serum of virtually all patients with HBV infection. Recently, radioimmunoassay and enzyme immunoassays have been developed to detect serum HB_cAg and both IgM and IgG antibodies to HB_cAg. Finally, HB_eAg or "e antigen" is a third immunologically distinct antigen associated with the completed HBV particle. HB_eAg, when found in HB_sAg-positive sera, correlates with infectivity and is probably an unprocessed component of the core region of the virion. The specific antibodies elicited after exposure to these three antigens are termed anti-HB_s, anti-HB_c, and anti-HB_e, respectively. DNA polymerase activity parallels the level of HB_eAg and may coincide with the period of peak HBV replication.[18] Because of the unique physical, chemical, and biological properties of HBV infecting man, woodchucks, and Pekin ducks, the group name Hepadnavirus has been proposed.[10]

The parenteral transmission of HBV infection is well established. Exposure to infectious serum can occur by transfusion, hemodialysis, vaccination, accidental needle-stick by laboratory workers, sharing of needles among drug abusers, tattooing, ear-piercing, acupuncture, gastrointestinal endoscopy, and dental examination. Various sexual practices in homosexual men that involve potential exposure to contaminated blood or plasma appear related to the high incidence of this infection (see page 118). Vertical transmission of HBV from mother to fetus or neonate has been documented and may be the predominant route of transmission in Third World countries. The virus is probably transferred transplacentally or during parturition.

Although exact details of transmission remain undetermined, there is considerable evidence that HBV is transmitted by nonparenteral or inapparent parenteral routes through close person-to-person contact. HB_sAg has been identified in practically every body secretion or excretion, and the presence of complete HBV particles can be inferred from the high degree of infectivity of HB_eAg-positive body fluids. Unlike HAV infection, fecal–oral spread was not considered an important route of transmission. Instead, HBV was thought to be transferred from acute or chronic carriers to other susceptible persons through shared toothbrushes, razors, or fomites. Quite the opposite now appears to be true in homosexual men. Oral–oral transmission may also occur if HBV gains entry through minute lesions in mucosal surfaces.

Sexual Transmission of HBV

HBV infection is now recognized as a sexually transmitted disease. Since 1946, several cases of HB in sexual partners of acute or chronic HB_sAg carriers have been reported. Of particular interest is the repeated finding that homosexual males tested at VD clinics in Britain and the United States have the highest prevalence of combined HBV seropositivity (HB_sAg or anti-HB_s) of any group thus far studied. The prevalence rate of HB_sAg ranged from 3.8% to 6.0% and that for anti-HB_s from 34% to 68%.[19-27] In another study,[28] 10 out of 14 HB_sAg-seropositive homosexual males were also positive for HB_cAg.

By comparison, the prevalences of HBV infections in other high-risk groups are as follows: volunteer blood donors, 4.4%; physicians, 18.5%[29]; dialysis technicians and nurses, 35.7%[30]; and spouses and household members of HB_sAg carriers, 40%.[31] The only other group with a comparable rate of prior HBV infection includes drug abusers, whose estimated HBV seropositivity is 55% to 65%.[32]

The largest study of HBV infection in homosexual males was recently conducted jointly by the Centers for Disease Control (CDC) in Atlanta and the HBMC.[33,34] This retrospective and prospective study was designed to investigate specific sexual practices as possible risk factors in the transmission of HBV and also to assess the prevalence of current and past HBV infection. The study population included 3694 homosexual males (mean age 29 years) attending STD clinics in San Francisco, Los Angeles, Denver, St. Louis, and Chicago. All patients were interviewed and tested for the presence of HB_sAg, anti-HB_s, anti-HB_c, and anti-HB_e in their sera. Patients seeking medical attention for acute hepatitis were excluded. The prevalence of combined HBV seropositivity was estimated to be 62%. Of all patients, 6.3% were HB_sAg-positive and 52.6% had detectable anti-HB_s. Furthermore, of the 233 patients who were HB_sAg-positive, 68% were also positive for HB_eAg and 23% had anti-HB_e in their sera. In contrast, only 2 of 138 anti-HB_s-positive specimens contained HB_eAg.[35]

The results of this study indicated that two variables were most significantly related to HBV infection: the duration of regular homosexual activity and the number of male nonsteady partners (where "nonsteady" is defined as not more than two contacts with the same person) in the previous four-month period. The data in Table 2 show that combined HBV seropositivity increases from 15.6% in those men with less than twelve months of regular homosexual activity to 73.8% in men who were active for ten or more years. While HBV seropositivity was positively related to age, the relation between age and HBV infection was not significant when the duration of homosexual activity was taken into account. When the number of male nonsteady sexual partners during the four-month period before the interview was examined (Table 3), HBV seropositivity increased from 48.9% in those men having less than four partners to 79.7% among men with 49 to 72 nonsteady partners. The relationship between number of nonsteady sexual partners and incidence of HBV infection was even more striking in the prospective study data (last column of Table 3). By contrast, the numbers of male steady partners (three or more contacts with the same person) and female steady partners were not related to seropositivity. Similarly, specific sex practices with steady partners were not significant.

Further analysis of sexual activity with nonsteady partners yielded five

TABLE 2.   HBV Prevalence Study: Duration of Regular
Homosexuality by HBV Seropositivity[a]

Duration (years)	No. HBV positive	Combined HBV seropositivity (%)
<1	12	15.6
1–2	130	32.3
3–5	360	48.8
6–9	341	64.6
≥10	933	73.8
TOTAL	1776[b]	59.5

[a] $\chi^2 = 335.5$, 4 d.f., $p < 0.0001$.
[b] 496 patients with no data excluded.

specific sexual practices strongly related to HBV seropositivity. In describing these practices, "active" means that the patient entered an orifice of his partner and "passive" indicates that the patient's orifice was entered by his partner. The relative risk factor (RRF) indicates the relative increased rate of seropositivity for persons practicing each particular activity, adjusted to the number of nonsteady partners. The practices in decreasing order of significance are as follows: passive anogenital intercourse with ejaculation (RRF = 1.42), active oroanal intercourse (anilinction) (RRF = 1.22), passive anogenital intercourse without ejaculation (RRF = 1.20), rectal douching prior to passive anogenital intercourse (RRF = 1.2), and passive manual–anal intercourse (insertion of hand into rectum or "fist-fucking") (RRF = 1.2).[34]

TABLE 3.   HBV Seropositivity by Number of Male
Nonsteady Partners in Last Four Months[a]

No. of nonsteady partners	Retrospective combined seropositivity			Prospective HB$_s$Ag+ incidence
	Total	No. HBV positive	Percent HBV positive	Relative risk factor
0–4	885	433	48.9	1.00
5–12	1052	581	55.2	1.40
13–24	620	421	67.9	1.63
25–48	688	504	73.3	1.83
49–72	513	409	79.7	2.24
TOTAL	3758	2348	62.5	

[a] $\chi^2 = 234.4$, 4 d.f., $p < 0.0001$.

Orogenital sexual activity, whether passive or active and whether or not ejaculation or swallowing of semen occurred, was not independently associated with increased risk of HBV seropositivity. On prospective study of HB_sAg seroconversion, the three most important risk factors were passive anogenital intercourse (RRF = 1.76), active oroanal intercourse (RRF = 1.73), and rectal douching (RRF = 1.56).

All of the sexual practices that appeared to be significantly related to retrospective HBV seropositivity and prospective HB_sAg incidence involve contact with the rectal mucosa, and the authors speculate that the trauma of the easily damaged columnar mucosa during sexual intercourse may provide both a source of HBV infectious blood and a portal of entry for HBV infection. Neither saliva nor semen appears to be efficient in the sexual transmission of HBV. The infectious dose of HBV via blood inoculation has been shown to be as little as 1 $\times$ 10^{-8} ml of HB_sAg- and HB_cAg-positive serum.[36] As mentioned earlier, HB_sAg and HB_cAg are also detected in most other excretions and secretions including urine, semen, and saliva.

The roles of other STDs found in the rectum, such as herpes, gonorrhea, and nonspecific proctitis, in providing portals of entry for HBV are not defined in the present study. Rectal gonococcal infection, however, is positively correlated with HBV seropositivity in a study performed on a random sample of homosexual men who were tested in a VD van in Chicago.[37] Recently, Reiner and associates have demonstrated rectal mucosal lesions positive for HB_sAg in a majority of chronically infected men with a positive recent history of receptive anal intercourse.[38] While the cause(s) of these lesions is unknown, they may provide portals for the parenteral injection into the receptive partner as well as provide HB_sAg-positive serum that could infect the inserting partner through microscopic penile lesions or the urethra.

Clinical Aspects of Hepatitis B

The averge incubation period for HB is seventy-five days, but it can range from fifty to one hundred and eighty days. The serologic diagnosis of acute HB is based on the detection of HB_sAg or HB_cAg by the following methods in order of decreasing sensitivity: radioimmunoassay, enzyme-linked immunosorption assays, hemagglutination inhibition, complement fixation, counterelectrophoresis, and agar gel diffusion. HB_sAg and HB_cAg titers are detectable by the time jaundice appears and often persist up to four months after exposure in a typical acute infection. The prolonged presence of the complete virus (Dane particle) in the blood and other body fluids presumably renders the patient infectious for a much longer time than are patients with HAV infection.

Unlike for HA, a prolonged carrier state for HB exists. Presence of serum HB_sAg for longer than six months usually constitutes chronic antigenemia. This is of epidemiologic significance since between 6% and 10% of HBV-infected persons become chronic carriers. There is an estimated reservoir of 120 million human carriers in the world who can effectively maintain HBV without the need for serial transmission.[39] Based on estimates from the HBMC of a 2% to 5% carrier rate in the homosexual male population in the United States, there are approximately 100,000 to 500,000 HBV carriers at any one time.

Figure 1 illustrates the clinical and laboratory findings in a typical case of an acute icteric HBV infection. In general, the clinical spectrum of acute HB ranges from subclinical presentation to severe debilitating disease. The presence of underlying liver disease from abuse of alcohol or other hepatotoxins increases the severity of the illness. Fortunately, most of the homosexually active males seen at STD clinics are young, healthy, and without alcoholic liver disease. Previous reports of an overall high incidence of severe HBV infections may be accounted for by the contribution of a population of older patients, in whom underlying alcoholic liver disease is much more prevalent. However, the recent emergence of acquired cellular immunodeficiency states in large numbers of homosexually active men (see Chapters 16 and 17) raises the possibility of an increased frequency of severe fulminant and/or chronic infections in the homosexual population.

The appearance of anti-HB_sAg normally occurs during convalescence, usually about one to two months after HB_sAg disappears. During this hiatus, a single serologic test of HB_sAg or anti-HB_s is negative. At this time, however, anti-HB_c is present and may be used as a marker for recent HBV infection. More recently, IgM anti-HB_c has shown promise as the most sensitive marker for evaluating HBV prevalence in epidemiologic studies.[40] Anti-HB_s is most suitable as a marker for remote HBV infections and to assure that the patient has developed active immunity to HBV. Some patients with HB_sAg-positive hepatitis never develop detectable levels of anti-HB_s. In the population studied at the HBMC, 85% of HBV-infected patients developed anti-HB_s within five months after the acute rise in serum transaminases.

Perhaps the most serious concern in a patient with HB is the increased tendency to develop serious complications, such as chronic active hepatitis, fulminant hepatic necrosis, cirrhosis, and hepatoma. The mortality rate nationally for HBV infection is between ten and twenty times that for HAV infections.[41] The long-term sequelae of chronic HB are discussed in an upcoming section.

Hepatitis Non-A/Non-B

The postulation of the existence of Hep NA/NB is based on epidemiologic and serologic evidence. Other specific viruses have not yet been identified, but at least two agents have been proposed to explain viral hepatitis cases that do not exhibit HAV or HBV seropositivity.[42,43] These infections are not due to other viruses such as cytomegalovirus or Epstein–Barr virus. Little information is available about Hep NA/NB. It appears, however, that the transmission, course of infection, and epidemiology of Hep NA/NB are more similar to those of HB than those of HA. Several studies have reported that Hep NA/NB is responsible for more than 90% of posttransfusion viral hepatitis,[44,45] and the disease is seen frequently in parenteral drug abusers, who may have multiple bouts of acute viral hepatitis.[46] Parenteral transmission appears to be the principal mode of transmission. To date, there is little evidence indicating fecal–oral spread or venereal transmission of Hep NA/NB, although no thorough epidemiologic studies of this infection have been performed because definitive testing techniques are not available.

The incubation period of Hep NA/NB ranges from fifteen to one hundred and fifty days and averages fifty days. Since no specific antigens or antibodies have been identified, the diagnosis is based on the absence of HAV and HBV seropositivity. The clinical severity of Hep NA/NB seems to be between that of HB and HA. Most importantly, acute Hep NA/NB infections may be at least as prone to progress to chronic liver disease as HBV infections.[47–49]

Complications of Acute Viral Hepatitis

The various outcomes of acute viral HB and their associated serologic findings are illustrated in Figure 3. Sequelae are discussed in terms of acute and chronic manifestations.

Acute Sequelae: Fulminant Hepatic Failure

Fulminant viral hepatitis is a rare but catastrophic outcome of acute viral hepatitis. Although the disease has been reported to occur in 1% to 2% of patients with HB and Hep NA/NB and in 0.01% of patients with HA,[50] this syndrome has not been seen in the approximately 1000 cases of acute hepatitis seen at the HBMC during the last four years. The reason may relate to the young age (mean 27 years) and the general good health of patients attending an STD clinic. Nevertheless, isolated cases of fulminant hepatic failure in homosexual men have been reported by private practitioners and in the medical literature.

The syndrome is characterized at onset by vomiting, progressive jaundice, and decrease in liver size and progresses to mental deterioration, coma, and death in 80% to 90% of patients. Along with markedly elevated SGOT and SGPT levels, there occur severe hypoalbuminemia and markedly prolonged prothrombin time, which often results in a hemorrhagic diathesis. Other findings consistent with this syndrome include fever, elevated white cell count, marked bilirubinemia (>40 mg/dl), and elevated serum ammonia levels. Pathological examination of the liver reveals extensive destruction of hepatocytes and resulting

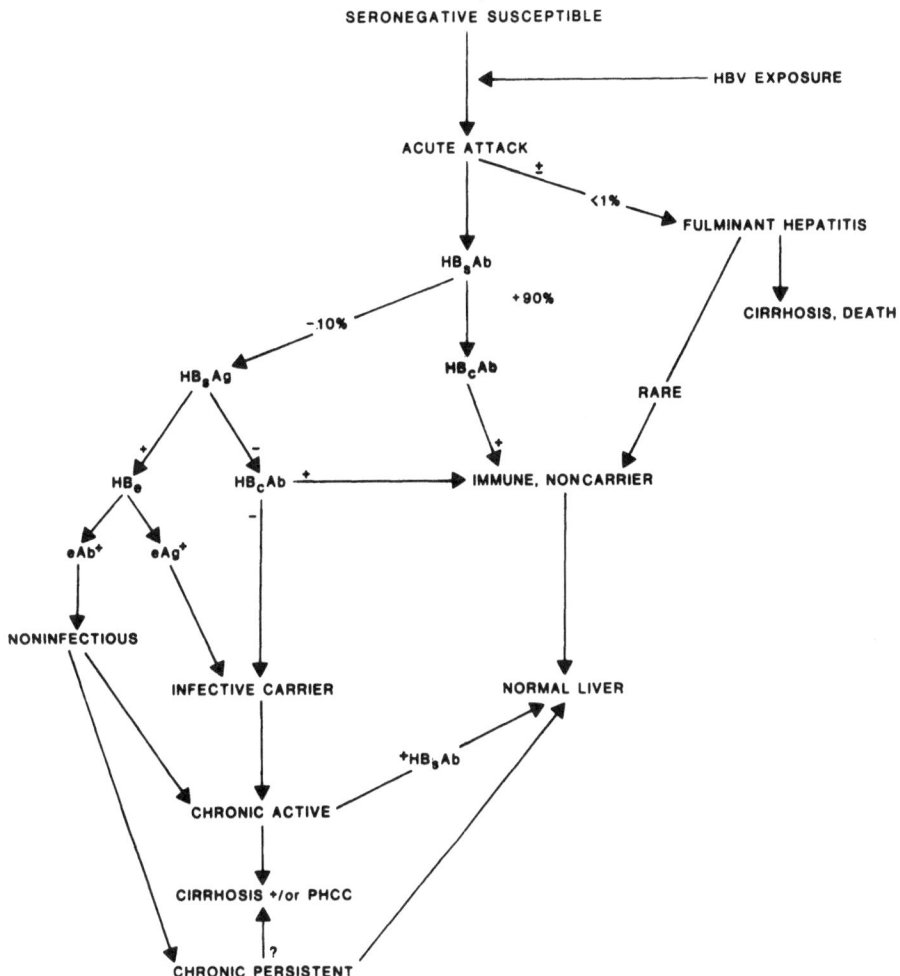

FIGURE 3. Sequelae of acute viral hepatitis B. PHCC, primary hepatocellular carcinoma.

collapse of the reticulum and obliteration of normal liver architecture. There is frequently an inflammatory reaction consisting of small round cells, plasma cells, polymorphonuclear leukocytes, and periportal ductular proliferation. Despite the apparent absence of significant numbers of viable hepatocytes at biopsy, persons recovering from this syndrome usually show minimal residual liver pathology, undoubtedly a testimonial to the regenerative capacity of the liver. The reasons why certain individuals develop fulminant hepatic failure are unknown, but defects in the immune system, such as those resulting from splenectomy and immunosuppressive therapy, have been associated with increased incidence of this syndrome.

Therapy is conservative and consists of supportive measures to sustain vital functions in the hope that the illness will subside spontaneously. Treatment of hepatic coma and cerebral edema is necessary in most cases, but there is no evidence that corticosteroids, exchange transfusions, or other heroic efforts can significantly alter the mortality of this rare complication of acute viral hepatitis.

Chronic Sequelae

Chronic hepatitis is defined as a continuing hepatic inflammation that lasts more than six months. There are two types of chronic hepatitis: persistent and active. The definitive diagnosis of chronic hepatitis is based on liver biopsies and laboratory evidence of persistent impairment of liver functions. As most young chronic patients are clinically well, one may delay biopsying HB_sAg-positive patients until elevated transaminases have been present for one year. Clinically ill or antigen-negative patients are biopsied earlier because of the increased likelihood of chronic active hepatitis in these patients.

Evidence for an association between HA and chronic liver disease is slight. Acute HB is a known frequent precursor of chronic hepatitis. Between 10% and 15% of patients with acute HB progress to chronic hepatitis,[51,52] but there may be an increased incidence of both chronicity and carrier state formation in homosexually active males attending STD clinics.[53] Chronic antigenemia may coexist with continuing liver inflammation but does not by itself constitute chronic hepatitis. Likewise, a patient with chronic hepatitis can have detectable anti-HB_s and a few patients have both HB_s and anti-HB_s circulating freely. The role of HB_e as a marker of chronic hepatitis is unclear. Chronic hepatitis can also be a sequel to Hep NA/NB.[47-49] Finally, chronic liver disease can follow anicteric, subclinical, and icteric bouts of acute infections.

Acute hepatitis in homosexual men mostly presents in the second and third decades of life. These men are otherwise healthy and recovery is without incident. The mortality and complications associated with acute viral hepatitis infections increase with age. Attempts to apply the same overall mortality rates would probably result in an overestimation in this group of healthy young men. It is useful to separate chronic HB into persistent and active hepatitis based on biopsy and clinical findings.

Chronic Persistent Hepatitis and the Carrier State

Most homosexual males who become chronic carriers of HB_sAg have chronic persistent hepatitis (CPH).[53-55] CPH is marked by mild liver enzyme abnormalities that may continue for years. The notable aspect of CPH is that it is almost always a benign and self-limited infection with a good prognosis for recovery. The serious complications of scattered lobular necrosis and cirrhosis are not seen. Laboratory findings can include persistent mildly elevated aminotransferases and bilirubinemia, normal serum albumin and prothrombin time, and normal or mildly elevated liver chemistries. Most patients are asymptomatic but some may complain of fatigue and anorexia. Hepatomegaly may be present but icterus is rare.

The definitive diagnosis is based on liver biopsy, which shows spotty panlobular inflammation characterized by infiltration of lymphocytes and plasma cells into normally sized portal tracts. Portal inflammation is focal and fibrosis is either absent or minimal. Any focal hepatocellular necrosis is scattered and spares the hepatic lobule.

Management of Chronic Persistent Hepatitis.   Most patients appear in good health and therefore do not need any specific medical treatment. Liver chemistries should be monitored until transaminases or serum bilirubin levels or both return to normal. Patients with Gilbert's syndrome also have mild bilirubinemia but it is unconjugated. Alcohol and known hepatotoxic drugs should be avoided. Patients who also exhibit chronic antigenemia should be appropriately counseled about their potential for hepatitis transmission to sexual partners. As greater than 65% of HB_sAg carriers at HBMC are also e-antigen carriers, one can assume that the majority of chronic carriers are infectious, and they should be counseled as such (see pages 131–133). There is no reason why these individuals cannot be involved in occupations—such as medicine, dentistry, or nursing—that involve close physical contact, as long as proper precautions to avoid blood contamination are taken.

Chronic Active Hepatitis

Chronic active hepatitis (CAH) is characterized by continued necrosis and inflammation with fibrosis, and in severe cases, postnecrotic cirrhosis and death owing to portal hypertension or hepatic failure. Up to 5% of patients with acute HB develop CAH.[51] Multiple etiologies have been suggested for the chronic active syndrome, including autoantibodies, HB, Hep NA/NB, idiopathic reactions, and toxic reactions to drugs known to include isoniazide, oxyphenacetin, α-methyldopa, methotrexate, phenothiazines (such as chlorpromazine, Thorazine®, salicylates, hydralazine), and sulfonamides. A serum antibody directed against liver membrane is found in the cryptogenic or "lupoid" type of CAH[46] but is absent in HB-associated disease. The histopathology presents as infiltrates of lymphocytes and plasma cells into portal tracts and scattered necrotic foci. The more serious hepatocellular damage can extend into the parenchyma and disrupt the lobular architecture. The commonly described "piecemeal necrosis" of CAH refers to foci of necrotic hepatocytes surrounded by inflammation. The extent of fibrosis is variable, but in severe cases portal fibrosis and lobular necrosis may result in bridging hepatic necrosis. The latter condition has a particularly poor prognosis because the patient can die of hepatic failure or subsequent cirrhosis and may be more prone to develop hepatocellular carcinoma. The diagnosis of CAH should be based on a liver biopsy and clear evidence of persistent hepatic injury over a period of at least six months.

Asymptomatic acute viral hepatitis may precede CAH. In fact, many cases begin insidiously and may be detected only if liver chemistries are measured during the course of a routine medical checkup. Antigen-negative CAH can follow HB_sAg-positive acute infections.[56]

Laboratory tests do not always differentiate between CAH and CPH. Serum transaminase levels may be persistently elevated or may fluctuate widely. Serum bilirubin and alkaline phosphatase levels may be increased. Increased prothrombin time and hypoalbuminuria are seen in cases with extensive liver damage and are usually signs of poor prognosis.

The most common symptoms are fatigue, anorexia, and vague abdominal complaints. A serum-sickness-like syndrome is occasionally observed. Clinical signs are generally more evident than in CPH and include hepatomegaly, splenomegaly, and abdominal tenderness. Severe cases may present with spider angiomas, ascites, and other signs of chronic liver disease.

Management of Chronic Active Hepatitis. The CAH patient should be restricted from alcohol and other known hepatotoxic drugs. The patient with chronic HB_sAg should be advised that he is potentially infectious. Liver chemistries should be measured several times a year. Patients can continue to lead normal lives within the limits of their tolerance of such restrictions. The use of corticosteroids in treating CAH patients who are symptomatic or HB_sAg-positive appears to be nonbeneficial and perhaps deleterious.[57,58] Research is currently being conducted on immunostimulating drugs such as levamisole and bacillus Calmette–Guérin (BCG) vaccine, as well as direct antiviral replication agents such as vidarabine and interferon,[59] but conclusive evidence for an efficacious treatment for CAH is not yet available.

Chronic Sequelae: Primary Hepatic Cell Carcinoma

The association of HBV and primary hepatic cell carcinoma (PHCC) was recognized in epidemiologic studies that showed a high incidence of HB_sAg and anti-HB_c in patients with liver cancer. The first studies were conducted in parts of Africa and Asia where hepatomas are more prevalent.[60-64] These findings have also been demonstrated in Caucasians.[65] Although proof of HBV as an etiologic agent for PHCC is not definite, it has been suggested that the correlation is higher in those patients who had HBV infections early in life, perhaps from carrier mothers.[66]

There have been no studies of the prevalence of liver cancer in homosexual males. Based upon the above reports, it is plausible that more PHCCs would be found among the members of a group with a higher rate of HBV infections, particularly when cirrhosis is present. Additionally disturbing is the possibility that potentially carcinogenic substances, such as amyl, butyl, and other volatile nitrites, may act synergistically on the induction of PHCC in homosexual males (see Chapter 18). The answer to these questions awaits more intensive investigation. In a recent study performed by Donald Francis, M.D., of the CDC, the risks of death due to PHCC and to cirrhosis in chronic HB carriers were estimated to be 30% and 7%, respectively.[67] Based on approximately 200,000 new cases of HB per year in the United States, this translates into an estimated 3500 deaths from cirrhosis and 870 from PHCC secondary to HB each year. Such figures are disturbing enough to give reason for hope that attention in the medical and scientific communities will be directed to the chronic hepatitis carrier and that there will be increased research into prophylaxis and treatment of this grave condition.

PROPHYLAXIS

Hepatitis A

Immune serum globulin (ISG) has been shown to be effective in preventing overt HAV infection in 80% to 90% of persons treated either before or within two weeks of exposure via intimate contact.[68] The usual dose is 0.02 ml/kg, or 1 ml to 2 ml in most adult males, given intramuscularly. Demonstrable anti-HAV is present for several months, unless subclinical or anicteric infection does take place, in which case lifelong immunity via passive–active immunization is acquired. We administer ISG to any person reporting sexual contact with a known case of HA within the prior two weeks and to persons reporting contact with viral hepatitis of unknown etiology. There are no data to suggest that periodic ISG administration, say every three months, is effective in preventing sexually transmitted HA, and the potential for adverse reactions to repeated injections of ISG argues against this practice.

Hepatitis Non-A/Non-B

There have not been any studies performed evaluating the efficacy of ISG prophylaxis in checking Hep NA/NB spread through intimate contact, and there is no information at present as to the possible presence in ISG of antibodies to the agent(s) responsible for Hep NA/NB. However, the recent identification of an antigen–antibody system associated with Hep NA/NB[69] and the increasing prevalence of this form of viral hepatitis in posttransfusion hepatitis may lead to the eventual detection of, and testing for the efficacy of, batches of ISG in Hep NA/NB prophylaxis.

Hepatitis B

Increasingly higher titers of anti-HB$_s$ have been found in commercial preparations of ISG during the past several years.[70] This discovery has led to the use of relatively large doses of conventional ISG, 5 ml to 10 ml, for the prophylactic treatment of persons exposed to HBV. Again, to be effective the ISG must be administered within fourteen days of the exposure, and protection is transient unless passive–active immunization occurs. The latter has been reported to occur in a significant number of persons receiving ISG for HBV exposure.[71] It has been suggested that STD clinics seeing large numbers of homosexual men screen various lots of commercial ISG and then reserve those lots with high titers of anti-HB$_s$ for individuals with a history of recent sexual exposure to viral hepatitis. A controlled study of this type of procedure has not been performed, but it would be of great value if it could validate a simple and relatively inexpensive form of prophylaxis against the two most common forms of sexually transmitted viral hepatitis.

A preparation of immune globulin prepared from persons with high titers of anti-HB$_s$, HBIG, has been marketed. The material costs $150 to $200 per 5-ml dose. The HBIG should be administered intramuscularly as soon after exposure as possible. The dose should be repeated in one month. HBIG is more efficacious than conventional ISG in single needle-stick exposures to HBV-contaminated blood.[72] The evidence concerning HBIG efficacy in the prevention of nonparenteral HB transmission is less clear, and no studies have been performed on sexually transmitted HB in homosexual men. In view of the expense of this material and its questionable margin of efficacy over conventional ISG in HB prophylaxis, we restrict its use to anti-HB$_s$-negative clinic personnel with accidental needle-stick exposures to HB$_s$Ag-positive blood and utilize large-dose ISG for sexual contacts of HB$_s$AB-positive individuals.

CONTROL

Hepatitis B Vaccine

The most significant development in the field of hepatitis since the discovery of the Australia antigen by Blumberg in the early 1960s has been the recent development of a vaccine for the active immunization of humans against HBV.

Developed independently by Ph. Maupas, M.D., at the Institute of Virology, Tours, France, and Maurice Hilleman, M.D., at the Merck Institute in the United States, the vaccine differs from classical viral vaccines in several important respects. Because HBV cannot be grown readily in tissue culture, there does not exist the opportunity for producing a live attenuated virus, as is the case for the other major antiviral vaccines presently in use. Instead, the vaccine is composed of purified and chemically inactivated HB_sAg obtained from the plasma of chronic HB_sAg carriers. Second, the recent demonstration that HBV infection is an STD in homosexually active men and perhaps other groups makes this the first vaccine to be developed against an STD. The significance of this latter aspect of the HBV vaccine is widely appreciated within the homosexual male community, with many of the major community STD clinics in the United States actively involved first in the clinical efficacy testing of the vaccine, then in supplying HB_sAg-positive plasma for vaccine production, and now in mounting large-scale HB vaccination programs.

The various HBV vaccine preparations are described in a recent symposium.[8] Both the Maupas and Hilleman vaccines have been shown to be antigenic in chimpanzees and humans, to be free of contaminating infectious HBV particles, and to protect both immunized chimpanzees challenged with live HBV and high-risk humans, such as hemodialysis patients and staff. Because of the homosexual male community's high incidence of sexually transmitted HB and its demonstrated motivation and willingness to participate to studies of HBV transmission such as the CDC-sponsored HBV prevalence study,[33] the major efficacy trials of the Merck vaccine have been undertaken in homosexual men.

The results of a Merck-sponsored study—performed by the New York Blood Center (NYBC) in collaboration with the New York Gay Men's Health Project (NYGMHP) under the direction of Wolf Szmuness, M.D., Cladd Stevens, M.D. (NYBC), and Daniel C. William, M.D. (NYGMHP)—were the first to be published.[73] That study showed a very high rate of protection (at least 92%) in persons receiving three vaccinations of 40 μg each over a six-month period. The only persons unprotected by the vaccine were those persons who failed to develop measurable anti-HB_s titers. A major federally sponsored trial of the Merck vaccine at the same STD clinics that participated in the HBV sexual transmission studies, utilizing 20-μg doses of vaccine administered at entry and one and six months later, gave similar results.[74] The Merck vaccine was subsequently licensed (under the trade name Heptavax B®) for clinical use in mid-1982.

Planning has already begun for the vaccination of groups at particularly high risk for HBV infection. These plans include those at risk for occupational reasons, such as health care personnel, dialysis patients and staff, and institutionalized persons. Those at risk because of parenteral exposure (drug addicts, hemophiliacs) and homosexual men are also included.[75] With our current knowledge concerning the epidemiology of HBV infection in homosexual men and the observation that postexposure vaccination may be efficacious in preventing clinical illness, vaccination of the sexual contacts of acute cases becomes a possibility, especially if the vaccination is offered at STD clinics, where acute cases and their identified sexual contacts are first presenting for STD testing and treatment. It has been suggested that patients at VD clinics in general represent a group with a tenfold increased risk of acquiring STDs and thus should be considered as a target group for vaccination programs aimed at high-risk groups. Similarly, we have recently suggested[37] that HBV serologic testing be used as an index of risk of exposure to the other STDs, such as gonorrhea and syphilis. Because of the cost of the vaccine ($100 per series of injections) and difficulties in reaching persons at highest risk for sexually transmitted HB, a task force was formed to provide specific guidelines and strategies for the most effective use of the vaccine in this area. The preliminary report of that task force and its recommendations have been published.[76]

Long-Term Safety of the Hepatitis B Vaccine

There is at present considerable discussion concerning the long-term safety of the Merck Hepatavax B Vaccine. This concern arises from the association between acquired immunodeficiency syndrome (AIDS) and the homosexually active males who might be donors of plasma for vaccine production. Since there is no serologic marker for the AIDS agent(s) at this time, it is impossible to screen blood donors for possible carriage of these putative agent(s). Further, the population with high titers of HS_sAg might be expected also to include individuals at risk of developing AIDS, owing to the similar epidemiology of the two illnesses. Unable to rule out contamination of the vaccine with such AIDS agent(s) definitively, many practitioners currently have been reluctant to recommend the vaccine, resulting in less than expected demand for it.

On the other hand, examination of the cohorts involved in both the vaccine efficacy studies by Merck (in New York City) and those by the CDC (in Chicago, San Francisco, and Denver) has shown that the incidence of AIDS in homosexual vaccinees is, if anything, below that of nonvaccinated comparison groups. However, the vaccine used in all the efficacy trials in homosexual men was manufactured in 1977, prior to the current AIDS outbreak. This controversy can only be resolved once a reliable marker for AIDS carriage and/or plasma contamination is discovered. In its absence, prospective studies of AIDS incidence levels in individuals receiving the commercial vaccine and matched groups at equal risk for developing AIDS are needed. Overall, the risk for acquiring chronic HB infection appears to outweigh any risk for AIDS in serosusceptible homosexually active males, and the vaccine should be recommended to such patients.[53,76]

Counseling Homosexual Males with Hepatitis and Their Sexual Contacts

The recent unfolding of knowledge regarding the sexual transmission of HB in homosexual males and the ready availability of HB_sAg testing pose several important questions for individuals found to be HB_sAg-positive, their sexual contacts, and the health care personnel seeing these patients at homosexual community STD clinics or elsewhere. The CDC study of HBV transmission established both that a sizable proportion of sexually active homosexual males had infectious HBV in their blood, either acutely (5% to 10%) or on a chronic basis (2% to 5%), and that sexual transmission could take place via inoculation of the mucosa of either the mouth or the rectum with contaminated serum, mucus, or feces. The mucosal inoculation of serum or secretions contaminated with HBV is among the most efficient mechanisms of HBV transmission,[77] and the efficiency of HBV transmission via these routes may be increased by microlesions produced during sexual intercourse, leading to direct percutaneous inoculation of virus particles.[38] Our findings that serosuceptible homosexual males had an approximately 25% to 30% risk of developing HBV infection during each year of prospective study[33] and that many individuals present to HBMC personnel for counseling regarding the sexual transmission of this disease are not surprising. These individuals include patients recently discovered to be HB_sAg-positive, sexual contacts of persons recently discovered to have clinical hepatitis or HB_sAg positivity, and known chronic HB_sAg carriers, as well as serosusceptible individuals.

Approximately half of the persons found to be HB_sAg-positive at screening are in the early stage of acute infection, with the other half being chronic antigenemic individuals. The work-up to distinguish between these two situations has been described previously, but initial counseling of the patient must be based on the assumption that he *is* infectious to others, regardless of the type of infection. These patients are therefore counseled to discontinue sexual activity and to advise known sexual partners during the previous month to obtain testing. As greater than 50% of their sexual contacts are already immune to HBV infection, the rapid determination of HBV serologies can quickly relieve anxiety in the majority of contacts. Identified serosusceptible contacts to HBV are then counseled on the risk of acquiring infection, which is based both on the types of sexual practices known to be important in sexual transmission of HBV and on the number of such contacts and their timing with respect to the index case's seroconversion. If the sexual contact occurred only within the last two weeks, then that person should be given passive prophylaxis with HBIG or ISG as described earlier, with initiation of vaccination with Heptavax B. These individuals need to be counseled that they still may acquire the disease and that they should refrain from sexual activity until they have been shown to be HB_cAg-

negative and HB_sAb-positive by serial testing. For sexual contacts of greater than two weeks past, little can be offered except for counseling concerning their risk of becoming ill or infectious themselves and the role of careful follow-up and serologic testing during the ensuing three to four months. This may change now that the HBV vaccine is available, as the Szmuness and Francis data suggest the possibility of significant postexposure protection in persons given the first vaccination during the incubation period.[73,74]

But what about chronic HB_sAg carriers, many of whom will be identified in the course of routine or epidemiologic screening of homosexually active males? Shikata[36] has shown that blood from persons whose blood is positive for both HB_s and HB_c antigens is highly infectious, in contrast to that of anti-HB_e-positive individuals, and the majority of homosexual males with HB_s antigenemia are positive for HB_e antigen.[35] Given these facts, we counsel all HB_sAg carriers that they are most likely infectious and ask that their sexual contacts be tested as described previously. The prohibition against further sexual activity for an indefinite period of time is, of course, difficult or impossible to enforce. It can only be hoped that lovers or other steady partners who are already immune to HBV can be identified. Those sexual contacts of the HB_sAg carrier who are serosusceptible can be given prophylaxis if indicated and monitored until they seroconvert to anti-HB_s positivity, at which time sexual activity can be resumed. With the HBV vaccine now available, such individuals should be offered the vaccine in the hope that immunity will develop with minimal or no evidence of clinical viremia or illness.

As for the carrier himself, counseling must stress the moral aspect of individual responsibility in halting the spread of HB in the homosexual population. The rapid progress being made in the application of active immunization to this problem means that carriers can look forward to a time in the not too distant future when many or all of the homosexual persons they might encounter will be immune to HBV infection. In the meantime, they are advised to limit sexual contact to persons known to be immune, which means that anonymous sexual activities as well as group sex in homosexual bathhouses should be avoided. Actively involving the individual in the identification and bringing to testing of sexual contacts and the offering of detailed education and counseling regarding sexually transmitted HBV infection may greatly increase compliance and successful limitation of disease transmission in the homosexual male population. It is our experience that this is possible only in a health care setting where homosexual males feel comfortable discussing their sexuality and sexual practices, such as community-sponsored STD clinics. However, a recent survey of chronic HB patients attending such support groups at the HBMC showed that the single most important factor in motivating persons to reduce their number of sexual contacts was the actual physical severity of the disease. No relationship was found between the patient's known e-antigen status and the perceived risk of disease transmission.[78]

The other major area of concern to HB_sAg carriers is the long-term health and occupational consequences of chronic antigenemia. Following the work-up described in the section on chronic hepatitis, many carriers will be found to have signs of no or minimal benign disease. The rate of spontaneous conversion to HB_sAg negativity with subsequent appearance of anti-HB_s is unknown in this population, but if it is similar to that in other populations, a significant proportion of such individuals may eventually become antigen-negative. Serial antigen and serum transaminase determinations at three-month intervals permit checking of this possibility as well as monitoring for chronic liver disease. If chronic liver disease is detected, the advisability of treatment with immunostimulating or antiviral agents must be determined on the basis of liver biopsy, clinical findings, and the relative risk-to-benefit ratios of the particular experimental treatment regimens. Chronic liver disease occurs in only a small proportion of chronic carriers, but it needs to be explained at the outset to all carriers. Finally, experimental protocols involving the use of BCG, adenine arabinoside, and interferon are under investigation for the therapeutically induced conversion of carriers to the immune state, but none of these studies has yet demonstrated a practical and efficacious treatment. While the widespread application of the HBV vaccine to the homosexual male population will resolve many of the problems discussed in this chapter, it will not eliminate the already existing large pool of chronic HBV carriers. Studies aimed at treating these persons, both to terminate antigenemia and to reduce the likelihood of long-term health consequences of chronic liver disease, must be made a major priority of hepatitis research in the "postvaccine" era.

There are no definite reasons for excluding HB_sAg carriers from any occupation, as the risk of carrier-to-contact transmission is minimal, provided that adequate hygienic precautions are taken. In a CDC study of hospital dialysis centers and operating rooms,[79] the overwhelming majority of cases of hospital exposure were patient-to-patient, with employees, regardless of HB_sAg status, participating only as passive vectors of contaminated patient blood. Therefore, patients need to be counseled that chronic HBV need not interfere with work— and health care personnel need to educate their colleagues on the irrationality of guidelines that exclude HB_sAg-positive individuals from certain occupations and work settings.

REFERENCES

1. Centers for Disease Control: Hepatitis. *MMWR* 27:29–35, 1979.
2. Bryan JA, Pattison CP: Viral hepatitis: A primer. *Postgrad Med* 59:66–84, 1976.

3. Tolsma DD, Bryan JA: The economic impact of viral hepatitis in the U.S. *Public Health Rep* 91:349–353, 1976.
4. Blumberg BS, Alter HJ, Visnich S: A "new" antigen in leukemia sera. *JAMA* 191:541–546, 1965.
5. Koff RS: *Viral Hepatitis*. Clinical Gastroenteroloy Monograph Series. New York, John Wiley & Sons, 1978.
6. Krugman S, Goecke DJ: *Viral Hepatitis*. Major Problems in Internal Medicine, vol 15. Philadelphia, WB Saunders, 1978.
7. Reed JS, Boyer JL: *Viral Hepatitis: Epidemiologic, Serologic, and Clinical Manifestations*, vol 25. Chicago, Yearbook Medical Publishers, 1979.
8. Vyas GN, Cohen SN, Schmid RR (eds): *Viral Hepatitis*. Philadelphia, Franklin Institute Press, 1978.
9. Szmuness W, Alter HJ, Maynard JE (eds): *Viral Hepatitis: 1981 International Symposium*. Philadelphia, Franklin Institute Press, 1982.
10. Melnick JS: Classification of hepatitis A virus as Enterovirus Type 72 and hepatitis B virus as Hepadnavirus Type 1. *Intervirology* 18:105–106, 1982.
11. Purcell RH: The hepatitis viruses: An overview, in Szmuness W, Alter HJ, Maynard JE (eds): *Viral Hepatitis: 1981 International Symposium*. Philadelphia, Franklin Institute Press, 1982, pp 3–12.
12. Centers for Disease Control: Hepatitis—United States, *MMWR* 26:177, 1977.
13. Dienstag JL, Feinstone SM, Karikian AZ, et al: Fecal shedding of hepatitis A antigen. *Lancet* 1:765–767, 1975.
14. Szmuness W, Dienstag JL, Purcell RH, et al: Distribution of antibody to hepatitis A antigen in urban adult populations. *N Engl J Med* 295:755–759, 1976.
15. William DC, Felman YM, Marr JS, et al: Sexually transmitted enteric pathogens in male homosexual population. *NY State J Med* 77:2050–2052, 1977.
16. Corey LC, Holmes KK: Sexual transmission of hepatitis A in homosexual men. Incidence and mechanism. *N Engl J Med* 304:435–438, 1980.
17. Judson F: Personal communication, 1981.
18. Krugman S, Hoofnagle JH, Gerety RJ, et al: Viral hepatitis, type B: DNA polymerase activity and antibody to hepatitis B core antigen. *N Engl J Med* 29:1331–1335, 1974.
19. Fulford KWM, Dane DS, Catterall RD, et al: Australia antigen and antibody among patients attending a clinic for sexually transmitted diseases. *Lancet* 1:1470–1473, 1973.
20. Heathcote J, Sherlock S: Spread of acute type B hepatitis in London. *Lancet* 1:1468–1470, 1973.
21. Jeffries DJ, James WH, Jefferiss FJG, Willcox RR: Australia (hepatitis-associated) antigen in patients attending a venereal disease clinic. *Br Med J* 2:455–456, 1973.
22. Szmuness W, Much MI, Prince AM, et al: On the role of sexual behavior in the spread of hepatitis B infection. *Ann Intern Med* 83:489–495, 1975.
23. Coleman JC, Waugh M, Dayton R: Hepatitis B antigen and antibody in a male homosexual population. *Br J Vener Dis* 53:132–134, 1977.
24. Dietzman DE, Harnisch JP, Ray G, et al: Hepatitis B surface antigen (HB$_s$Ag) and antibody to HB$_s$Ag prevalence in homosexual and heterosexual men. *JAMA* 238:2625–2626, 1977.
25. Lim KS, Wong VT, Fulford KWM, et al: Role of sexual and non-sexual practices in the transmission of hepatitis B. *Br J Vener Dis* 53:190–192, 1977.
26. Ostrow DG, Shaskey DM: The experience of the Howard Brown Memorial Clinic of Chicago with sexually transmitted diseases. *Sex Transm Dis* 4:53–55, 1977.
27. Ellis WR, Coleman JC, Fluker JL, et al: Liver disease among homosexual males. *Lancet* 1:903–904, 1979.

28. Sagnelli E, Vernace SJ, Paronetto F: Dane particle associated hepatitis B core antigen in patients with HB₈Ag positive chronic hepatitis. *Gastroenterology* 75:864–868, 1978.

29. Denes AE, Smith JL, Maynard JE, et al: Hepatitis B infections in physicians—Results of a national survey. *JAMA* 239:210–212, 1978.

30. Szmuness W, Prince AM, Grady GF, et al: Hepatitis B infection—A point prevalence study in 15 U.S. hemodialysis centers. *JAMA* 227:901–906, 1974.

31. Szmuness W, Prince AM, Hirsch RL, et al: Familial clustering of hepatitis B infection. *N Engl J Med* 289:1162–1166, 1973.

32. Seff LB, Kiernan T, Zimmerman HJ, et al: Hepatic diseases in asymptomatic parenteral narcotic drug abusers: A Veterans Administration collaborative study. *Am J Med Sci* 270:41–47, 1975.

33. Schreeder MT, Thompson SE, Hadler SC, et al: Epidemiology of hepatitis B infection in gay men. *J Homosexuality* 5:307–310, 1980.

34. Schreeder MT, Thompson SE, Hadler SC, et al: Hepatitis B in homosexual men: Prevalence of infection and factors related to transmission. *J Infect Dis* 146:7–14, 1982.

35. Murphy BL, Schreeder MT, Maynard JE, et al: Serological testing for hepatitis B infection in male homosexuals: Special emphasis on Hepatitis B e antigen and antibody by radioimmunoassay. *J Clin Microbiol* 11:301–303, 1980.

36. Shikata T, Karasawa T, Abe K, et al: Hepatitis B e antigen and infectivity of hepatitis B virus. *J Infect Dis* 136:571–576, 1977.

37. Altman N, Ostrow, DG: Risk factor identification for STDs in gay men. *Sex Transm Dis* (submitted).

38. Reiner NE, Judson FN, Bond, WW, et al: Asymptomatic rectal mucosal lesions and hepatitis B surface antigen at sites of sexual contact in homosexual men with persistent hepatitis B virus infection: Evidence for de facto parenteral transmission. *Ann Int Med* 96:170–173, 1982.

39. *World Health Organization Technical Report* series 602, 1977.

40. Gerlich WH, Luer W, Thomssen R, et al: Diagnosis of acute and inapparent hepatitis B virus infections by measurement of IgM antibody to HBᶜAg. *J Infect Dis* 142:95–101, 1980.

41. Szmuness W: Recent advances in the study of the epidemiology of hepatitis B. *Am J Pathol* 81:629–649, 1975.

42. Mosley JW: Hepatitis types B and non-B. Epidemiologic background. *JAMA* 235:967–969, 1975.

43. Shimizu YK, Feinstone SM, Purcell RH, et al: Non-A, non-B hepatitis: Ultrastructural evidence for two agents in experimentally infected chimpanzees. *Science* 205:197–200, 1979.

44. Prince AM, Brotman B, Grady GF, et al: Long-incubation post-transfusion hepatitis without serological evidence of exposure to hepatitis-B virus. *Lancet* 2:241–246, 1974.

25. Feinstone SM, Kapikian AZ, Purcell RH, et al: Transfusion-associated hepatitis not due to viral hepatitis type A or B. *N Engl J Med* 292:767–770, 1975.

46. Mosley JW, Redeker AG, Feinstone SM, et al: Multiple hepatitis viruses in multiple attacks of acute viral hepatitis. *N Engl J Med* 296:75–78, 1977.

47. Rakela J, Redeker AG: Chronic liver disease after acute non-A, non-B viral hepatitis. *Gastroenterology* 77:1200–1202, 1979.

48. Iwarson S, Lindberg J, Lundin P: Progression of hepatitis non-A, non-B to chronic active hepatitis: A histological follow-up of two cases. *J Clin Pathol* 32:351–355, 1979.

49. Knodell RG, Conrad ME, Ishak KG: Development of chronic liver disease after acute non A, non B post-transfusion hepatitis: Role of gamma globulin prophylaxis in its prevention. *Gastroenterology* 72:902–909, 1977.

50. Rakela J, Redeker AG, Edwards VM, et al: Hepatitis A virus infection in fulminant hepatitis and chronic active hepatitis. *Gastroenterology* 74:879–882, 1978.

51. Redeker AG: Viral hepatitis: Clinical aspects. *Am J Med Sci* 270:9–16, 1975.

52. Nielson JO, Dietrichson O, Elling P, et al: Incidence and meaning of persistence of Australia antigen in patients with acute viral hepatitis. *N Engl J Med* 285:1157–1160, 1971.
53. Ostrow DG, Altman N, Shah N, et al: Chronic hepatitis B in homosexually active men: Prospective risk and preventive factors. Proceedings of the Fifth International STD Congress, 1983 (in press).
54. Skinhøj P, Høybye G, Hentzer B, et al: Chronic hepatitis B infection in male homosexuals. *J Clin Pathol* 32:783–785, 1979.
55. Hopf U, Meyer Zum Buschenfeld KH, Arnold W: Detection of a liver membrane auto-antibody in HB$_s$Ag-negative chronic active hepatitis. *N Engl J Med* 294:578–582, 1976.
56. Galbraith RM: Chronic liver disease developing after outbreak of HB$_s$Ag-negative hepatitis in haemodialysis unit. *Lancet* 2:886–889, 1975.
57. Gregory PB, Knauer CM, Kempson RL, et al: Steroid therapy in severe viral hepatitis. A double-blind, randomized trial of methyl-prednisolone versus placebo. *N Engl J Med* 294:681–687, 1976.
58. Lam KC, Lai CL, Trepo C, et al: Deleterious effect of prednisolone in HB$_s$Ag-positive chronic active hepatitis. *N Engl J Med* 304:380–386, 1981.
59. Damjanovic V, Brumfitt W: Prophylaxis and treatment of viral hepatitis. *J Antimicrob Chemother* 6:11–32, 1980.
60. Simmons MJ, Yap EH, Yu M, et al: Australia antigen in Singapore Chinese patients with hepatocellular carcinoma and comparison groups: Influence of technique sensitivity on different frequencies. *Int J Cancer* 10:320–325, 1972.
61. Furuta S, Nagata A, Kiyosawa K, et al: Anti-HB$_c$ titer in relation to the etiological role of hepatitis B virus in primary hepatocellular carcinoma. *Acta Hepato-Gastroenterol* 24:3–6, 1977.
62. Kubo Y, Okuda K, Shimokawa Y, et al: Hepatitis B surface antigenemia in patients with hepatocellular carcinoma in relation to clinical course and alpha-fetoprotein. *Gastroenterology* 72:1212–1216, 1977.
63. Kubo Y, Okuda K, Hashimota M, et al: Antibody to hepatitis B core antigen in patients with hepatocellular carcinoma. *Gastroenterology* 72:1217–1221, 1977.
64. Van den Heever A, Pretorius FJ, Falkson G, et al: Hepatitis B surface antigen and primary liver cancer. *S Afr Med J* 54:359–361, 1978.
65. Trichopoulos D, Gerety RJ, Sparros L, et al: Hepatitis B and primary hepatocellular carcinoma in a European population. *Lancet* 1:1217–1219, 1978.
66. Szmuness W: Hepatocellular carcinoma and the hepatitis B virus: Evidence for a causal association. *Prog Med Virol* 24:40–69, 1978.
67. Francis D: Personal communication.
68. Landrigan PJ, Huber DHM, Murphy GD, et al: The protective efficacy of immune serum globulin in hepatitis A. A statistical approach. *JAMA* 223:74–75, 1973.
68. Kabiri M, Tabor E, Gerety RJ: Antigen–antibody system associated with non-A, non-B hepatitis detected by indirect immunofluorescence. *Lancet* 1:221–224, 1979.
70. Grady GF, Rodman M, Larsen LH: Hepatitis B antibody in conventional γ-globulin. *J Infect Dis* 132:474–477, 1975.
71. Hoofnagle JH, Seef LB, Bales ZB, et al: Passive active immunity from hepatitis B immune globulin. Reanalysis of a Veterans Administration cooperative study of needle-stick hepatitis. *Ann Int Med* 91:813–818, 1979.
72. Seef LB, Wright EC, Zimmerman HJ, et al: Type B hepatitis after needle-stick exposure: Prevention with hepatitis B immune globulin. Final report of the Veterans Administration Cooperative Study. *Ann Int Med* 88:285–293, 1978.
73. Szmuness W, Stevens CE, Harley EJ, et al: Hepatitis B vaccine. Demonstration of efficacy in a controlled clinical trial in a high risk population in the United States. *N Engl J Med* 303:833–841, 1980.

74. Francis DP, Hadler SC, Thompson SE, et al: The prevention of hepatitis B with vaccine. Report of the CDC Multi-center efficacy trial among homosexual men. *Ann Int Med* 97:362–366, 1982.

75. Centers for Disease Control, Immunization Practices Advisory Committee: Inactivated hepatitis B virus vaccine. Recommendations of the Immunization Practices Advisory Committee. *Ann Int Med* 97:379–383, 1982.

76. Ostrow DG, Behar M, Baker AE, et al: Preliminary report of the Task Force on Vaccination Strategies for Sexually Transmitted Hepatitis B Infection. *Sex Transm Dis* 9:151–153, 1982.

77. Favero MS, Maynard JE, Leger RT, et al: Guidelines for the care of patients hospitalized with viral hepatitis. *Ann Int Med* 91:872–876, 1979.

78. Ostrow DG, Chene D, McMillen H: Attitudes of chronic hepatitis B patients towards risk of disease transmission. Presented at the 1982 American Public Health Association Meeting, Montreal, Nov 15, 1982.

79. Maynard JR: Health care risk factors of hepatitis B. Presented at "Prevention and Control of Viral Hepatitis Type B," CME Program of the 1979 APHA Convention, New York, Nov 5, 1979.

80. Niermeijer P, Gies CH: Natural history of acute hepatitis B in previously healthy patients: A prospective study. *Acta Hepato-Gastroenterol* 24:317–325, 1977.

IV

Anal Disorders

Hemorrhoids, Anal Fissure, and Condylomata Acuminata

HERAND ABCARIAN

Although the occurrence of anorectal disorders in the young is not uncommon, the incidence of these diseases is more common among homosexual men, and because of sexual practices in this population these problems assume additional importance. Of all benign anorectal disorders, hemorrhoids, anal fissure, and condylomata acuminata are most frequently encountered.

HEMORRHOIDS

Etiology

Hemorrhoids are esentially dilations or varicosities of the hemorrhoidal venous plexus of the anal canal. Their etiology is unknown but occasional familial predisposition has been observed. Diarrhea, constipation, and straining during defecation are considered contributing factors. Repeated trauma to the anal canal in homosexual males may not especially increase the likelihood of the disease but could lead to increasing symptoms.

Epidemiology

Hemorrhoids are quite rare during childhood and adolescence; the incidence increases with age. After age 55, approximately 50% of the population have

HERAND ABCARIAN • Section of Colon and Rectal Surgery, Cook County Hospital, and Department of Surgery, University of Illinois College of Medicine at Chicago, Chicago, Illinois 60612.

signs and symptoms of hemorrhoids. Contrary to former beliefs, there is no evidence for increased incidence of hemorrhoids in homosexual men.

Clinical Aspects

Classification

Hemorrhoids are classified into two major categories: internal (those covered with columnar mucosa) and external (those covered with skin). Based on clinical presentation, internal hemorrhoids can be grouped into four grades:

Grade 1: Hemorrhoid enlargement without protrusion.
Grade 2: Hemorrhoid enlargement with occasional protrusion during defecation.
Grade 3: Continuous protrusion of internal hemorrhoids, recurrent after manual reduction.
Grade 4: Prolapsed, strangulated irreducible hemorrhoids, which may be associated with ulceration, gangrene, or tissue slough.

Symptoms of Internal Hemorrhoids

Classical symptoms of internal hemorrhoids are bleeding and protrusion. Bleeding is infrequent and related to trauma to the anal canal (e.g., passage of hard stool, anal coitus, use of enemas). As the disease progresses, however, even passage of soft normal stool causes bleeding. Similarly, protrusion in early stages is associated with defecation only, but could occur with lifting, coughing, prolonged standing, or even passage of flatus in more advanced stages. Chronic intermittent protrusion of hemorrhoids causes anal discharge, perianal wetness, and pruritus ani.

Development of pain in internal hemorrhoids usually heralds a complication, commonly thrombosis, during which the hemorrhoid becomes acutely swollen and indurated, causing perivascular neural pressure. Should thrombosis resolve spontaneously, the pain also subsides in a few days. However, if edema persists and increases in intensity, arterial obstruction ensues with resultant ulceration, gangrene, tissue slough, and abscess formation.

Symptoms of External Hemorrhoids

External hemorrhoids are usually asymptomatic unless they become acutely thrombosed. During such an attack, the patient complains of constant burning and pain associated with sudden appearance of a small nodule near the anal opening. If small, the thrombosis may recede spontaneously, but larger lesions produce severe pain. Spontaneous rupture with excessive bleeding may occur. After the acute phase subsides, external hemorrhoids usually persist as small perianal skin tags. Recurrent attacks are not infrequent.

Diagnosis

Uncomplicated internal hemorrhoids are difficult to diagnose with digital examination. The small venous varicosity usually collapses under digital pressure and diagnosis may be missed. Anoscopic examination aids in making the correct diagnosis and rules out other causes of anal disease such as fissure, pruritus, and anal warts. Proctosigmoidoscopy is essential to exclude inflammatory bowel disease, polyps, or cancers within the reach of the instrument. If there is any suspicion, a barium enema should be performed to exclude neoplastic or inflammatory diseases above the reach of the sigmoidoscope. However, if the patient is also being evaluated for infectious diarrhea or dysentery, any procedures that require barium laxatives or antibiotics should be postponed until all tests for bacteria as well as ova and parasites have been completed.

Internal hemorrhoids complicated by thrombosis, prolapse, and their sequelae are usually easily diagnosed. Chronically prolapsed hemorrhoids may undergo epithelialization and ulceration; the epithelium and ulcers at times need to be biopsied to exclude epidermoid carcinomas. Anoscopic and protosigmoidoscopic examinations must be performed whenever possible to exclude other disorders.

The diagnosis of thrombosed external hemorrhoids usually is made by identification of a 7-mm to 10-mm purplish tender nodule at or near the anal opening. The nodule is immediately subcutaneous, easily movable, and quite firm. Occasionally, thrombosed external hemorrhoids are multiple. In the quiescent phase, tags should not be painful, and any degree of pain may indicate the presence of anal fissure immediately cephalad to the tag.

Treatment

Treatment of uncomplicated internal hemorrhoids includes correction of bowel habits, high-roughage diet, avoidance of hot spices, avoidance of anal trauma (including anal intercourse), and the taking of warm sitz baths. Bulk-producing stool softeners such as psyllium preparations are helpful in relieving constipation, provided they are taken with large quantities of water. Various suppositories, preparations, and ointments are usually not helpful. The majority of patients respond to this conservative management.

Alternatives in the treatment of hemorrhoids have been recently reviewed.[1] Injection of sclerosing agents into hemorrhoids can be accomplished as an office procedure with good results when hemorrhoids are small, internal, and uncomplicated. When prolapse and bleeding occur concomitantly, the best method of treatment is ligation with a rubber band, utilizing the Barron or McGivney ligators.[2] Hemorrhoidectomy should be reserved only for extensive, complicated hemorrhoids that do not respond to conservative medical management.

ANAL FISSURE

Anal fissure is the most common painful anal lesion. The majority of anal fissures occur as a result of trauma to the anal canal, e.g., passage of hard stool or anal coitus.

Clinical Aspects

Symptoms of anal fissure include pain initiated by defecation and associated with bright red bleeding of varying quantities. The characteristic symptom is severe anal pain lasting minutes to hours following defecation. Consequently, patients often become fearful of defecation and resort to laxatives and enemas to soften the stool, a practice that serves to aggravate their symptoms by causing explosive or frequent loose bowel movements.

Diagnosis

Diagnosis can be made by digital inspection of the anus during gentle separation of the buttocks. The fissure always can be seen in the midline, with over 90% of the fissures located posteriorly. Digital examination may be too painful to perform but sometimes can be accomplished with the use of local anesthetic ointments.

Differential diagnosis of anal fissure from other anal lesions is quite important, especially among homosexual men. The most common lesion, other than anal fissure in homosexual males, is a syphilitic chancre. This lesion is most often located in the lateral anal walls and has rolled edges with a dirty base. Anal syphilitic chancres are painful due to the spasm of the internal sphincter. Darkfield examination usually reveals the spirochetes.

The second most common nonmidline lesion in homosexual males is that caused by Crohn's disease. This disease usually manifests as a purplish ulcer hidden by thick, rolled edges (hooded ulcer). Should an anal ulcer be associated with a history of diarrhea, Crohn's disease must be suspected. Proctosigmoidoscopy, biopsy of the lesion, and contrast gastrointestinal X rays are usually diagnostic. Stool cultures and examinations for ova and parasites should precede any contrast studies in patients who practice receptive anal coitus or anilinction. Finally, acute proctitis in men should be differentiated from anal fissure. With acute proctitis, anal pain associated with tenesmus and passage of blood, mucus, and pus during defecation is a telltale sign of rectal, rather than anal, involvement. Diagnosis is often established by careful inspection of the anal canal, which rules out the presence of midline fissures. Gentle proctosigmoidoscopy reveals the typical acute inflammation with purulent or bloody mucoid discharge in the lumen. The disease is usually limited to the distal 10 cm to 15 cm of the rectum and is characterized by edema, erythema, friability, and frank ulceration of the rectal mucosa. Biopsy reveals nonspecific ulceration and cultures may show nonspecific or gonococcal infection.

Treatment

Almost 50% of adults presenting with anal fissure respond to conservative therapy. The fissure may be cauterized with a 10% solution of silver nitrate on a cotton-tipped applicator. Sitz baths and psyllium preparations to promote soft stools are often quite helpful. Anal coitus, use of enemas, and insertion of medication with gloved fingers should be avoided. Local anesthetic or steroid ointments are often not helpful and may sensitize the patient.

If the patient responds to medical management and the fissure heals in three to four weeks, conservative therapy is gradually withdrawn. If the fissure becomes intractable or recurs after an apparently successful medical management, the patient should be referred for surgery. The appropriate operation and surgical alternatives have been discussed in the literature.[3]

All nonmidline fissures should be considered suspect for a systemic disease (e.g., Crohn's disease, syphilis, tuberculosis, lymphoma, leukemia) and patients should undergo appropriate work-up before any surgical treatment is contemplated. Even when patients go to surgery undiagnosed, a nonmidline fissure should only be biopsied to establish the diagnosis. More extensive operations (e.g., sphincterotomy) should be avoided.

CONDYLOMATA ACUMINATA (VENEREAL WARTS)

Venereal warts are viral in origin and are commonly seen in the anorectal and urogenital regions. Like many other venereal diseases, the incidence of venereal warts is on the rise, and because of extreme difficulty in eradicating this disease increasing numbers of chronic, recurrent, or persistent cases are being seen at the present time.

Etiology

The causative agent in venereal warts is human papilloma virus (HPV) a 52-nm to 55-nm DNA virus. There are seven types of HPV, and Types 2 and 6 are usually associated with condylomata acuminata. Transmission of warts by cell-free filtrate was first reported by Ciuffo in 1907.[4] Lewis and Wheeler[5] cited the autoinoculability of warts and noted that the inoculation of ground suspension of warts into volunteers results in the transmission of the disease. The intranuclear inclusion bodies suggestive of virus particles were discovered in 1949.[6] Electron microscopic studies of condyloma cells have shown evidence of viral agents,[7,8] and the use of fluorescein-tagged anti-human-wart antiserum has demonstrated the presence of viral antigen in the nuclear areas of skin papillomas in man.[9] Finally, Oriel and Almeida,[10] using the electron microscope technique of negative staining, discovered that intranuclear virus particles resembled those found in human cutaneous warts caused by papovavirus.

Epidemiology

The virus is transmitted by sexual contact. Thus, condylomata acuminata are commonly referred to as "venereal warts." The anorectal and urogenital areas offer a warm and continuously moist environment, which is necessary for growth of the virus.

Although the true incidence of this disease remains unknown, the highest incidence of condylomata is in the anorectal region of homosexual men. In Marino's report[11] on anorectal lesions found in homosexual men, 25% presented with condylomata acuminata, and, in a previous publication by Abcarian et al.[12] 91% of the men either were homosexually oriented or had a history of anal intercourse previous to the diagnosis. In Oriel's series,[13] 83% of the men and 62% of the women with anal condylomata acuminata had a history of anal intercourse. In an attempt to prove the venereal transmission of anal warts, Oriel examined all sexual contacts of patients before and after the appearance of warts. None of the examined contacts, however, had penile warts.

Anal warts are not exclusively seen in homosexual males, but are found in heterosexual males and females as well. The presence of warts elsewhere on the body, especially the fingers, may cause genital and anal warts by autoinoculation. The incidence of common cutaneous warts in patients with anal warts is between 15% and 25%.[12,14] Appearance of perianal warts in children with cutaneous warts may be interrelated. Young[15] has suggested that the wart virus may be a normal inhabitant of the anorectum in some people and that anal intercourse may allow its entry into the anoderm because of repeated trauma. However, the absence of warts in patients with anal abrasions or fissures refutes this theory.

Clinical Aspects

A common early symptom of anal warts is itching, which at times is quite intense and disproportionate to the actual number of warts present. As anal warts grow and multiply, rectal bleeding on defecation or intercourse may occur. Because of its insidious onset and the presence of symptoms frequently seen with other anal disorders, especially hemorrhoids, patients either ignore the symptoms or use over-the-counter hemorrhoidal remedies. Physicians may also miss the diagnosis if only rectal examination is performed. When warts grow larger and protrude through the anal canal, the patient usually seeks medical attention and the diagnosis is made easily.

The incubation period of wart virus is not known but can be as long as many weeks or months. Condylomata may begin as perianal disease and remain localized in this area without anal involvement. Unfortunately, as a rule, anal involvement precedes perianal lesions by a few weeks or months, and, when the disease is diagnosed on the basis of perianal lesions, extensive condylomata acuminata are often already present in the anal canal. Extensive perianal warts can produce a malodorous discharge that is quite offensive and disturbing to the patient. At this stage, the diagnosis is easily made by identification of few scattered or extensive grapelike clusters of condylomata varying in size from a few millimeters to a few centimeters. There may be extensions to the perineum and scrotum or concomitant presence of pubic, penile, scrotal, labial, or vaginal warts. Proctosigmoidoscopy should be performed if there is any doubt as to other causes of rectal bleeding.

Diagnosis

Diagnosis of anal warts in homosexual males calls for anoscopic examination. The lesions may cover the anoderm and extend up to or a few millimeters above the dentate line, but frank involvement of rectal mucosa is uncommon.

The characteristic appearance of anoperianal warts is so typical that biopsy of the lesion for confirmation of diagnosis is rarely necessary. The only differential diagnosis to be considered is condylomata lata, which can be diagnosed by the typical pearly white appearance of the lesion and the strongly positive serologic test for syphilis present in all cases. Careful examination of the external genitalia is important to rule out the presence of warts in these areas. Inguinal lymph nodes are not enlarged in patients with anal warts.

Treatment

Numerous methods have been used for the treatment of anal warts but none has been universally successful. In a study by Abcarian et al.,[12] 40 patients treated with surgical excision, fulguration, podophyllum, and bichloracetic acid were studied. Eighteen of the 40 patients had only one of these forms of therapy while 22 had a combination of all three. In only one-fourth of the patients were these treatments quickly effective in eradication of the disease, while 75% of the patients needed repeated treatments in one form or another for prolonged periods ranging from four months to two years. Consequently, it is difficult to predict the number of treatment sessions or the length of time treatment will require. Of all the therapeutic methods, podophyllum, a resin from May apple used in liquid or ointment form, is still the most popular. It can be utilized as a 10% to 25% solution in tincture of benzoin or in petrolatum jelly in the same concentration. Podophyllum is most successful in the treatment of perianal warts. The application is associated with a sensation of burning or stinging (worse when applied in the anal canal) which subsides within a few minutes. After a quiescent period of twelve to twenty-four hours, the chemical caustic reaction of podophyllum produces intense tissue swelling with reappearance of throbbing pain and tenesmus. This phase is associated with softening and enlargement of warts, followed by tissue slough, purulent-appearing discharge, and removal of warts. Smaller warts may disappear totally and larger warts may shrink to a great extent. Depending on the initial response of the patient and the severity of tissue reaction, the treatment should be repeated in one to two weeks. Podophyllum is extremely caustic and should be applied only by the physician. It should be removed from the skin by means of a thorough sitz bath six to eight hours after application. The first application should be followed by a bath two hours later, as some patients have idosyncratic reactions. Longer contact or injudicious use of podophyllum may result in second-degree burn with blistering.

Bichloracetic acid is a caustic acid used for removal of cutaneous warts. Its use in anal warts was suggested in 1971 by Swerdlow and Salvati.[16] Application of this chemical to warts produces coagulation necrosis with instant blanching of tissues associated with an extensive burning sensation that usually lasts from thirty to forty-five minutes. The necrotic tissue is sloughed in three to five days with clinical evidence of anal discomfort and bleeding. Bichloracetic acid is extremely caustic and should be used with great care. Occasionally, even with careful application, it produces severe chemical burns and is unsuitable for further application in some patients. Consequently, this treatment should be avoided unless tolerance is established. This treatment can be repeated within one to two weeks based on the patient's tolerance and tissue healing.

Cryotherapy with carbon dioxide and especially with liquid nitrogen is effective and often succeeds where podophyllum fails.[17] Liquid nitrogen cryotherapy produces intensely cold temperatures that cause tissue freezing and destruction as the nitrogen evaporates. The frozen tissue subsequently sloughs and the skin wound heals with good cosmetic results. Repeated application is usually necessary for persistent warts.

Antitumor preparations—especially parenteral injections of Thiotepa®, 5-

fluorouracil, and bleomycin—have been tried for extensive condylomata acuminata. Slight reduction in size of these lesions is the rule, but no cure can be expected from the use of these agents. 5-Fluorouracil cream has been reported to be effective in meatal warts, but no more so than liquid nitrogen.

Surgical excision and fulguration of warts either as an outpatient or inpatient procedure under local, regional, or general anesthesia still remains the mainstay of wart therapy for patients unresponsive to topical application of caustic agents. It is unfortunate to note, however, that the incidence of recurrence after surgical excision is also high.[18]

Possible causes of the high recurrence rate in venereal warts are that patients may resume sexual activity before completion of therapy, that treated patients may change sexual partners and become reinfected with either the same or a different strain of virus, and that incubating warts may appear after completion of apparently successful treatment.

Immunotherapy has also been tried in the treatment of venereal warts. This process was originally suggested in 1944 by Biberstein,[19] who reported beneficial results in 90% of patients with condylomata acuminata treated by wart vaccine. Immunotherapy, however, remained dormant for over a quarter of a century until Powell and his associates[20] reported the use of autogenous vaccine in 24 patients with anorectal and urogenital condylomata. In this study, excellent treatment results were seen in 20 patients, good results in three patients, and poor results in one patient. Nel and Fourie[21] reported 70% complete and 10% partial regression in a small series of patients. In all these reports, immunotherapy was associated with no adverse systemic effects.

The largest series of anal condylomata acuminata in homosexual men was reported in 1977 by Abcarian and Sharon.[22] In this study, 58 of 70 vaccinated patients had excellent response with total disappearance of warts and remained free of disease, while in eight patients the bulk of condylomata disappeared, leaving a small asymptomatic residual. Only four patients did not benefit from immunotherapy. The result of immunotherapy was not different in patients with primary disease with no previous treatment and in patients with recurrent disease in whom immunotherapy was utilized after failure of other treatment modalities. However, a more recent double-blind controlled study by Malison et al.[23] claimed that autogenous vaccine was no more effective than placebo when duration of disease was taken into account. They therefore concluded that autogenous vaccine should still be considered experimental treatment and used as such in patients refractory to other treatments.

REFERENCES

1. Abcarian H: Anorectal disorders: When is conservate care enough? *Mod Med (Minneapolis)*, January 1980, pp 15–30.

2. Shub H, Salvati F, Rubin R: Conservative treatment of fissure. *Dis Colon Rectum* 21:582–583, 1978.

3. Abcarian H: Surgical correction of chronic anal fissure. *Dis Colon Rectum* 23:31–36, 1980.

4. Ciuffo G: Inesto positive confitrato di vercuca vulgane. *Bior Ita Mal Ven Pelle* 48:12, 1907.

5. Lewis GM, Wheeler CE Jr: *Practical Dermatology*, ed 2. Philadelphia, WB Saunders, 1967, p 679.

6. Strauss MJ, Shaw EW, Bunting H, et al: "Crystallite" virus-like particles from skin papillomas characterized by intranuclear inclusion bodies. *Proc Soc Exp Biol Med* 72:46–54, 1949.

7. Morgan HR, Balduzzi PG: Propagation of an intranuclear inclusion-forming agent from human condyloma acuminatum. *Proc Natl Acad Sci USA* 52:1561–1569, 1964.

8. Smith KO, Dougherty E, Melnick JL, et al: Fine structure of unassembled viral subunites from human warts. *J Bacteriol* 90:278–289, 1965.

9. Walter EL Jr, Walker DL, Cooper GA: Localization of specific antigen in human warts. *Arch Pathol* 79:419–428, 1965.

10. Oriel JD, Almeida JD: Demonstration of virus particles in human genital warts. *Br J Vener Dis* 46:37–46, 1970.

11. Marino AW Jr: Proctologic lesions observed in male homosexuals. *Dis Colon Rectum* 7:121–127, 1964.

12. Abcarian H, Smith D, Sharon N: The immunotherapy of anal condyloma acuminatum. *Dis Colon Rectum* 19:237–244, 1966.

13. Oriel JD: Anal warts and anal coitus. *Br J Vener Dis* 47:373–378, 1971.

14. Oriel JD: Natural history of genital warts. *Br J Vener Dis* 47:1–9, 1971.

15. Young HM: Viral warts in the anorectum possible precluding rectal cancer. *Surgery* 55:367–374, 1964.

16. Swerdlow DB, Salvati EP: Condyloma acuminatum. *Dis Colon Rectum* 14:226–232, 1971.

17. Gold JD: Liquid air and carbonic acid snow: Therapeutic results obtained by the dermatologist. *NY J Med* 92:1276–1280, 1960.

18. Lyell A: Management of warts. *Br Med J* 2:1576–1579, 1966.

19. Biberstein H: Immunization therapy of warts. *Arch Dermatol* 50:12–21, 1944.

20. Powell LC Jr, Pollard M, Jenkins JL Sr: Treatment of condyloma acuminatum by autogenous vaccine. *South Med J* 63:202–208, 1970.

21. Nel WS, Fourie ED: Immunotherapy and 5 percent topical 5-fluorouracil ointment in the treatment of condylomata acuminata. *S Afr Med J* 47:45–50, 1973.

22. Abcarian H, Sharon N: The effectiveness of immunotherapy in the treatment of anal condyloma acuminataum. *J Surg Res* 22:231–236, 1977.

23. Malison MD, Morris R, Jones LW: Autogenous vaccine therapy for condyloma acuminatum— A double-blood controlled study. *Br J Vener Dis* 58:62–65, 1982.

Trauma to the Rectum
Colorectal Foreign Bodies and Manual–Anal Intercourse

HERAND ABCARIAN

Foreign bodies of the colon and rectum are being seen with increasing frequency within the bisexual and homosexual male population. The introduction of these foreign bodies is seen as a result of criminal assault against a variety of victims, and this situation is usually associated with serious and life-threatening complications. The circumstances under which foreign bodies are introduced into the rectum and colon can be grouped under five categories:

1. Diagnostic or therapeutic introduction (e.g., thermometers, rectal tubes, disposable enema tips, irrigation catheters, barium for upper or lower gastrointestinal X-ray examinations[1]).
2. Self-administered treatment to alleviate symptoms of anorectal disease (e.g., insertion of short broomsticks to relieve itching or reduce prolapsed hemorrhoids[2,3]).
3. Criminal assault (e.g., glass bottles[4] or broomsticks).
4. Accidental introduction (e.g., ingestion of chicken or fish bones[4]).
5. Autoeroticism (e.g., vibrators—by far the most common cause of retained colorectal foreign bodies).

An additional major source of rectal trauma in a subgroup of homosexual men is the use of hands, fists, and entire forearms for anal stimulation.

HERAND ABCARIAN ● Section of Colon and Rectal Surgery, Cook County Hospital, and Department of Surgery, University of Illinois College of Medicine at Chicago, Chicago, Illinois 60612.

COLORECTAL FOREIGN BODIES

Clinical Aspects

Owing to the diverse nature and causes of the colorectal foreign bodies, symptoms and signs may be quite varied. Diagnostic or therapeutic introduction resulting in a retained foreign body is usually diagnosed quite early and attempts to retrieve the object are also begun soon afterward. The only exception in this category is the presence of inspissated, rock-hard barium in the upper rectum or rectosigmoid following gastrointestinal contrast X rays in the elderly or mentally retarded patients. Under these circumstances, the evolution of constipation and occasionally obstipation is insidious and only a careful examination of the patient, which includes digital rectal examination, proctosigmoidoscopy, and abdominal X rays, will reveal the diagnosis.

Accidental ingestion of sharp objects (e.g., chicken bones, beef bones, fish bones, toothpicks) may initially be dismissed or disregarded by the patient. Should these sharp objects lodge in the rectum, they might lacerate the rectal mucosa and lead to formation of anorectal abscesses. The patient may have forgotten the accidental ingestion or actually be totally unaware of the presence of a foreign body that may be found impacted in the rectal ampulla, in the base of an infected fistulous tract, or in an abscess cavity.[5] Clinical presentation varies from rectal pain and bleeding to perirectal infection and abscess.

By and large the majority of foreign bodies are introduced for autoerotic purposes or by the sexual partner. The patient usually seeks help after exhausting all attempts to remove the foreign body. By this time the object is usually either impacted in the rectum or has been pushed up into the rectosigmoid. Although perforation of the rectosigmoid during futile efforts at removal of a foreign body is quite possible, this complication and the ensuing peritonitis are usually seen following criminal assaults or attempted suicides.[6] Should these patients go untreated even for a few hours, purulent peritonitis and septic shock may cause multiple complications or death.

Diagnosis

Diagnosis of colorectal foreign bodies primarily relies on a careful history and physical examination. Clinical history is especially important in suicidal or assault patients in whom the foreign body has already been removed by the patient or the assailant and when the patient presents with peritonitis. In all cases, the time of introduction of the foreign body should be ascertained whenever possible. During rectal examination, care must be taken not to push the foreign body further into the colon.

Biplane abdominal and pelvic X rays should be performed in all patients to elucidate the number, type, and location of the foreign bodies as well as to rule out perforation of the colon and rectum. The location of the foreign body might well dictate the final therapeutic approach. Therefore, a simple classification was proposed in 1977 by Eftaiha et al.[7] to assist in definitive treatment. In this classification, "low-lying" foreign bodies were described as palpable in the rectal ampulla and "high-lying" foreign bodies were diagnosed at or proximal to the rectosigmoid junction. Utilizing this classification, a total of 42 foreign bodies were removed from 41 patients during a seven-year period (1970–1977) at Cook County Hospital in Chicago. Thirty-two were classified as low-lying and ten were high-lying foreign bodies.

Treatment

The use of enemas or cathartics in cases of retained colorectal foreign bodies is contraindicated as they may increase the degree of impaction and surrounding tissue edema.[7,8] Only when inspissated barium causes the impaction is a small retention enema (1% dioctyl sodium sulfosuccinate followed by gentle saline enemas) indicated to break up the concretion and relieve the impaction. The patient should be examined under anesthesia, preferably regional (spinal or caudal), for maximum muscle relaxation. Every attempt should be made to remove the foreign body transanally before subjecting the patient to laparotomy.

Almost all low-lying foreign bodies can be removed transanally following appropriate anesthesia, which insures adequate sphincter relaxation and allows gentle manipulation. Most high-lying foreign bodies can be manipulated and delivered into the upper rectum for their transanal removal. If a preexisting anorectal disease (e.g., anal fissure) inhibits the dilation of the anus, a lateral internal sphincterotomy is indicated and should be performed without hesitation. A grasping forceps or tenaculum may be used whenever there is no risk of breaking or splintering the foreign body.

Foreign bodies made of glass require special attention. Every effort should be made to remove these objects intact. Accidental breaking of a glass object could lacerate or perforate the rectum, necessitating a major surgical procedure with proximal colostomy. If the open end of the glass is directed cephalad, a negative pressure develops within the glass, drawing the mucosa into the mouth of the container. In such cases, and also whenever there is mucosal edema at the distal end of the foreign body, prohibiting easy maneuvering of objects, two to four well-lubricated Foley catheters may be introduced around the object. After inflation of the Foley catheter balloons, injection of air into the catheters will help overcome the suction effect, and gentle traction on the catheters will assist in the caudad displacement and removal of the glass object.

The majority of high-lying foreign bodies can be manipulated downward into the rectal ampulla under appropriate anesthesia. These can then be managed according to the principles outlined previously. After removal of foreign bodies, an immediate proctosigmoidoscopy should be performed to rule out mucosal lacerations, bleeding, perforation, or additional foreign bodies. Proctosigmoidoscopy can be accomplished easily and needs no preparation. If the mucosa is intact, the patient should be observed in the hospital for twenty-four to forty-eight hours for the development of bleeding or delayed symptoms and signs of perforation or perirectal infection.

If a high-lying foreign body cannot be delivered transanally, an elective laparotomy should be planned and the colon should be prepared both mechanically (i.e., laxatives, enemas, clear liquid diet) and with antibiotics so that the bowel can be closed primarily after colostomy and removal of the foreign body are accomplished.

An emergency laparotomy for the removal of a foreign body is rarely indicated. However, when a glass foreign body shatters during an attempt at transanal removal or when an impacted high-lying foreign body produces partial or complete colonic obstruction, emergency surgery may be necessary. In such cases, when adequate mechanical preparation of the colon cannot be accomplished, systemic combination antibiotics (penicillin, clindamycin, and an aminoglycoside) are administered preoperatively, a diverting colostomy is mandatory, and the antibiotics should be continued for at least seven to ten days postoperatively.

By following the aforementioned principles, a retained foreign body can be removed with maximum safety and morbidity can be reduced to a minimum.

MANUAL–ANAL INTERCOURSE

An increasing number of homosexual men are presenting to private practitioners, venereal disease clinics, and hospital emergency rooms with rectal trauma related to a history of insertion of hands (fists) or forearms into the anus for sexual stimulation. Occasionally, foreign objects such as dildos, vibrators, or round balls may also have been used, resulting in a combination of rectal trauma and a retained foreign body. In these instances, a careful history, taken in complete privacy, followed by a meticulous physical examination, including proctosigmoidoscopy without preparation, is essential for proper diagnosis and management.

Rectal trauma secondary to manual–anal insertion ranges from minor abrasions of the anus or exacerbation of fissures or hemorrhoids to potentially fatal transmural colonic perforation, peritonitis, and sepsis. Minor abrasions of the anus are treated conservatively with symptom-relieving measures such as stool softeners and sitz baths, and patients should be advised that abstinence from rectal intercourse or manual–anal practices will accelerate the healing process.

More serious problems include partial perforations, prolapsed hemorrhoid or rectum, and torn sphincters. These conditions must be evaluated as to the degree of severity and urgency.

Clinical Aspects

Patients presenting with a complaint of abdominal pain, rectal bleeding, retained foreign body, or other signs of trauma to the rectum as the result of manual–anal intercourse must be evaluated immediately. Vital signs, with close attention to orthostatic blood pressure and pulse changes, indicate the degree of blood loss through rectal bleeding. Bowel sounds, if present, are a reliable indicator that the trauma has not caused bowel wall perforation, thus lessening the chance of peritonitis or serious bleeding. Finally, anoscopic and sigmoidoscopic examinations indicate the degree of bleeding, and often the site(s) of injury can be visualized directly during these procedures.

Treatment

In the absence of active bleeding or signs of peritonitis at the time of initial evaluation, most rectal traumas can be managed conservatively on an outpatient or clinic basis. The major problems are pain owing to mucosal or perineal tears, and traumatic proctitis, which begins one to two days following the initial injury. Stool softeners, e.g., dioctyl sodium sulfosuccinate (Colace®) or psyllium hydrophilic mucilloid (Metamucil®), and a clear liquid diet are prescribed for two to five days or longer to reduce pain on defecation. The patient is also advised to take hot baths two to three times a day.

If there is any question of infection developing in patients without peritonitis or transmural perforation, but with signs of mucosal edema or exudate or both upon examination, then oral antibiotic therapy is indicated. Oral ampicillin or tetracycline, 0.5 g four times a day, should be prescribed until symptoms resolve.

Surgical Intervention

Any patient presenting with active rectal bleeding or signs of peritonitis must be hospitalized immediately for control and monitoring of these problems. Practitioners who have managed a number of patients with injuries resulting from manual–anal intercourse generally agree that the management and outcome of these injuries differ little, if at all, from those of lower gastrointestinal bleeding from other causes. In most cases, bleeding subsides without surgery if peritonitis does not develop. Hospital management of major gastrointestinal bleeding involves immediate type and cross matching of the patient's blood. Blood loss is monitored by central venous pressure (CVP), orthostatic blood pressure, and pulse. Blood is replaced to maintain a hematocrit greater than 35% with minimum CVP and orthostatic blood pressure changes. Patients who have required as many as 20 to 30 units of blood have healed spontaneously without the need for laparotomy.

Treatment must always be tailored to the injury present. If peritonitis, uncontrolled bleeding, or major sphincter lacerations occur, antibiotic coverage and immediate repair are indicated. Perforation of the rectum is a surgical emergency and is handled with laparotomy, closure of the perforation, and proximal colostomy, together with drains and administration of antibiotics. While not enough patients have been followed in this last group, it appears that most patients recover, and at least half are eventually reoperated upon for removal of colostomy.

REFERENCES

1. ReBell FG: Problems of foreign bodies of the colon and rectum. *Am J Surg* 76:678–684, 1948.
2. Gillespie WF: Vaseline bottle in the rectum. *Can Med Assoc J* 31:302–303, 1934.
3. Lucas MA, Ryan JE: An unusual case report of foreign body in the rectum and sigmoid. *Ky Med J* 45:289–290, 1947.
4. Macht SH: Foreign body (bottle) in the rectum. *Radiology* 42:500–501, 1944.
5. Moreira CA, Wogpakd S, Gennar AR: A foreign body (chicken bone) in the rectum causing extensive peri-rectal and scrotal abscess. *Dis Colon Rectum* 18:407–409, 1975.
6. Bretters AG: An unusual rectal injury. *Br Med J* 2:602–603, 1955.
7. Eftaiha M, Hambrick E, Abcarian H: Principles of management of colorectal foreign bodies. *Arch Surg* 112:691–695, 1977.
8. McCaffery TD Jr, Lilly JO: Management of foreign affairs of the GI tract. *Dig Dis* 20:121–126, 1975.

V

Dermatologic Disorders

Scabies

MILTON ORKIN and HOWARD I. MAIBACH

Uncommon in the 1950s, scabies has increased in frequency since 1964 to epidemic proportions worldwide.[1,2] In the United States, scabies accounts for 2% to 4% of all visits to dermatologists.[3]

The socioeconomic characteristics of patients with this infestation are representative of those of the general population. Scabies, in recent years, is being seen frequently in homosexually active males. The frequency of scabies in black Americans appears to be significantly lower than that in white Americans and in some other racial groups.[4]

In the current cycle, typical scabies is seen less frequently. Special forms, especially minimal scabies in clean persons, are common and difficult to diagnose.[2]

In the early stages of the cycle, there was a low index of suspicion for the diagnosis of scabies. Currently, there is a tendency to overdiagnose this infestation.

ETIOLOGY

The adult female itch mite, *Scarcoptes scabiei,* has a rounded body and four pairs of legs and measures 400 μm in length. The mite walks rapidly on a human being, covering 2.5 cm/min.[5] Finding a suitable location, it burrows into the horny layer to the boundary of the stratum granulosum. The burrow provides its home for life, approximately thirty days. Within hours of burrowing, the mite

MILTON ORKIN ● Department of Dermatology, University of Minnesota Medical School, Minneapolis, Minnesota 55422.   HOWARD I. MAIBACH ● Department of Dermatology, University of California School of Medicine, San Francisco, California 94143.

begins laying two or three eggs a day that are half the size of adult mites. The eggs progress through larval and nymphal stages to form adult mites in ten days. The average number of adult female mites on an infested patient is 11.[6]

The mites concentrate in special sites, two-thirds on the hands and wrists. Since the eruption may be caused in part by immature stages of the mite and by sensitization, the distribution of adult female mites does not parallel that of the typical scabietic lesions. In primary infestation, itching or eruption does not occur for several weeks, the time required for sensitization.

CLINICAL ASPECTS

Classic Scabies

Itching is characteristically nocturnal. Lesions are roughly symmetrical. The hands are often the first areas involved; lesions (frequently eczematous) occur mainly on the finger webs and the sides of the digits. The flexor surfaces of the wrist are commonly involved, as are the extensor surfaces of the elbows (lesions may be nodular but more commonly they are dry and eczematous) and the anterior axillary folds.[7] The female breasts may have eczematous lesions resembling those of Paget's disease. Papular lesions are usually present on the abdomen, particularly around the umbilicus in a spokelike arrangement. Penile involvement is characteristic, and nodules may dominate or chancriform changes may be present. The disease may also affect the lower portion of the buttocks in the gluteal crease where they join the upper part of the thighs; impetiginous crusting on the buttocks should always make one suspicious of the diagnosis of scabies. In adults, the upper back, neck, face, scalp, palms, and soles are seldom involved.

The pathognomonic burrow is a short, wavy, dirty-appearing line. At most sites, small, erythematous, often excoriated papules are encountered; many of these may be "larval papules,"[8] which we believe are important morphological components of the current cycle. Secondary eczematization and infection may overshadow other features, making diagnosis more difficult. Many dermatoses present with monomorphous lesions; scabies is usually a polymorphous disease. An exception is the occasional patient with scabies in whom urticaria is the only cutaneous manifestation.

Scabies is a great imitator. Differential diagnosis includes nearly all pruritic dermatoses,[9] including atopic eczema, contact dermatitis, prurigo, papular urticaria, pyoderma, pruritus caused by systemic disease, infectious eczematoid dermatitis, insect bites, excoriations, lichen planus, dermatitis herpetiformis, mastocytosis, urticaria, and pediculosis, as well as syphilis, keratosis follicularis, and vasculitis.

Special Forms of Scabies

Scabies in the Clean

There has been a definite increase in the incidence of scabies in clean persons. The disease is easily misdiagnosed in these cases because lesions may be barely observable and burrows difficult to find.[2] The person presumably removes many mites with frequent bathing (soap destroys many life forms). In these cases, larval papules may be significant. Meticulous physical examination will suggest the diagnosis, which is confirmed by identification of the mite.

Scabies Incognito[2]

Corticosteroid administration (topical or systemic) may ameliorate symptoms and signs of scabies while the infestation and transmissibility persist. Corticosteroid therapy frequently results in unusual clinical presentations, atypical distribution, and an unusual extent of involvement, in some instances closely simulating a variety of other entities. It will be of interest to see if scabies incognito occurs after use of the recently released hydrocortisone (0.05%) over-the-counter preparations.

Nodular Scabies

The ratio of nodular to other forms of scabies is 1 : 15 or greater. The nodules are reddish-brown and pruritic and occur on covered parts (male genitalia, groin, and axillary regions most frequently). Mites are seldom identified in nodules present for more than a month. The disease frequently remains misdiagnosed for long periods; histiocytosis X and lymphoma are considered clinically. The histological features are similar to those of lymphoma, especially Hodgkin's disease, and arthropod bites.

Diagnosis is facilitated by the overlapping occurrence or recent history of more typical scabies (usually responding to scabicides). The nodules probably develop as a hypersensitivity reaction.

The nodules clear spontaneously, although they may persist for months to more than a year despite antiscabietic therapy. They frequently subside with nightly application of tar gel (Estar®) for two or three weeks. They also may improve or clear with careful intralesional injection of corticosteroid (triamcinolone acetonide).

Scabies in Infants and Young Children

Misdiagnosis is frequent in children because of a low index of suspicion, secondary eczematous changes (possibly widespread) suggesting other conditions, and atypical distribution to include head, neck, palms, and soles.[10] Vesicles are common. Secondary bacterial infection is not uncommon, particularly on the hands and feet. Children recently adopted from foreign countries, especially Korea and Vietnam, have a high frequency of scabies, which often appears after the children arrive at their destination.[2]

Animal-Transmitted Scabies

This condition is not uncommon in the United States. Although persons may be infested with mites from various animals, dogs (usually puppies) are the major source. Animal mites do not differ morphologically from human mites but do differ biologically. Humans are infested inadvertently by direct or indirect contact. The condition often goes undiagnosed.

The frequency of scabies in dogs has increased greatly since 1963 throughout the United States. The external surface of the ears is the most frequent site of predilection, corresponding to the high frequency of hand involvement in human scabies. In the United States and Canada in the past decade, an increasing number of regional outbreaks of canine scabies transmitted to humans have been reported. Canine-transmitted scabies in humans differs from human scabies in that the former is characterized by a greater ease of transmission, a different distribution pattern, an absence of burrows, and a shorter incubation period.

Animal-transmitted scabies is self-limited (several weeks). The animal should be treated by a veterinarian skilled in veterinary dermatology. Symptomatic family members may be treated with supportive measures. It is unnecessary to treat asymptomatic members of the household or sexual contacts outside the household, since the condition usually is not contagious between humans.

Crusted (Norwegian) Scabies

This rare condition is highly contagious, even on casual contact, because of the myriad of mites in the exfoliating scales. Local or regional epidemics of more typical forms of scabies frequently result, usually in hospitals or other institutions. Crusted scabies is a psoriasiform dermatosis of the hands and feet, with dystrophy of the nails and a variable erythematous, scaling eruption that may become generalized. Pruritus is minimal. The disease shows a predilection for persons who are mentally retarded, physically debilitated, or immunologically deficient (from congenital or iatrogenic cause). Crusted scabies is a rare complication in renal transplant patients receiving immunosuppressive therapy.

An abortive papular form of scabies, probably the result of infestation with immature forms (without adult females), has been noted in fellow patients and particularly in medical, nursing, and support staff exposed to patients with crusted scabies. This eruption consists of irritating papules, similar to papular urticaria, on the arms and legs.

Therapy for crusted scabies is similar to that for the more common types, although this type responds more slowly and may require repeated applications of scabicides. Use of a keratolytic agent before application of the scabicide may facilitate resolution.

Scabies with Other Sexually Transmitted Diseases

Sexual transmission of scabies, particularly in sexually active young adults, is common. This infestation is frequently seen at venereal disease clinics and may coexist with gonorrhea, syphilis, pediculosis pubis, and other sexually transmissible conditions. The frequency of asymptomatic gonorrhea is high in female patients with scabies, particularly in the 15- to 29-year-old age group.[11]

Secondary Infections and Their Complications

Secondary bacterial infections may complicate scabies. Nephritogenic streptococcal strains may colonize scabietic lesions and lead to acute glomerulonephritis. This condition has been reported mainly in tropical areas but also recently in Canada and France; its potential is universal.

EPIDEMIOLOGY

Although it is unwise to be dogmatic about the way in which a particular patient contracted scabies, close personal contact is usually involved.[12] The long incubation period usual in individuals infested for the first time may make it difficult to trace the source. If one member of the household becomes infested, multiple members or the entire family may eventually be affected unless specific treatment is instituted. When several members of a family or group complain of a pruritic eruption, scabies is the likely diagnosis.[7]

In young adults, sexual transmission is likely. Although syphilis and gonorrhea are frequently transmitted by brief sexual contact, scabies is more likely to be transmitted when the partners spend the night together. Scabies is one of the few sexually transmitted diseases that is also commonly transmitted nonsexually in households, to individuals of all ages.

The greater the "parasite rate" in an individual, the greater the likelihood of transmission; the importance of those few individuals with high parasite rates, as with patients with crusted scabies, in transmitting scabies is obvious. Immature mites are capable of causing infestation, although the usual cause is probably the newly fertilized adult female.

Scabies is frequent in school-age children but is unlikely to be transmitted in schools.[13] Outbreaks are not uncommon in nursing homes, hospitals, and other institutions. Nosocomial outbreaks of scabies have been reported[14]; presumably many more instances have not been reported.

The cause of the current pandemic of scabies is not clear. Although a number of factors (poverty, poor hygiene, sexual promiscuity, misdiagnosis, increased travel, and demographic and ecological considerations) promote development of scabies, the cause is likely multifactorial. Increasing information suggests that immunologic factors are important.

DIAGNOSIS

If an undamaged burrow is visible to the naked eye, the mite usually can be picked out with a needle or scalpel blade and transferred to a glass slide for microscopy.

Skin Scrapings

Recently developed, unexcoriated papules or burrows are located with the help of a hand lens or head loupe. Mineral oil is placed on a sterile scalpel blade and allowed to flow onto the lesions.[15] Vigorous scraping with the blade about six or seven times removes the top of burrows or papules. The oil and scraped material are transferred to a glass slide, and a coverslip is applied. Diagnosis is confirmed by the presence of the mite (in any stage) or of the typical fecal pellets, which outnumber the living organisms.

Biopsy

Dermatopathologists have noted increased opportunity to make the diagnosis, even in unsuspected cases, by identifying the mite in tissue sections.

TREATMENT[16]

The choice of a drug for treatment of scabies must take into account efficacy and potential toxicity. There has been limited interest in comparative, controlled efficacy trials of scabicides.

Patients tend to apply the drugs more frequently and over longer periods (sometimes weeks or months) than prescribed. Limiting the quantity prescribed prevents overtreatment dermatitis (which the patient may mistake for persistence of the scabies) and minimizes percutaneous penetration. Approximately 30 g (1 oz) of a topical preparation is required to cover adequately the trunk and extremities of an average adult; proportionately less is needed for children and infants. The scabicide should be applied thinly but thoroughly from the neck downward to all areas, with special attention to the hands, feet, and intertriginous areas.

All members of the household and sexual contacts of infested persons may be treated; however, some pbysicians prefer to treat only infested persons. Since symptoms may not develop for as long as two months after initial exposure, asymptomatic persons may harbor mites and transmit the disease.

Twenty-four hours after effective therapy the patient can no longer transmit the disease. However, symptoms and signs may not clear for weeks since the hypersensitivity state does not cease immediately on mite destruction. The patient should be alerted to this possibility so that he or she will know what to expect. Systemic use of antibiotics is seldom required unless there is objective evidence of bacterial infection. At the conclusion of therapy intimate apparel and bed linen should be washed and dried by machine (hot cycle in each), washed and ironed, or boiled.

Treatment can fail if the patient does not follow instructions. Reinfestation from an outside source does not occur commonly except with sexual transmission. Dermatitis, generally from too frequent use of a scabicide, is usually irritant in nature. Resistance to scabicides has not been proven. Resistance can be proved only by demonstrating the mites again in patients in whom there is reasonable assurance that the medication has been properly applied. Parasitophobia is not uncommon with or without scabies; diagnosis should not be made until examination fails to show infestation.

Specific Agents

The most commonly used scabicides and instructions for their use are presented in Table 1.

Lindane cream or lotion (gamma benzene hexachloride; Kwell®; Scabene®) is easy to use and effective. Allergic contact dermatitis from this agent has not been documented; irritant contact dermatitis from too frequent use is not uncommon. Nine percent of a single dose of lindane in acetone applied to the forearm can be accounted for in the urine[18]; this cutaneous absorption has been verified in scabietic and normal children.[19] Studies of acute toxicity have shown central nervous system (CNS) toxicity.[20] Careful studies to determine the presence or absence of subclinical CNS toxicity have not been performed, nor has CNS toxicity from appropriately used topical therapy been proven.[21] Clinical CNS toxicity has been limited to misuse situations.

TABLE 1. Treating Scabies: What to Tell the Patient[a]

Lindane[b]	Crotamiton[b]	Precipitated sulfur, 6%[b,c]
1. Apply one thin layer to entire trunk and extremities after bathing and leave on for 12 h.	1. Bathe and massage medication into skin from neck downward nightly for two nights.	1. Bathe and apply preparation to trunk and extremities nightly for three nights.
2. At end of 12 h, shower or bathe to remove medication thoroughly; change intimate apparel and bed linens.	2. Twenty-four hours after second application, wash off medication thoroughly; change intimate apparel and bed linens.	2. Twenty-four hours after last application, bathe to remove medication thoroughly; change intimate apparel and bed linens.

[a] From ref. 17.
[b] Nonrefillable prescription should be made out for only amount needed: about 30 g (1 oz) for adults.
[c] Precipitated sulfur is messy and odoriferous.

Until appropriate pediatric toxicologic data are available, we prefer not to use lindane in infants and young children or in pregnant women. In older children and nonpregnant adults, an application of the lotion is left on for twelve hours and then washed off thoroughly; the lotion should be kept away from the eyes and mucous membranes. A second application is appropriate only when there is evidence of failure of compliance (the family should be instructed again), reinfestation, or apparent resistance.

Kramer et al.[22] reviewed the reports of adverse drug reactions to lindane cream or lotion. They concluded that this scabicide was safe to use in infants and small children, as long as the manufacturer's instructions were followed, but they suggested additional precautions: Hot bath or shower should be avoided before application; the application should be for six hours (rather than twelve hours); repeat treatments should be limited to a maximum of two applications separated by at least one week; and the infant or young child should be fully clothed or under the direct observation of a responsible adult to prevent his licking or mouthing the drug during the application period.

Crotamiton (N-ethyl-O-crotonotoluidide; Eurax®) is a satisfactory scabicide; whether it is more or less efficacious than lindane is not known. Sensitization occurs rarely but not in scabies therapy. Crotamiton cream should be thoroughly massaged into the skin from the neck downward, with particular attention to the hands, feet, and intertriginous areas; a second application should be administered twenty-four hours later.

Sulfur, used for centuries, is generally prescribed as precipitated sulfur (5% to 10%) in petrolatum. The ointment is applied nightly for three successive nights. Patients find it less acceptable than modern scabicides because of odor, messiness, and staining.

Accompanying Medications

An oral antipruritic medication, such as an antihistamine or salicylate, may be used simultaneously with the scabicide. For the pruritus that characteristically lingers after adequate antiscabietic therapy, a hydrocortisone preparation may provide symptomatic relief in adults and a lubricating agent or emollient may be helpful in infants and small children. In a rare instance of incapacitating posttreatment itching in an adult, a short course of systemic corticosteroid therapy, such as a seven- to ten-day course of prednisone at an initial dosage of 40 mg/day, gives prompt, dramatic relief.

REFERENCES

1. Orkin M: Resurgence of scabies. *JAMA* 217:593–597, 1971.
2. Orkin M: Today's scabies. *JAMA* 232:882–885, 1975.
3. Shaw PK, Juranek DD: Recent trends in scabies in the United States. *J Infect Dis* 134:414–416, 1976.
4. Alexander AM: Role of race in scabies infestation. *Arch Dermatol* 114:627, 1978.
5. Mellanby K: Biology of the parasite, in Orkin M, Maibach, HI, Parish LC, et al (eds): *Scabies and Pediculosis.* Philadelphia, JB Lippincott, 1977, pp 8–16.
6. Mellanby K: *Scabies,* ed 2. London, EW Classey, 1972.
7. Epstein E Sr, Orkin M: Scabies: Clinical aspects, in Orkin M, Maibach HI, Parish LC, et al (eds): *Scabies and Pediculosis.* Philadelphia, JB Lippincott, 1977, pp 17–22.
8. Shelley WB, Wood MG: Larval papule as a sign of scabies. *JAMA* 236:1144–1145, 1976.
9. Orkin M, Maibach HI: Current concepts in parasitology: This scabies pandemic. *N Engl J Med* 298:496–498, 1978.
10. Hurwitz S: Scabies in babies. *Am J Dis Child* 126:226–228, 1973.
11. Nielsen AO, Secher L, Sier K: Gonorrhea in patients with scabies. *Br J Vener Dis* 52:394–395, 1976.
12. Mellanby K: Epidemiology of scabies, in Orkin M, Maibach HI, Parish LC, et al (eds): *Scabies and Pediculosis.* Philadelphia, JB Lippincott, 1977, pp 60–63.
13. Juranek D, Schultz MG: Epidemiologic investigations of scabies in the United States, in Orkin M, Maibach HI, Parish LC, et al (eds): *Scabies and Pediculosis.* Philadelphia, JB Lippincott, 1977, pp 64–72.
14. Gooch JJ, Strasius SR, Beamer B, et al: Nosocomial outbreak of scabies. *Arch Dermatol* 114:897–898, 1978.
15. Muller GH, Jacobs PH, Moore NE: Scraping for human scabies: A better method for positive preparations. *Arch Dermatol* 107:70, 1973.
16. Orkin M, Epstein E Sr., Maibach HI: Treatment of today's scabies and pediculosis. *JAMA* 236:1136–1139, 1976.

17. Orkin M, Maibach HI: Scabies: A current pandemic. *Postgrad Med* 66:52–62, 1979.
18. Feldman RJ, Maibach HI: Percutaneous penetration of some pesticides and herbicides in man. *Toxicol Appl Pharmacol* 28:126–132, 1974.
19. Ginsburg CM, Lowry W, Reisch JS: Absorption of lindane (gamma benzene hexachloride) in infants and children. *J Pediatr* 91:998–1000, 1977.
20. American Medical Association Council on Pharmacy and Chemistry: Toxic effects of technical benzene hexachloride and its principal isomers. *JAMA* 137:571–574, 1951.
21. Maibach HI, Orkin M: Adverse reaction to treatment, in Orkin M, Maibach HI, Parish LC, et al (eds): *Scabies and Pediculosis*. Philadelphia, JB Lippincott, 1977, pp 117–124.
22. Kramer MS, Hutchinson TA, Rudnick SA, et al: Operational criteria for adverse drug reactions in evaluating suspected toxicity of a popular scabicide. *Clin Pharmacol Ther* 27:149–155, 1980.

Pediculosis Pubis

MILTON ORKIN and HOWARD I. MAIBACH

Pediculosis pubis* is epidemic in the United States and Western Europe.[1] The increase occurred without restriction to lower socioeconomic levels.

Cases of pediculosis pubis are seen more commonly in venereal disease clinics and student health services, and by family physicians, than in dermatologists' offices. The recent sexual revolution played a vital role in this epidemic, particularly among young unmarried individuals, since the condition is readily transmitted by sexual contact.[2] As is gonorrhea, pediculosis pubis is more common in females than males aged 15 to 19 years. The sex distribution is reversed over age 20.[3]

CLINICAL ASPECTS

As the name implies, the most common site affected is the pubic region. Although the organisms, *Phthirus pubis,* do not move much from the initial site of contact, involvement may occur, especially in hairy individuals, on the short hairs of the thighs and trunk, and occasionally on the beard and mustache. Involvement of the eyelashes and the periphery of the scalp occurs mainly in children, with transmission likely from close contact with an infested mother; however, such involvement can occur rarely in adults of all ages.[4] Pruritus, probably in large measure the result of allergic sensitization, is the common

---

* Pediculosis capitis and pediculosis corporis are not discussed in this chapter.

MILTON ORKIN ● Department of Dermatology, University of Minnesota Medical School, Minneapolis, Minnesota 55422.   HOWARD I. MAIBACH ● Department of Dermatology, University of California School of Medicine, San Francisco, California 94143.

symptom. Excoriations may lead to pyoderma (which may mask the parasites) with lymphadenitis and febrile episodes. This is probably less common in developed countries, because the discomfort frequently leads to early diagnosis and effective therapy prior to the development of secondary manifestations.[5]

Characteristic, but not common, are the maculae caeruleae (sky-blue spots), unique, asymptomatic, bluish or slate-colored macules located on the trunk and thighs, which fade within a short period. They are probably due to altered blood pigments of the infested human, or to an excretion product from the louse's salivary gland.

When pediculosis pubis involves portions of the body other than the pubic region, the diagnosis may be difficult. This infestation should be suspected in any pruritic eruption of a hairy area. Diagnosis, at times, may be established more easily by examination of the axillae and other locations than the pubic region, since the patient may have already eradicated the pruritic groin problem with self-medication, prior to consulting the physician, but will be less likely to treat other sites.

Eyelash infestation is particularly difficult to diagnose, since seborrheic or infectious eczematous blepharitis may be simulated; careful examination reveals that the "crusts" consist of parasitic organisms.

Pediculosis pubis frequently coexists with other sexually transmitted diseases (STDs), particularly gonorrhea and trichomonas, and to a lesser extent scabies, nongonococcal urethritis, genital warts, candidiasis, and syphilis.[3]

DIAGNOSIS

Adult organisms are few; they are easily distinguished from head and body lice. Although initially difficult to diagnose on the patient, the parasites become more discernible after a blood meal, when they become rust-colored. The diagnosis is more frequently made by identifying the more numerous nits attached by a cement substance to the pubic hair, initially at its junction with the skin. Since the ova grow out with the hair, the approximate duration of the infestation can be judged by the distance of the ova from the cutaneous surface. Although the nits can be seen with the naked eye, they can be confused with kinks and knots in the hair, or flakes of seborrheic dermatitis (which can be brushed off); it is desirable to confirm the diagnosis by plucking the hair, placing it on a slide, and demonstrating the nit under the microscope. Differential diagnosis includes impetigo, pyoderma, infectious eczema, seborrheic dermatitis, psoriasis, and contact dermatitis.

The diagnosis of pediculosis pubis should initiate a search for coexisting STDs, beginning with a culture for gonorrhea and a serologic test for syphilis.

TREATMENT

Lindane cream or lotion (gamma benzene hexachloride; Kwell®; Scabene®) is extensively used.[6] Therapy is preceded by a bath followed by drying with a towel. A thin layer of lindane lotion is applied to the infested and adjacent hairy areas, with particular attention to the pubic mons and perianal region. In hairy individuals therapy should include the thighs, trunk, and axillary regions. The lindane lotion is left on for twelve hours and then washed off thoroughly in a second bath similar to the first. Some physicians prefer lindane shampoo lathered into affected sites for five minutes, rinsed thoroughly, and towel dried. The authors believe that the lindane lotion is more effective than the lindane shampoo regimen. Remaining nits may be removed with a fine-tooth comb or forceps. One application is usually sufficient; a second application is repeated in one week if viable eggs persist, or if new eggs appear at the hair–skin junction. Translucent empty (no embryo) nits are signs of inactive infestation and need not be further treated; if in doubt examine the hairs under the microscope. Shaving the areas is not necessary.

Synergized pyrethrins (RID® and others) are over-the-counter products which appear to be safe and effective in the treatment of lice infestations.[7] They are applied undiluted until the infested areas are entirely wet and allowed to remain in place for ten minutes; then the area is washed thoroughly with warm water and soap or shampoo and dried. A fine-tooth comb, provided in some trade packages, permits removal of dead lice and eggs. One application is usually sufficient; the second application is repeated in one week if viable eggs persist or new eggs appear at hair–skin junctions.

Although extensive comparative studies of pediculocides have not been done, a study comparing Lindane and synergized pyrethrins produced similar results in patients with pubic lice.[8]

Sexual contacts should be examined when possible and treated simultaneously. Other uninfested household members need not be treated.

Therapy of eyelash involvement formerly consisted of applications of yellow oxide of mercury (still effective) and more recently of the use of anticholinesterase preparations (effective, but ocular symptoms and signs may be associated with the therapy). A simpler method is the use of petrolatum applied thickly twice daily for eight days, followed by mechanical removal of any remaining nits. If there is scalp involvement, the scalp should be treated concomitantly with lindane shampoo.

At the conclusion of therapy, infested individuals and sexual partners should use clean underclothing, pajamas, sheets, and pillowcases; these articles should be washed by machine or automatically dried (hot cycle in each) or laundered and ironed.

Resistance

No resistance of pubic lice to insecticides has been noted. Therapeutic inefficacy is usually due to failure to follow instructions completely, neglecting to treat sexual contacts, or reinfestation. Persistent pruritus may be caused by irritation by the pediculicide (usually from too frequent use), irritation by or sensitization to previous medications, or patient anxiety. Parasitophobia is not uncommon, with or without pediculosis, and is difficult to manage.

REFERENCES

1. Gratz NG: The current status of louse infestations throughout the world: The control of lice and louse-borne diseases, in *Proceedings of the International Symposium on the Control of Lice and Louse-borne Diseases*, Pan American Health Organization, 1973, p 23.
2. Felman YM, Nikitas JA: Pediculosis pubis. *Cutis* 25:482–489, 1980.
3. Fisher L, Morton RS: Phthirus pubis infestation. *Br J Vener Dis* 46:326–329, 1970.
4. Witkowski JA, Parish LC: Phthiriasis capitis. *Int J Dermatol* 18:559–560, 1979.
5. Epstein E Sr, Orkin M: Pediculosis: Clinical aspects, in Orkin M, Maibach HI, Parish LC, et al (eds): *Scabies and Pediculosis*. Philadelphia, JB Lippincott, 1977, pp 153–156.
6. Orkin M, Epstein E Sr, Maibach HI: Treatment of today's scabies and pediculosis. *JAMA* 236:1136–1139, 1976.
7. Orkin M, Maibach HI: Scabies and pediculosis, in Gellis SS, Kagan BM (eds): *Current Pediatric Therapy*. Philadelphia, WB Saunders, 1982, pp 453–454.
8. Newsom JH, Fiore JL Jr, Hackett E: Treatment of infestation with *Phthirus pubis:* Comparative efficacies of synergized pyrethrins–benzene hexachloride. *Sex Transm Dis* 6:203, 1979.

Venereologic Dermatology in Homosexual Men

ALEXANDER A. FISHER

HERPES SIMPLEX (GENITAL AND ORAL)

GENERAL CONSIDERATIONS

Genital herpesviral infections are almost always sexually acquired. Rarely, genital herpes may be acquired by autoinoculation with any cutaneous site; by medical personnel who are exposed to oral or genital lesions during the physical examination of, specimen collection from, or management of patients with herpes; and by wrestlers, who may acquire "herpes gladiatorum" by direct nonvenereal contact with infected individuals. Herpes simplex may occur on the wrestler's hands and then be transmitted to his genitals. Similarly, masseurs may acquire nonvenereal genital herpes.

ETIOLOGY

Herpes simplex is caused by two antigenically distinct viruses: herpes simplex virus type 1 (HSV1) and herpes simplex virus type 2 (HSV2).[1-4] Originally,

ALEXANDER A. FISHER ● Department of Dermatology, New York University Postgraduate Medical School, New York, New York 10003.

each virus was presumed to produce herpes infections on different sites, i.e., herpetic infections present above the waist were associated with HSV1 and those present below the waist were associated with HSV2. It is now apparent that genital herpes can be caused by HSV1, which usually presents orally. However, HSV1 and HSV2 do show a predilection for specific sites. Overall, about 16% of genital lesions are caused by HSV1 and the remainder by HSV2. Genital herpes caused by HSV1 may be becoming more prevalent as a result of increased orogenital sex play.[5]

Both HSV1 and HSV2 are transmissible and most people harbor these viruses, although few individuals become symptomatic. When a person has been infected by herpes simplex virus, the virus persists within the infected individual for life.[6] Some estimates place the number of people in the United States who harbor the virus at over 5 million.

Sexual abstinence is advisable while the lesions are active, that is, in the vesicular or papular state, when they appear on the mouth or genitalia. Once the acute infection has cleared (usually in about two weeks), the latent stage begins. The location and state of the virus during latency are not known. In the case of genital herpes, the most probable site is the neurons of the sacral ganglia.[7] The factors determining the induction and maintenance of the latent state are also not known. The immunologic state of the host is probably the most significant factor underlying the reactivation of latent virus. Attention is now being focused on cell-mediated immunity because humoral antibody appears ineffective in preventing recurrences.

The underlying latent infection is punctuated by periodic episodes of active viral replication. When the quantity of active viruses reaches a certain threshold level, shedding of infectious virus occurs, and recurrent or reactivated clinical disease may result. It is likely that both the cytocidal effects of acute viral replication and the immunopathological consequences of the host's immune response are involved in disease production.[8]

One of the problems of herpes genitalis is the unpredictability of recurrences and the possibility of asymptomatic recurrences with viral shedding. Even though virus cannot be isolated between recurrences from the cutaneous sites of infection, the female pattern of asymptomatic cervical recurrences and the possibility of asymptomatic urethral infection in the male raise the question of whether there is a safe period in the absence of active lesions, as suggested by Chang.[1]

Many patients presenting with initial genital HSV infections have sexual partners without recent signs or symptoms of infection. These contacts usually have serum antibody to HSV, but no clinically detectable HSV infections are present when they are examined. Perhaps these sexual partners may have had unnoticed lesions or transient shedding of HSV from the genitalia or other sites without lesions. About 0.5% of the general population and perhaps as many as 15% of males attending clinics for sexually transmitted diseases (STDs) excrete virus in the genital secretions.[2,9]

There are probably wide variations in the duration of virus shedding. HSV has been recovered from the mouth in 5% of asymptomatic adults sampled at random.[7] Brown et al.[10] stated that recurrent lesions in women appeared to be symptomatic longer than those in men (appreciable pain for six to eight days compared with three to four days) and to excrete virus longer (six to eight days compared with three to four days). In one study, HSV2 was isolated from the cervix of five of 50 women with a history of genital herpes during the preceding six months, but who, at the time of isolation, demonstrated no signs or symptoms of the illness.[11] In a smaller study, Adam et al.[12] took daily cultures between recurrences from three women with a history of genital herpes and detected, repeatedly in all three, infectious virus or viral antigens in exfoliated cells. Rattray et al.[13] studied women with recurrent disease and found both asymptomatic herpetic lesions and transient shedding of HSV from the cervix or vulva without obvious herpetic lesions.

In males, data are conflicting. One hundred ninety randomly selected males showed a 15% incidence of HSV2 in various genitourinary cultures from the urethra, prostatic fluid, prostate, and vas deferens.[14] However, in another study no virus was isolated from 144 random vasectomy specimens.[15] Also, no virus was isolated from the semen between recurrences of 30 patients with a history of recurrent herpes genitalis.[16] The latter study would seem to be extremely significant since semen is the most likely vehicle of transmission in the absence of overt cutaneous lesions.

The true extent of asymptomatic carriage at various sites is not known and, for any one individual, probably fluctuates. In the meantime, with a high incidence of infection and no absolutely effective treatment or prophylaxis, patients are concerned about the spread of disease to their sexual partners. It is the task of physicians to help prevent new infections by advising individuals how long an active infection may be potentially contagious to another person.

EPIDEMIOLOGY

Man is the only host to, and the exclusive reservoir of, HSV1 and HSV2. No arthropod vectors have been implicated in transmission of herpesvirus infections, which occur only by human contact. Serologic surveys among various populations and age groups demonstrate a widespread prevalence of herpetic infections. Prevalence tends to be higher among lower socioeconomic groups, undoubtedly a consequence of living in close quarters.[17] As noted previously, herpes simplex is an occupational hazard among medical personnel, wrestlers,[18] and masseurs.

About 50% of newborns possess herpes antibody as a result of transplacental transfer. This figure declines to virtually zero by the age of ten months. HSV1 antibody begins to rise from the first year and increases most rapidly during the first four years of life. In the 10- to 14-year-old age group, almost 70% of children in some populations show serologic evidence of exposure to HSV1.[1]

HSV2 antibodies appear after about 14 years of age and their frequency increases more than that of HSV1 antibodies from about this age. This phenomenon is undoubtedly correlated with the onset of sexual activity. By 50 years of age, over 90% of individuals show evidence of infection with HSV.

The age difference in the prevalence of antibodies to HSV1 and HSV2 are also reflected in the age differences as correlated with the sites of infection. Genital herpes, which is generally considered to be an STD, is most prevalent in the 15- to 30-year-old age group, a highly sexually active population. The attack rate of sexual contacts to infected individuals is estimated at about 75%.

CLINICAL DIAGNOSIS

Herpes simplex usually is readily diagnosed clinically, particularly in patients with vesicular lesions and a history of recurrence at or near the same site.

In men, the primary infection is usually accompanied by fewer than 10 to 12 vesicles and sometimes by a single shallow ulcer known as a herpetic chancre. The lesions usually appear on the prepuce, glans, or sulcus, and occasionally in the urethra. Urethral infection causes dysuria and a urethral discharge. In rare instances the herpetic lesions heal with cicatrices.[3]

The vesicles are usually present for three to five days or more (longer and more severe with primary infection) before rupturing to form shallow, nonindurated ulcers. The primary infection may be accompanied by inguinal pain, lymphadenopathy, and constitutional symptoms, such as fever, malaise, and headache. Recurrent attacks occur in about two-thirds of all cases during the year following the initial episode of herpes genitalis. These recurrent attacks are restricted to a small area, usually at the same site, and are characterized by fewer, less painful lesions, a shorter duration, and a shorter period of viral shedding.

Anorectal herpes is characterized by anal vesicles and ulcers. The infection spreads to the cleft; inguinal adenopathy often occurs. Pruritis ani and rectal pain may be severe. In most instances of anal herpes there is a history of anal intercourse. This statement applies to both the heterosexual woman and the homosexual man.

Herpetic ulcers above the level of the anal ring may produce marked inflammation and induration, which may mimic rectal carcinoma. Biopsy through proctoscopic examination may be necessary to achieve the diagnosis.

HSV2 may occasionally cause systemic infection with meningoencephalitis. It may cause abortion if the mother is infected early in pregnancy or generalized, often fatal infection of the newborn if she contracts the disease late in pregnancy.

LABORATORY DIAGNOSIS

Laboratory tests that may assist diagnosis fall into the following categories:

1. Demonstration of morphological changes in infected cells.
2. Detection of viral antigen in infected cells and isolation of the virus.
3. Serologic methods to identify and quantitate HSV antibodies.

A diagnosis of herpes progenitalis is made by demonstrating the characteristic multinucleated giant cell on a Tzanck smear. This smear is prepared by scraping the lesions, particularly unruptured vesicles, and staining the scrapings with Wright's or Giemsa stain after fixing the preparation with methanol for several minutes. Characteristic multinucleated giant cells with large intracellular inclusions are then seen.

However, the histopathological changes do not differentiate primary from recurrent infections, nor do they differentiate between HSV1 and HSV2 infections. In addition, they are not specific for herpes simplex, since similar changes can be seen in chickenpox and herpes zoster (shingles). However, laboratory tests are available for the identification and typing of HSV1 and HSV2.

Antibodies to both types of virus can be identified and quantitated by a variety of techniques. However, since HSV infections are common, the results of laboratory tests are difficult to interpret. Virus can be isolated from the mouth and genital secretions of asymptomatic individuals. Therefore, the diagnostic significance of virus isolation must always be considered in conjunction with the clinical presentation.

Similar limitations apply to serologic tests because of the common prevalence of antibodies to herpes simplex. Recurrences are rarely associated with antibody increases. However, a fourfold increase in antibody titer between acute and convalescent sera, if found, is significant.

DIFFERENTIAL DIAGNOSIS

Canker Sore versus Herpes

It is important to distinguish "aphthous" stomatitis (canker sores) from herpes in homosexual males because of the frequency of oropenile contact and because canker sores are not infectious.

Ulcerations that come and go in different parts of the movable buccal mucosa are probably canker sores. Blisters that recur on the hard palate and lip margins are more likely herpes simplex. A burning sensation one to two days before blisters appear usually indicates herpes. Stress and certain medications may precipitate canker sores, which appear as a shallow ulcer with a white base and flat, even borders. Herpes simplex manifests typically as grouped blisters on a red base. Enlarged lymph nodes in the neck favor a diagnosis of herpes. HSV is a cause of urethritis in 1% of men with nongonococcal urethritis and has been reported to be a cause of proctitis in homosexual men.

Behçet's Syndrome

Behçet's syndrome, of unknown etiology, is characterized by recurring genital and oral ulcerations that may be associated with eye lesions and pyoderma. In late stages, neurological, gastrointestinal, pulmonary, or cardiac lesions may develop.

Behçet's syndrome ulcers on the genitalia and in the mouth are extremely tender, 5 mm to 20 mm in diameter, with a yellowish slough and an erythematous periphery. Single lesions, which are most common, are usually found on the scrotum or penis. Oral lesions of the aphthous type are usually seen on the lower lip, but they may be found anywhere in the buccal cavity. Ophthalmic findings include conjunctivitis, keratosis, or iritis with hypopyon. The disease is likely progressive and ultimately fatal.

Concurrent Syphilis

Particularly in such high-risk groups as homosexual men, there is a concurrence of herpes simplex and primary syphilis. Therefore, all cases of herpes genitalis, including those with negative darkfield examinations and initial non-reactive serologic tests for syphilis, should be followed in two to four weeks by a repeat serologic test for syphilis.[19]

TREATMENT

There is no specific treatment for herpes simplex. Drying agents such as rubbing alcohol, ether, or 1% zinc sulfate solutions help promote drying of the lesions.[3] These drying agents are applied with a cotton-tipped applicator three times a day. Rectal herpes pain can be reduced by the use of cold sitz baths and stool softeners.

Treatment with photoinactivation of the virus with a dye and ultraviolet light is no longer used because of its suspected carcinogenic potential.[8,9] If, in fact, the virus resides in nerve cells and not in the skin cells, topical agents, dyes, and light cannot effectively eradicate the virus. These types of therapy may possibly render the virus noninfectious on the skin, thereby preventing its spread from one skin cell to another.

Recently, new highly selective nucleoside analogs have been discovered that are extremely active against some HSV. The only one currently available is acyclovir [9-(2-hydroxyethoxymethyl) guanine] (Zovirax®). The initial step in the metabolism of this drug is the conversion to nucleotides by phosphorylation, which is accomplished by a virus-specific enzyme, thymidine kinase.[20] This nucleoside analog is a poor substrate for cellular enzymes; thus the drug accumulates only in virus-infected cells. The monophosphate forms of the compounds are rapidly converted to the deoxynucleotide triphosphates, and these molecules interfere with the action of a second virus-induced enzyme (DNA polymerase) and thus inhibit virus replication.[21]

In the study by Corey et al.[22] topical acyclovir in initial genital disease (seven to ten days) significantly reduced the duration of virus shedding, hastened the resolution of lesions, and decreased the scope of symptoms over the period when the drug was applied. Two trials of intravenous acyclovir (Zovirax IV infusion) in severe initial genital herpes indicate that the therapeutic effect is more marked than that seen with the use of the topical preparation,[23,24] and the drug is now available.

In cases of recurrent genital lesions, Corey and his colleagues[22] also demonstrated that acyclovir shortened the duration of virus shedding in men but did not produce resolution of the lesions or relief of symptoms. The most serious potential adverse effect of topical acyclovir is the emergence of herpes simplex strains resistant to the drug. The recommended use of topical acyclovir is to cover all lesions with the ointment six times a day for seven days, using a rubber glove to avoid autoinoculation of the virus. Although the use of topical acyclovir might cut down the transmission of the disease, it would not change the practical advice to the patient to avoid sexual intercourse while the lesions appear active and to have sexual partners wear condoms if unsure.

If the lesion is painful, a topical anesthetic may be applied. However, benzocaine, a notorious sensitizer, should be avoided. Instead, nonsensitizing topical anesthetics such as lidocaine (Xylocaine®), or pramoxine (Pramosone®) should be prescribed.[4] These topical medications are applied in a 1% concentration with a cotton-tipped applicator three times a day. The patient should wear gloves when applying any topical preparation to active lesions of cutaneous or genital herpes simplex to prevent herpetic infections of the hands, fingers, or fingernails.

PREVENTION

At present there is no available successful immunization against HSV. With respect to the transmission of genital herpes, avoidance of direct contact with persons who have active lesions is advised. The use of a condom substantially reduces the risk of transmission and is strongly recommended during the week after the lesions resolve. However, condoms occasionally break, so the most prudent course is to avoid completely direct sexual contact, particularly with a casual partner, while active lesions are present. The use by women of spermicidal foams—which have been shown to be potent viricidal agents in vitro[25,26]—is an additional prophylactic measure.

Recurrences are usually of relatively brief duration.[5] Patients must be advised to avoid sexual intercourse as long as erosions, blisters, or ulcers are present. In addition to contact–contact spread, patients should be counseled regarding the risk of spread from one site (lips or penis) to other sites (e.g., anus or scrotum) by autoinoculation. Finally, patients with recurrent infections can be taught to recognize the prodromal symptoms (tingling, mild itching warmth) and to reduce irritation/heat at the site of recurrence to lessen the frequency/ severity of attacks.

Recently, a self-help group of individuals suffering from genital herpes, called HELP, has been formed.* The purpose of the organization is to provide support in dealing with the pain, suffering, sexual inactivity, and moral questions that are the consequences of the disease. It also attempts to disseminate new information regarding prevention and treatment of herpes simplex. In addition, *The Herpes Book* by Richard Hamilton, M.D. (Los Angeles, J. P. Tarcher, Inc., 1980) is an excellent source of information for the worried patient.

MOLLUSCUM CONTAGIOSUM

GENERAL CONSIDERATIONS

Molluscum contagiosum is a sexually transmitted dermatosis of viral etiology that is commonly seen in homosexual males. The lesions are located principally on the inner thighs, pubis, penis, scrotum, and lower abdomen. Since the lower trunk and genitalia are the most commonly affected areas of the body, and a history of sexual transmission from an infected partner can usually be obtained, in adults genital molluscum contagiosum should be considered an STD. While molluscum contagiosum has been reported to occur rarely in the anal area in heterosexual patients,[27] this site of infection is not uncommon in homosexual male patients.

---

* Interested readers may learn more about this special service for people who have herpes by contacting the American Social Health Association, 260 Sheridan Avenue, Palo Alto, California 94305. Annual membership is $8.00 per year and the subscriber receives four issues of the Association's newsletter, which publishes the latest scientific information about herpes.

ETIOLOGY

The molluscum contagiosum virus is the largest member of the poxvirus group, which also includes several other DNA viruses. The most important poxviruses that cause human diseases are smallpox and vaccinia. On electron microscopy the molluscum contagiosum virus is brick-shaped and measures 230 nm × 240 nm. It cannot be grown either in egg culture (chorioallantoic membrane) or in laboratory animals. However, it can be cultured on both human epidermis and amnion epithelium.

Transmission by direct contact is always assumed for molluscum contagiosum, despite failure to produce the disease by experimental inoculation of volunteers with viral filtrate. Unlike HSV, the molluscum contagiosum poxvirus is unassociated with neural involvement and nerve root dormancy. However, individual molluscum lesions can persist for as long as three and even five years. There is thus the theoretical possibility of a clinically inapparent molluscum lesion persisting for several years until a proper stimulus reactivates clinical infection.[28-30]

CLINICAL MANIFESTATIONS

The incubation period of molluscum contagiosum is about four to six weeks. The lesions begin as smooth-surfaced pinhead-sized discrete papules, which slowly increase in size to a circumscribed nodule of up to 10 mm in size. The average size is 3 mm to 5 mm. These nodules have a characteristic waxy whitish-pink appearance. Their outstanding diagnostic feature is central umbilication, a dimpled depression on the top surface of the lesion. Closer examination reveals an opening cutout of which milky-white material can easily be expressed. Several lesions are usually found, sometimes distributed widely over the skin surface.

Untreated, the lesions may remain for months and even years, but they rarely grow above the size of 10 mm. Unlike warts, molluscum contagiosum often becomes secondarily infected, usually with staphylococci, producing painful lesions that require antibiotic therapy. These lesions may be confused with pyoderma. Rarely, "giant" lesions of molluscum contagiosum may occur, which simulate furuncles, particularly when they are secondarily infected.

COMPLICATIONS

The most common complication of molluscum contagiosum is the development of an inflammatory reaction in one or more of the individual lesions.

Secondary eczematous dermatitis resulting from scratching may also occur. Molluscum contagiosum of the eyelids may produce a follicular or papillary conjunctivitis. Occasionally, a superficial punctate keratitis may develop.

DIAGNOSIS

Molluscum contagiosum is usually diagnosed clinically by the presence of flesh-colored or pink pearly papules with umbilicated centers from which a plug of caseous material may be extruded. In those instances in which the umbilicated center is not obvious, spraying the suspected lesions with ethyl chloride turns the entire molluscum lesion white except for the center, which remains dark.

If there is any doubt as to the correct diagnosis, punch biopsy easily demonstrates the characteristic histopathological appearance of molluscum contagiosum. The cells of the stratum malpighii of the epidermis become filled with an eosinophilic hyaline spherical mass, known as the molluscum body, which enlarges until it occupies almost the entire cytoplasm, pushing the nucleus to the cell periphery. The molluscum body consists of a large mass of DNA virus, "elementary bodies," embedded in a gelatinous matrix. In early lesions, elementary bodies are scattered at random throughout the cytoplasm. As the lesions grow, the elementary bodies cluster together to form the large molluscum body.

Microscopic examination of the white caseous material from the lesion confirms the diagnosis. Material for examination is obtained by squeezing out or curetting the globule of infected cells, crushing the material on a slide, and staining with Giemsa stain. The cells are then examined for the presence of large characteristic cytoplasmic inclusion bodies.

DIFFERENTIAL DIAGNOSIS

While the clinical picture of molluscum contagiosum is absolutely typical in most cases, a secondarily infected lesion can sometimes be confused with pyoderma. Flat warts and syringomas may resemble molluscum contagiosum, but the central umbilication helps differentiate molluscum from these two diseases. Multiple keratoacanthomas are most easily confused with molluscum contagiosum. However, the former usually occur in patients above age 40, whereas molluscum primarily affects those in the 15- to 35-year-old age group. More deceptive is the rare giant molluscum contagiosum, which simulates furuncles, particularly when secondarily infected. Occasionally, molluscum contagiosum has been confused with varicella, lichen planus, and epitheliomas (basal cell type).

Pappillae coronae glandis or pearly penile papules are tiny swellings on the coronal sulcus or glans penis that can look like early molluscum lesions. These papules appear as parallel rows of lesions around the coronal sulcus, or they may be scattered over the glans penis. They are considered innocuous congenital anomalies, while molluscum lesions are usually of recent origin.

TREATMENT

Treatment of molluscum contagiosum consists of removal of all the lesions by physical or chemical means. Curettage using a sharp dermal curette is quite effective. Local anesthesia, with either lidocaine (Xylocaine) or ethyl chloride spray, is often helpful in anxious patients. One can also simply express out the contents of small molluscum lesions with a curved forceps. When using this approach, the clinician should also destroy the base of the lesion by lightly touching it with phenol or silver nitrate. Other treatment consists of the application of 25% trichloroacetic acid or liquid nitrogen. Healing usually occurs with minimal scarring since the lesions are superficial.

Careful examination of the patient is important to make certain that every single lesion has been extirpated. Pubic hair, in particular, is often the hiding place of an unnoticed lesion that later causes recurrence. All patients with molluscum contagiosum are scheduled for follow-up about a month after initial therapy to treat any new lesions that have occurred owing to viral shedding, before a whole new crop of lesions form. Sexual partners with lesions should be treated simultaneously to prevent "ping-pong" reinfection. All patients with genital molluscum contagiosum should be screened for syphilis and gonorrhea, since there is a tendency for several STDs to occur in the same patient at the same time.

BACTERIAL AND FUNGAL ANOGENITAL INFECTIONS

While such viral skin conditions as herpes, molluscum contagiosum, and condylomata acuminata are more common in homosexual men than in heterosexual men, pyogenic and fungal infections occur at about the same rate in both groups and are usually not sexually transmitted. Their confusion with STDs and their frequent occurrence in patients visiting venereal disease clinics necessitate their consideration in those patients who present with skin lesions.

PYOGENIC LESIONS

Pyogenic skin infections are particularly common in the anogenital region for anatomic reasons, i.e., the presence of numerous glandular structures, hair, skin and flexures, and proximity to the anus. Septic penile lesions may cause local edema and adhesions may form between the glans penis and the prepuce where pockets of infection may occur. Impetigo, furunculosis folliculitis, and abscesses may also be seen. Inguinal adenitis with local tenderness may also be present. Most of these infections are caused by staphylococci or streptococci. Poor hygiene and localized trauma (scratching) that results in breaks on the skin surface, or chronic disease states, may encourage overgrowth of the skin flora. Care must be taken to distinguish scabies and pediculosis pubis from pustular pubic folliculitis. Fellatio among homosexual men exposes them to teeth scratches and bites (heterosexual men are not immune), and these may lead to extensive lesions of mixed aerobic and anaerobic organisms.

BULLOUS IMPETIGO

Bullous impetigo is most frequently caused by a Group II Type 71 staphylococcus that liberates an epidermolysin. Infection results in large blisters containing fluid that is initially clear but may quickly become purulent. Cultures taken from bullous impetigo usually show the growth of only *Staphylococcus aureus*. Over 30% of all staphylococci recovered from the lesions of bullous or nonbullous impetigo are penicillin-resistant.

Therapy. Systemic antibiotics given orally are the treatment of choice. Treatment should be initiated with a penicillinase-resistant penicillin (50,000 units daily), erythromycin (250 mg three times a day), or cephalosporin.[31] The duration of antibiotic therapy will depend on the site and extent of infection, but is usually one to two weeks.

Topical therapy with antibiotics such as neomycin and bacitracin has been shown to be ineffective against staphylococci. However, cleansing the skin with povidone–iodine (Betadine Skin Cleanser®) and the application of erythromycin ointment (Ilotycin®) expedites the healing process after the bullous lesions have broken and crusts have formed.

BACTERIAL FOLLICULITIS

Bacterial folliculitis is most frequently caused by *S. aureus*. Occasionally, other gram-positive and gram-negative bacteria have been isolated from these lesions. Demonstration of the causative bacteria by gram stain smear and culture is important for appropriate therapy, since a similar folliculitis may be induced by fungi, drugs (iodides and steroids), or lubricating oils.

Therapy. Systemic antibiotics are frequently required to treat bacterial folliculitis. The antibiotics and doses used are similar to those used for treating bullous impetigo if *S. aureus* is the causative organism. Culture and susceptibility should be performed whenever bacteria are suspected.

WHIRLPOOL FOLLICULITIS

Frequenters of bathhouses or health clubs who take Jacuzzi® or whirlpool baths may acquire a *Pseudomonas* folliculitis. This dermatosis is characterized by the abrupt onset of itchy papules and pustules on the trunk and extremities; the head and neck are spared.[32–34] Cultures from the pustules and the water of the Jacuzzi or whirlpool are positive for *Pseudomonas aeruginosa*. The condition is self-limiting, usually healing without treatment in about a week. The condition must be differentiated from an atypical viral syndrome, streptococcus or staphylococcus folliculitis, iododerma, bromoderma, or swimmer's itch. Diagnosis is established by culture of the lesion and the taking of a history.

Therapy. As a rule, antibiotics are not needed and a simple drying lotion such as calamine lotion is all that is required. In the presence of severe inflammation or markedly pustular lesions, a topical antibiotic ointment, such as erythromycin (Ilotycin) is useful.

RINGWORM INFECTIONS AND CANDIDIASIS

Tinea Cruris

This type of ringworm (dermatophytosis) of the inguinal area (popularly known as "jock itch") is sometimes sexually acquired, but is often self-inoculated from accompanying ringworm infection of the nails and feet. Tinea cruris can be caused by *Epidermophyton floccosum, Trichophyton rubrum,* and *Trichophyton mentagrophytes.*

Vesicular Ringworm

This type of ringworm, often accompanied by small blisters, is usually caused by *T. mentagrophytes.* The eruption tends to be moist, eczematous, and pruritic. Almost invariably there is also a vesicular eruption of the soles or toe webs.

Chronic Ringworm

The chronic form of ringworm is due to *T. rubrum*, which produces a dull red, rather sharply demarcated, dry, nonpruritic eruption. The toenails and feet are usually also infected with this organism.

Candidiasis (Moniliasis, Oidomycosis)

This groin and anal eruption is caused by *Candida albicans*, a pathogenic yeast not related to the fungi that cause ringworm infections. The eruption is usually acute, pruritic, macerated, and rather sharply defined, and may be accompanied by involvement of the fingernails (candidal paronychia). Obese and immunosuppressed individuals and those suffering from diabetes mellitus are most likely to acquire this type of infection.

Differential Diagnosis

Tinea cruris and candidiasis are differentiated by potassium hydroxide examination and culture from intertrigo caused by prickly heat, seborrheic eczema, and psoriasis.

Treatment

Such recently introduced elegant creams as clotrimazole (Lotrimin®), tolnaftate (Tinactin®), haloprogin (Halotex®), and miconazole nitrate (Micatin®) are often effective against ringworm, while nystatin and miconazole creams or lotions are usually effective in the treatment of candidiasis. Feet involved with tinea infection are treated at the same time.

If tinea cruris does not respond to topical medication, the systemic administration of griseofulvin may be indicated. Griseofulvin (Grisactin®) is administered as a 500-mg tablet once daily with the main meal for three weeks. Occasionally, the patient will experience a gastric upset with the medication. Photodermatitis is a rare complication.

ALLERGIC DERMATITIS

TOPICAL MEDICATIONS

Not infrequently, homosexual men use strong soaps, detergents, or irritating topical medications on the genitals to prevent or treat an eruption. These strong agents often produce a superimposed irritant dermatitis. In addition, to alleviate burning or itching sensations, sensitizing topical anesthetics are used that can produce severe allergic reactions.

The following four topical medications are the most common causes of allergic contact dermatitis resulting from sensitizing topical medications. Moreover, since homosexual men acquire various infections of the genital and anal area more frequently than heterosexual men, a great many cases of allergic contact owing to these agents are seen in the anogenital areas of this population.[35,36] Benzocaine and the topical antihistamines are over-the-counter drugs and are used to relieve itching and pain. Neomycin and Mycolog® Cream are used for presumably infected lesions. All these agents are potent and common sensitizers.

Benzocaine Dermatitis. The use of benzocaine as a local anesthetic to retard ejaculation is a common cause of allergic contact dermatitis. Marked itching and swelling may occur from the use of this notorious sensitizer. Benzocaine is also used topically in over 600 products to alleviate burning and itching of the anogenital area. This topical anesthetic often produces a superimposed allergic contact dermatitis upon the original cause of the burning and itching.

Furthermore, benzocaine-containing medications should be avoided because they cross-react with hair dyes and sunscreens containing para-aminobenzoic acid.

Nonsensitizing topical anesthetics such as lidocaine (Xylocaine) or pramaxine (Tronothane® Lotion or Cream) should be used instead of benzocaine if a topical local anesthetic agent is desired.

Mycolog Cream Dermatitis. This popular cream has produced so many instances of allergic contact sensitization to ethylenediamine, a preservative in the cream, that its use is forbidden in the New York Skin and Cancer Clinic. The findings of the North American Contact Dermatitis Research Group confirm the fact that Mycolog Cream is a common cause of allergic contact dermatitis.

Once sensitized to ethylenediamine, the asthmatic patient must avoid the use of aminophylline, which contains ethylenediamine, and all sensitized individuals must avoid the use of antihistamines that are ethylenediamine derivatives (e.g., pyribenzamine).

Topical Antihistamine Dermatitis. The topical antihistamines Caladryl®, Benadryl®, Pyribenzamine®, and Surfadil® are also common and potent sensitizers that produce allergic contact dermatitis when used in the anogenital area. Corticosteroid creams should be used instead.

Neomycin Dermatitis. This widely used antibiotic often produces an allergic reaction when applied to eroded or ulcerated lesions in the anogenital region. A safe, effective topical antibiotic such as erythromycin ointment (Ilo-tycin) is preferable.

Irritant Dermatitis Resulting from the Inhalation of Volatile Nitrites. In recent years, we have encountered at least three cases of allergic contact dermatitis resulting from the inhalation of butyl or amyl nitrite ("poppers," see Chapter 18). This produced an erythema, edema, and yellow crusting of the tip and alae of the nose. Patch testing in these patients showed that butyl nitrite cross-reacted with amyl nitrite but not with nitroglycerine.

Irritant Dermatitis Resulting from Topical Application

Chemical injury may result from the application of irritating chemical agents to the genital area. Strong soap solutions and detergents, benzalkonium chloride, potassium permanganate, or Lysol® self-administered as a measure of prophy-laxis against venereal infection may result in tissue damage. These strong, ir-ritating solutions produce redness, burning sensations, swelling, and, in severe cases, blisters or erosions.

Irritant versus Allergic Reactions

Irritant reactions from strong medications occur in most individuals without previous exposure. Allergic reactions occur only in those who have been pre-viously exposed to the agent when sensitization has occurred. Proper patch test procedures identify contact allergens.

CONSORT CONTACT DERMATITIS

Consort contact dermatitis is an allergic dermatitis acquired by one sexual partner from contact with a substance that the other partner has applied or is wearing.[37] The following are examples of cases proven by patch test procedures.

Perfumes. One homosexual male patient acquired dermatitis from a per-fume that his partner was using. In another instance, the perfume dermatitis was photoallergic in nature from musk-ambrette, the symptoms appearing after sun exposure.

Lubricants. One patient acquired an allergic dermatitis of the penis from propylene glycol in K-Y® Jelly that his partner had applied as a rectal lubri-cant.[38,39]

Deodorant Sprays. One patient acquired an allergic dermatitis on the penis, scrotum, and lower abdomen from a deodorant spray that his consort used.

Condoms. One patient acquired a perianal dermatitis from allergic hypersensitivity to his partner's condom. Routine patch testing revealed a positive reaction to rubber chemicals. A positive patch test was also obtained to the rubber condom.

Contact Dermatitis from Condoms

Several health authorities consider the condom the single most important prophylactic agent against venereal disease in homosexual males. The condom has the following advantages: It can be conveniently kept on the person for quick use when needed and it is inexpensive, easily within the limits of even teenagers' financial capabilities. The condom places the responsibility for prophylaxis on the initiator and can actually enhance the sexual pleasure of both partners by delaying orgasm.

Since allergic hypersensitivity to rubber condoms occurs occasionally, rubber-sensitive men should be informed that nonrubber condoms such as Fourex® (Schmidt) and Lambskin® (Young's Rubber), which are made of processed sheep's intestine, are available.

TRAUMATIC DERMATOLOGIC PROBLEMS

LESIONS CAUSED BY PHYSICAL INJURY

Anal sexual eroticism is a fact of modern life. Injuries to the anus and genitalia from various manipulations and contact with "erotic" objects have to be considered in homosexual men who present with abrasions, fissures, erosion, or ulcers in the genitalia and perirectal areas. Lesions that are linear or angular rather than round should be suspected of being due to physical trauma.

In addition to biting, a sexual partner may produce ulcers of the penis by scratching, burning the penis with a lighted cigarette, or injuring the penis with an instrument. Deep lacerations of the perianal area and the rectum itself can occur from "fisting"—insertion of the partner's hand into the rectum (see Chapter 12).

Balanoposthitis, an inflammation of the membrane covering the glans penis and the prepuce, occurs most frequently in uncircumcised males. The amount and type of involvement depend on the presence or absence of the redundant prepuce, the degree of phimosis, and the severity of the irritation.

Irritant balanitis, involving only the glans, is usually mild, but it can progress to erosive balanitis, with edema, hyperemia, and bleeding of the glans. The patient should be cautioned to avoid excessive trauma and irritation from strenuous intercourse or fellatio.[40,41]

The management of contact balonoposthitis involving both glans penis and prepuce consists of retraction of the foreskin two or three times daily, with careful cleansing with soap and water. The prepuce must not be left in the retracted position, because paraphimosis may result. The penis is soaked for fifteen minutes in Burrows solution diluted 1 to 10 in water three times daily; 1% hydrocortisone cream or lotion is then applied.

Uncorrected paraphimosis may produce linear ulcerations along the constricting prepuce. These linear erosions may become secondarily infected with accompanying tender lymphadenitis.

TRAUMATIC PENILE ULCERS

Small ulcerations may result from the trauma of sexual intercourse; these range from superficial abrasions and fissures to deeper lesions. The patient and the referring physician are often concerned about the possibility of venereal disease. Diagnosis is based on the sexual history and the exclusion of other disorders.

Patients do not always admit the origin of penile ulcers caused by human bites. Occasionally, patients mistakenly attribute a penile lesion to arthropod bites, zippers, or some fanciful form of traumatic insult, when in reality the ulcer is a syphilitic chancre.

Dequalinium R, a quaternary ammonium compound with antimicrobial and antifungal properties, is a recently recognized cause of penile ulcerations. Most cases have been recognized in Europe, but the antiseptic may be acquired by travelers abroad and brought into this country. The patients are usually uncircumcised men who have been treated with dequalinium because of preexisting balanitis. The resultant ulcers may be deep and necrotic, with sites of predilection on the glans and prepuce. Unexplained ulcers of the penis that do not correspond to well-defined disease may be of factitial origin.[42] Patients have produced ulcers of the penis from a wide range of objects, including lighted cigarettes and razor blades.

Treatment. Traumatic ulcers should be cleansed with a solution consisting of half water and half hydrogen peroxide. An erythromycin ointment (Ilotycin) is then applied. Painful lesions can also be treated by applying such nonsensitizing topical anesthetics as lidocaine (Xylocaine).

SCLEROSING LYMPHANGITIS OF THE PENIS[42-44]

Homosexual males on rare occasions exhibit a specific type of edema of the glans penis and coronal area that is doughy and plastic-appearing. The disease appears suddenly about twenty-four to forty-eight hours after a sexual exposure as a mild swelling of the prepuce with a nontender cordlike lesion in and around the coronal sulcus and sometimes encircling the entire penis. In mild cases, the patient has no pain, and the edema subsides in one to two days. In more severe cases, twenty-four hours or so after excessive sexual activity, sudden swelling of the penis appears, particularly at the coronal area. The swelling may or may not be painful. A cordlike structure may appear that is purplish in color and runs down the shaft of the penis or around the coronal sulcus, encircling it partially or totally. On palpation, the cordlike structure is tense, and the edematous area feels doughy and plastic. There may or may not be tenderness. The lesion disappears spontaneously and no medical intervention is required. Mild pain on erection of the penis may occur, but there is no pain on walking or from pressure of tight jockey shorts. Sclerosing lymphangitis is self-limiting and no active treatment is necessary. Differential diagnosis usually includes insect bites and Peyronie's disease.

LYMPHOCELE

This condition may occur following excessive sexual intercourse or masturbation. The lymphatics in the coronal sulcus temporarily become blocked. Clinically, the patient presents with wormlike translucent masses, in contrast to sclerosing lymphangitis, in which the lesion is purplish and not translucent.

EDEMA OF THE PENIS

Striking edema of the penis is a common reaction pattern of injury. The thin epithelium and loose subepithelial tissues of the penile shaft and prepuce permit large amounts of fluid to accumulate in this area, sometimes as a consequence of relatively minor insults.

A "friction" edema of the penis may occur in circumcised individuals several hours after repeated vigorous intercourse. Diagnosis is based on history and the absence of ulceration, adenopathy, urethral discharge, paraphimosis, or a significant incubation period, which are characteristic of edema caused by venereal infection. Rapid recovery occurs following sexual abstinence. Medical intervention is unnecessary.

Marked edema of the penis may also occur after intercourse in homosexual men who have dermatographism, a condition in which light friction of the skin anywhere on the body produces a linear wheal. These individuals often show a band of erythema in the belt line. Tight jeans produce redness and swelling of the thighs and anogenital area. Antihistamine prevention therapy, such as taking 50 mg Benadryl® one hour before intercourse, may prove effective in ameliorating dermatographism.

SEXUAL TRAUMA IN PRECIPITATING PSORIASIS OF THE ANOGENITAL AREA

Psoriasis is a common chronic inflammatory disorder of unknown etiology. Lesions of psoriasis may be found on the penis, scrotum, pubic region, and perineum and are generally asymptomatic. The uncomplicated lesion is dull red in color and is covered with fine, silvery scales. If these scales are scratched off, fine punctate bleeding points are noted (Auspitz's sign). On moist surfaces (the glans penis in uncircumcised males), the lesions are red, shiny, and nonscaly. Diagnosis is usually easy because of the presence of psoriasis elsewhere on the body, such as the knees, elbows, sacrum, or scalp. Pitting and irregularity of the nails may be present. The course of the disease is marked by spontaneous remission and relapse. Biopsy is diagnostic.

Homosexual men with psoriasis have been observed who never had any evidence of psoriasis of the perianal area until they engaged in anal intercourse. The trauma of rectal intercourse was capable of precipitating psoriasis in previously unaffected areas. This phenomenon is called Kobner's phenomenon.

REFERENCES

1. Chang TW: Genital herpes and type 1 herpes virus hominis. *JAMA* 238:155–158, 1977.
2. Chang TW, Fiumara NJ, Weinstein L: Genital herpes. Some clinical and laboratory observations. *JAMA* 22:544–548, 1974.
3. Wolontis S, Jeansson S: Correlation of herpes simplex virus type 1 and 2 with clinical features of infection. *J Infect Dis* 135:28–34, 1977.
4. Nahmias A, Dowdle W, Naib Z, et al: Genital infection with type 2 herpes virus hominis: A commonly occurring venereal disease. *Br J Vener Dis* 45:294–298, 1969.
5. Ferrer R, Felman YM, Nikitas JA: Genital herpesvirus infections. *Sex Transm Dis Newslett* (City of New York) 1:01–04, 1978.
6. Felman YM: Anorectal herpes virus infection. *Med Asp Human Sexuality* 15(3):32E–32F, 1981.
7. Steven JG: Herpetic latency and reactivation, in Rapp F (ed): *Oncogenic Herpes Viruses*. Boca Raton, Florida, CRC Press, 1980, vol 2, pp 1–11.
8. Overall JC Jr: Dermatologic diseases, in Galasso GJ, Merigan TC, Buchanan RA (eds): *Antiviral Agents and Viral Diseases of Man*. New York, Raven Press, 1979, pp 305–384.
9. Jeansson S, Molin L: Genital herpes virus hominis infections: A venereal disease? *Lancet* 1:1064, 1970.
10. Brown ZA, Kern ER, Spruance SL, et al: Clinical and virologic course of herpes simplex genitalis. Medical progress. *West J Med* 130:414–421, 1979.
11. Adam E, Kaufman RH, Mirkovic RR, et al: Persistence of virus shedding in asymptomatic women after recovery from herpes genitalis. *Obstet Gynecol* 54:171–173, 1979.
12. Adam E, Dreesman G, Kaufman RH, et al: Asymptomatic virus shedding after herpes genitalis. *Am J Obstet Gynecol* 137:827–830, 1980.

13. Rattray MC, Corey L, Reeves WC, et al: Recurrent genital herpes among women. Symptomatic v. asymptomatic viral shedding. *Br J Vener Dis* 54(4):262–265, 1978.
14. Centifanto YM, Drylie DM, Deardourff SK, et al: Herpes type 2 in the male genitourinary tract. *Science* 178:318–319, 1971.
15. Traub RG, Madden DL, Fuccillo DA, et al: The male as a reservoir of infection with cytomegalovirus, herpes, and mycoplasma. *N Engl J Med* 289:697–698, 1973.
16. Deture FA, Drylie DM, Kaufman HE, et al: Herpes virus 2. Study of semen in male subjects with recurrent infections. *J Urol* 120:449–451, 1978.
17. Nahmias AJ, Starr SE: Infections caused by herpes simplex virus, in Hoeprich PD (ed): *Infectious Diseases*, ed 2. Hagerstown, Maryland, Harper & Row, 1977.
18. Allen HB, Davis RG: Herpes gladiatorum. *Cutis* 13:822–824, 1974.
19. Chapel TA, Jeffries CD, Brown WJ: Simultaneous infection with *Treponema pallidum* and herpes simplex virus. *Cutis* 24:191–192, 1979.
20. Fyfe, JA, Keller PM, Furman PA, et al: Thymidine kinase from herpes simplex virus phosphorylates the new antiviral compound, 9-(2-hydroxymethyl) guanine. *J Biol Chem* 253:8721–8727, 1978.
21. Furman PA, St Clair MH, Fyfe JA, et al: Inhibition of herpes simplex virus-induced DNA polymerase activity and viral DNA replication by 9-(2-hydroxymethyl) guanine and its triphosphate. *J Virol* 32:72–77, 1979.
22. Corey L, Nahmias AJ, Guinan ME, et al: A trial of topical acyclovir in genital herpes simplex virus infections. *N Engl J Med* 306:1313–1319, 1982.
23. Fyfe KH, Corey L, Keeney RE, et al: Double-blind placebo-controlled trial of intravenous acyclovir for severe primary genital herpes. Presented at the 21st Interscience Conference on Antimicrobial Agents and Chemotherapy, Chicago, Nov 4–6, 1981.
24. Mendel A, Adler MW, Sutherland S, et al: Intravenous acyclovir treatment for primary genital herpes. *Lancet* 1:697–700, 1982.
25. Singh B, Postic B, Cutler J: Viricidal effect of certain contraceptives on type 2 herpesvirus. *Am J Obstet Gynecol* 126:422–425.
26. Postic B, Singh B, Squeglia NL, et al: Inactivation of clinical isolates of herpes virus hominis, type 1 and 2 by chemical contraceptives. *Sex Transm Dis* 5:22–24, 1978.
27. Felman YM, Nikitas JA: Genital molluscum contagiosum. *Cutis* 26:28–32, 1980.
28. Johnson ML: Molluscum contagiosum reactivation. *JAMA* 243:2529, 1980.
29. Brown ST, Weinberger J: Molluscum contagiosum: Sexually transmitted disease in 17 cases. *J Am Vener Dis Assoc* 1:35–38, 1974.
30. Cobbold RJC, MacDonald A: Molluscum contagiosum as a sexually transmitted disease. *Practitioner* 204:416–419, 1970.
31. Hernandez AD, Burnett JW: *Current Therapy 1979*. Philadelphia, WB Saunders, 1979, pp 654–655.
32. Sausker WF, Aeling JL, Fitzpatrick JE, et al: Pseudomonas folliculitis acquired from a health spa whirlpool. *JAMA* 239:2362–2364, 1978.
33. McCausland WJ, Cox PJ: Pseudomonas infections traced to motel whirlpool. *J Environ Health* 37:455–457, 1975.
34. Burkhard GC, Shapiro R: Pseudomonas folliculitis. *Cutis* 25:642–643, 1980.
35. Fisher AA: Allergic reaction to topical (surface) anesthetics. *Cutis* 25:584–625, 1980.
36. Fisher AA: Antihistamine dermatitis. *Cutis* 18:329–336, 1976.
37. Fisher AA: Consort contact dermatitis. *Cutis* 24:595–668, 1979.
38. Fisher AA, Brancaccio RR: Allergic contact sensitivity to propylene glycol in a lubricant jelly. *Arch Dermatol* 115:1451, 1979.
39. Fisher AA: Propylene glycol dermatitis. *Cutis* 21:166–178, 1978.

40. Wide H, Canby JP: Penile venereal edema. *Arch Dermatol* 108:263, 1973.
41. Wright RA, Judson FN: Penile venereal edema. *JAMA* 241:157, 1979.
42. Gorlick G: Chronic rash of the glans penis: A differential diagnosis. *JAMA* 242:469–471, 1979.
43. Fiumara NJ: Nonvenereal sclerosing lymphangitis of the penis. *Arch Dermatol* 111:902–903, 1975.
44. Lassus A, Niemi KM, Valle S-L, et al: Sclerosing lymphangitis of the penis. *Br J Vener Dis* 48:545, 1972.

VI

Acquired Immune Disorders

Kaposi's Sarcoma and Other Rare Malignancies in Homosexual Men

YEHUDI M. FELMAN, DAVID G. OSTROW, and TERRY ALAN SANDHOLZER

Kaposi's sarcoma (KS) is named after the Austrian dermatologist Moritz Kaposi Kohn (1837–1902), who first recognized the disease in 1872.[1] Its synonym is multiple idiopathic hemorrhagic sarcoma, and it is described histologically in Robbin's text on pathology as having four essential diagnostic components:

1. Endothelial proliferations, sometimes as cellular sheets, sometimes as multiple thin-walled new vessel formations.
2. Hemorrhage, recent or old, manifested by extravascular red blood cells or hemosiderin.
3. Fibroblastic proliferation.
4. An inflammatory reaction composed of lymphocytes.

YEHUDI M. FELMAN • Departments of Dermatology, Preventive Medicine, and Community Health, State University of New York Downstate Medical School, Brooklyn, New York 11203.   DAVID G. OSTROW • Biological Psychiatry Program, Lakeside Veterans Administration Medical Center, and Departments of Psychiatry and Community Medicine, Northwestern University Medical School, Chicago, Illinois 60611; and Howard Brown Memorial Clinic, Chicago, Illinois 60616.   TERRY ALAN SANDHOLZER • San Francisco, California 94117.

EPIDEMIOLOGY

Until recently, KS was an extremely rare malignant neoplasm, with an incidence of 0.02 to 0.05 per 100,000 population, usually seen in elderly men of Jewish and Mediterranean descent and young men from equatorial Africa. Geographic clustering is characteristic of the disease. Heretofore, KS has been seen most commonly in the African cluster, where it has an equatorial distribution (in contrast to the north–south distribution of Burkitt's lymphoma[2]) and where it accounts for 9% of all malignancies and follows an aggressive course. In the United States until 1981, KS followed the pattern of being present in men of Jewish and Mediterranean ancestry and in three other types of patients: patients with terminal cancer, patients receiving immunosuppressive medication (e.g., kidney transplant recipients), and patients with inherited immune disorders.[3] Classical KS is not common in American blacks.[4]

Classical KS occurs mostly in men, with a male/female ratio of 15 : 1. One study showed that 37% of patients with KS developed other primary malignancies and a twenty times greater rate of lymphoreticular disease, as opposed to non-KS malignancies.[5]

Review of the New York University Coordinated Cancer Registry for KS in men under age 50 revealed no cases from 1970 to 1979 at Bellevue Hospital and only three cases at New York Hospital from 1961 to 1979. In June 1981, the Centers for Disease Control (CDC) reported five cases of *Pneumocystis carinii* pneumonia (PCP) in five homosexual men in the Los Angeles area.[6] A month later, in July 1981, the CDC was to publish the report that 26 homosexual men had been diagnosed with biopsy-proven Kaposi's sarcoma during the prior thirty-month period.[7] These cases of KS included 20 patients from New York City and six from California, as reported to the CDC by physicians from these areas. This new cluster of patients with KS in the United States represented a 35-fold increase in incidence as compared to KS in nonhomosexual patients. Patients who comprise the recent cluster in the New York City area range in age from 15 to over 60 years, with a mean of 31 years.[8] Table 1 summarizes the epidemiologic, clinical, and treatment response characteristics of classical European and African and the current United States forms of KS.

KAPOSI'S SARCOMA AND ACQUIRED IMMUNODEFICIENCY SYNDROME

KS may be considered an "opportunistic neoplasm" resulting from an underlying acquired immunodeficiency syndrome (AIDS) and the failure of the cellular immune surveillance system to detect and eliminate spontaneously arising KS cells. However, this view of KS would not explain why this particular

TABLE 1. Characteristics of Three Clusters of Kaposi's Sarcoma[a]

	Classical European	African (Bantu)	Current U.S. cases
Age	Elderly	Under 40	Mean 35
Sex	Predominantly male (M/F = 15 : 1)	Male = female	Predominantly male (M/F = 12 : 1)
Ethnic background	Jewish or Mediterranean descent	Bantus	Diverse, 20% to 25% Italian descent
Appearance	Swollen limbs, plaques, red/blue patches in all forms		
Location	Legs, feet	Lymph nodes, trunk, gut, extremities	Lymphatics, trunk, legs, oral cavity
Time to death	13 years	Less than 5 years	50% dead in less than 2 years
Cause of death	Not KS	KS	KS or OI
Responds to radiotherapy	Yes	Poorly	Poorly
Responds to chemotherapy	Yes	Poorly	Poorly

[a] Abbreviations: KS, Kaposi's sarcoma; OI, opportunistic infection.

neoplasm is occurring as an epidemic at this time, and any proposed etiology must ultimately explain the predilection for malignant transformation of the presumed endothelial KS precursor cells. The recent reports of observations of areas of vascular proliferation resembling KS in lymph node biopsies of homosexual patients with lymphadenopathy syndrome[9] suggest a common defect leading to both KS and opportunistic infection (OI) in AIDS. OIs known to be associated with AIDS include the aforementioned PCP, systemic candidiasis, mycobacteriosis, cryptospiridiosis, and cryptococcosis (see Chapter 17). Currently, about 1300 cases of AIDS have been diagnosed and now account for 2% to 3% of all deaths in homosexual men ages 25 to 45 in the New York City, San Francisco, and Los Angeles areas.[10] Approximately 95% of patients are men and 75% are homosexually or bisexually oriented (Tables 2 and 3).

Epidemiologically the problem is further complicated by CDC reports of 50 new cases of AIDS in young Haitian men between the ages of 25 and 45 who admit to only heterosexual activity.[11] In this cluster of Haitian men (10 cases in Brooklyn, New York; 20 cases in Miami, Florida) have been victims of PCP, central nervous system toxoplasmosis, progressive herpes, and disseminated tuberculosis. Further, 19 cases of KS have been reported to the CDC from Port-au-Prince, Haiti.[12] All patients deny IV drug abuse, and there are no recorded cases of KS in Haiti prior to 1969.[10] The connection between these Haitian cases and the homosexual and IV drug user cases is as yet unexplained. What is obvious is that new clusters of KS and OI are occurring and that

TABLE 2.   Distribution of 1025 AIDS Cases Reported to the Centers for
Disease Control as of 2 February 1983[a-c]

Group	KS only	PCP only	KS + PCP	OIs	Totals
Homosexual males	273 (26.6)	322 (31.4)	82 (8.0)	68 (6.6)	745 (72.6)
Undetermined sex preference	5 (0.5)	4 (0.4)	0	4 (0.4)	13 (1.3)
IV drug abusers	4 (0.4)	126 (12.3)	2 (0.2)	29 (2.8)	161 (15.7)
Haitians	2 (0.2)	19 (1.9)	0	29 (2.8)	50 (4.9)
Hemophiliacs	0	6 (0.6)	0	1 (0.1)	7 (0.7)
No-risk patients[d]	11 (1.1)	29 (2.8)	0	9 (0.9)	49 (4.8)
Totals	295 (28.8)	506 (49.4)	84 (8.2)	140 (13.6)	1025 (100)

[a] From Centers for Disease Control, AIDS Activity Surveillance Data, 2 February 1983.
[b] Abbreviations: KS, Kaposi's sarcoma; OI, opportunistic infections, not KS, not PCP; PCP, *Pneumocystis carinii* pneumonia.
[c] Females are not reported in this analysis under a separate category but are included in this table. They comprised 59 (5.8%) patients: 29 IV drug abusers, 5 Haitians, and 25 heterosexuals.
[d] No-risk patients means that the patients were not IV drug abusers, nor Haitians, nor homosexual men, nor hemophiliacs.

TABLE 3.   Distribution of AIDS Cases by Disease in Homosexual Men in
Eleven American Cities as of 2 February 1983[a,b]

Geographic area	KS only	PCP only	KS +PCP	OIs	Totals
New York	122	137	41	38	338
San Francisco	55	48	19	0	122
Los Angeles	31	26	4	3	64
Chicago	2	10	1	3	16
Houston	5	9	2	0	16
Miami	4	4	1	4	13
Philadelphia	4	4	1	2	11
Washington, D.C.	1	9	1	0	11
Newark	4	4	0	2	10
Atlanta	2	6	0	1	9
Boston	0	5	1	1	7
Totals	230	262	71	54	617[c]

[a] From Centers for Disease Control, AIDS Activity Surveillance Data, 2 February 1983.
[b] Abbreviations: KS, Kaposi's sarcoma; OI, opportunistic infections, not KS, not PCP; PCP, *Pneumocystis carinii* pneumonia.
[c] Not inclusive of all AIDS cases.

TABLE 4. Racial/Ethnic
Characteristics of KS and OI Cases
in New York City[a]

Group	KS cases (%)	OI cases (%)
Caucasian	71	40
Black	14	25
Hispanic	11	37
Haitian	0	6
Other	0	0.5
Unknown	4	7.5
Total no.	106	173
Mean age	37 years	34–35 years

[a] From ref. 8.

these entities are not restricted exclusively to men, homosexual or bisexual, although homosexual men comprise the majority of cases reported. KS in homosexual men develops later in life than the lymphadenopathetic form of disease seen in African children and young men, but much earlier than in previously reported patients with KS in the United States and Europe. A summary of the cases reported to the CDC and New York City Department of Health KS-AIDS task forces is given in Tables 2–4.

ETIOLOGY

In the present epidemic in homosexual men, KS is now considered to be a consequence of AIDS. The etiology and cell of origin of KS have not yet been determined. However, the outbreak in certain endemic areas would suggest that genetic, infectious, and/or environmental factors are potentially important. Such factors could explain the tenfold greater incidence of KS among South African Bantus than among whites of the same region, or the high incidences found in certain ethnic groups. The current outbreaks among young homosexual males living in New York City, San Francisco, and Los Angeles could in part reflect the large homosexual male populations in these areas. However, the epidemiologic pattern being seen currently resembles point-source infectious disease outbreaks observed for infectious agents with long (four- to eighteen-month) incubation periods, such as with hepatitis B. Table 3 summarizes the distribution of AIDS cases in homosexual men in eleven American cities.

Several associations between patients with KS and their histories of various sexually transmitted diseases (STDs), number of sexual partners, and use of recreational drugs are currently under investigation. Primary among these associations is the observation that all patients with KS have a history of prior and repeated classical STDs—gonorrhea, syphilis, amebiasis, hepatitis B, and PCP were commonly reported.[13] The hypothesis that these patients already had faulty immune systems as a result of these infections, as well as other factors, currently prevails. In a study by Marmor et al., recreational use of amyl and butyl nitrites and sexual promiscuity have been indicted as possible factors in the breakdown in the immune systems of homosexual men that "might then be indicator variables for exposure to multiple sexually transmitted disease. These STDs, or a subset of them, might eventually have caused immunosuppression and subsequent development of Kaposi's sarcoma."[14] (For a discussion of nitrite use, see Chapter 18.) This research, however, does not explain the occurrence of KS in persons who admit to only monogamous relationships.

Recent studies suggest that cellular immunodeficiency is present in substantial proportions of asymptomatic homosexual men.[15–17] These individuals have decreased numbers of helper T lymphocytes and/or increased numbers of suppressor T lymphocytes. (Helper T lymphocytes promote the immune response, suppressor T lymphocytes inhibit effector B and T lymphocytes.) Normal individuals have a helper cell/suppressor cell ratio of between 1.5 and 2.5, whereas 30% to 80% of homosexually active men demonstrated ratios of less than 1.0. Although low ratios, even associated with lymphadenopathy, do not automatically foretell of impending immunodeficiency, five cases of KS appeared within the first year of surveillance of 34 homosexually active males with lymphadenopathy and decreased ratios.[9] The percentage of patients with low helper/ suppressor T lymphocyte ratios and/or lymphadenopathy who will progress to KS or life-threatening OI is presently unknown. It seems apparent that such individuals are at extremely high risk and should be monitored closely.

LYMPHADENOPATHY SYNDROME

A possibly related lymphadenopathy syndrome has been observed in homosexual men who do not have apparent KS, PCP, or other OI at the time of identification. In February–March 1982, 57 homosexual men with lymphadenopathy involving two or more extrainguinal sites with a median duration of eleven months were reported by the CDC.[18] These patients were not suffering from illness or using drugs that are thought to produce lymphadenopathy. Biopsies revealed reactive hyperplasia.

These patients had histories of STDs (gonorrhea, 58%; syphilis, 47%; amebiasis, 42%). Immunologic evaluation of 21 patients with persistent generalized lymphadenopathy showed that 38% had helper/suppressor T lymphocyte ratios of less than 0.9. One patient in the group of 57 studied by the CDC has since developed KS. As mentioned above, at least five of a similar group of 34 lymphadenopathy patients followed in New York City developed KS within the first year of observation,[9] and two cases of KS and one of PCP developed in 30 patients with lymphadenopathy syndrome followed in Chicago for six months.[19]

Generalized lymphadenopathy is seen in many varied situations, including viral infections, tuberculosis, syphilis, bacterial and fungal infections, connective tissue disorders, drug hypersensitivity, heroin use, and neoplastic disease (including leukemia and lymphoma).[20] The cause of lymphadenopathy in these patients has not yet been specifically diagnosed. However, in light of the above findings, the presence of unexplained lymphadenopathy syndrome is of great concern and is included, along with unexplained fevers, nightsweats, wasting diarrhea, and severe malaise, in a group of conditions termed "pre-AIDS."[21]

NON-HODGKIN'S LYMPHOMA

The possible appearance of a second unusual malignancy among young homosexual males has surfaced. Diffuse undifferentiated non-Hodgkin's lymphoma has been reported in five homosexual men to the CDC.[22] This report suggests that more than one kind of tumor may occur in association with the AIDS syndrome. There have also been case reports of other malignancies affecting homosexual males, including cloacogenic carcinoma of the rectum[23] and squamous cell carcinoma.[24] Anecdotal reports of increased incidences of these and other rare dermatologic malignancies in association with the AIDS outbreak have begun to appear.[25]

HLA PHENOTYPE (DR-5) AND KAPOSI'S SARCOMA

An interesting and possibly significant finding is the association in both heterosexual and homosexual KS patients with common HLA phenotype DR-5. The frequency of this phenotype in the entire normal population, including homosexual men, is 12%. In one study, 10 of 12 patients with KS were found to have this HLA phenotype.[26] Such individuals demonstrate not only a specific HLA type but also a defective immune surveillance system, rendering them susceptible to infection and possibly the growth of malignant cells, which, in immunologically normal individuals, would be suppressed and prevented from proliferating. The incidence of PCP has increased and is currently seen as an underlying complication, and it is often the cause of death in homosexual patients with KS. However, in a recent review of patients with KS and OI in New York

City, several significant epidemiologic differences between the two groups of patients were noted. On the whole, KS was more specifically found in white homosexually active men while OIs were relatively more common among men of black, Spanish, and Haitian descent (Table 4).[8]

VIRAL INFLUENCES

The association of herpes-type viruses with human malignancies such as Burkitt's lymphoma, nasopharyngeal carcinoma, and cervical carcinoma has already been established.[27] In addition, herpes-type viruses have been shown to suppress specifically T-lymphocyte function aimed at recognizing and mounting an immune response toward the viral antigens.[28] In light of the fact that 90% of homosexually active men demonstrate chronic or recurrent viral infections with herpesvirus, cytomegalovirus (CMV), and hepatitis B, it is possible that these recurrent or chronic infections may themselves be triggering factors for the development of acquired immunodeficiency. The possible connection of viral infection has become more prominent in speculation concerning the etiopathogenesis of the disease since the demonstration of the CMV genome within the cells of KS biopsy specimens.[29] However, CMV infection is extremely common in homosexual men. In one study, 94% of patients with KS had positive CMV antibody titers and 19% had positive urine CMV cultures.[30] As high as these figures are, they may not be significantly higher than in heterosexually active individuals with multiple partners. The CMV infection and even the insertion of the genome into the host chromosomes may be only an indication of the high rate of infection found in homosexually active men, rather than having any etiopathogenetic implications. Disseminated infection by viruses, *P. carinii, Candida,* atypical mycobacteria, and other opportunistic organisms, as well as the malignant conditions, may then be seen as a logical consequence of the immunodeficient state. This combination of factors—including the possibility that drugs such as volatile nitrites and marijuana are cofactors in the suppression of cellular immune function—is schematically summarized in Figure 1.[31]

PROGNOSIS

KS in older patients runs a prolonged course and has demonstrated a survival period of eight to thirteen years.[32] The prognosis for young homosexual patients is varied though not as favorable. The cause of death of KS patients in one study was either toxoplasmosis, disseminated CMV infection, or bacterial sepsis. Severe immunodeficiency was evident by the course of the disease in many of these patients.[33] It is not known if the underlying cellular immunodeficiency

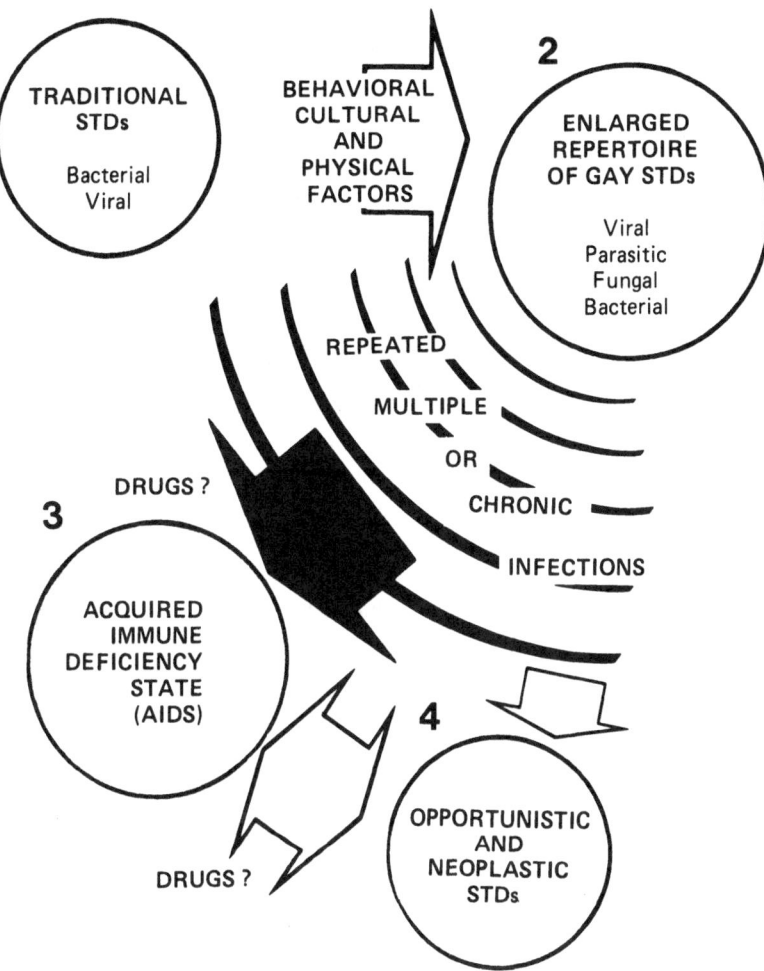

FIGURE 1. Overall model of emerging "gay STD" problems.

contributes to the aggressive clinical course (including lymph node involvement) of KS in these patients, as it does in renal transplant patients receiving immuno-suppressive therapy.[34] Also, the relationship of CMV infection to the pathogenesis of KS in general, and specifically in the young homosexual male, has not yet been ascertained. It has been postulated that prolonged and insidious exposure to CMV and repeated antigenic stimulation may be causative of KS initiation and development.[30] However, the contribution of immune defects originated by CMV to the outbreak of KS in unclear. Young homosexual men with KS have not yet developed secondary neoplasms as do older patients with KS, but this may be due to the extremely short life expectancy of patients with KS and AIDS.

DIAGNOSIS

KS is characterized by the appearance of multicentric red-blue to brown violacious skin nodules or plaques over the skin and sometimes in the internal viscera. Individual tumors usually reach a diameter of 10 mm to 30 mm and then stop growing. Since the process is multifocal, the adjacent areas may fuse, forming a plaque or tumor.[35] Involvement of visceral organs, including lymph nodes[36] and lungs,[37] has been observed without skin lesions in both the homosexual and classical forms of the disease. In nonhomosexual patients with KS, one or more lesions frequently occur on the extremities without additional lesions elsewhere. In the current cluster of homosexual men, skin lesions on the face, scalp, trunk, and upper extremities have been noted.

Histopathological diagnosis of KS may be difficult because the changes in some lesions of the aggressive form of KS seen in homosexual men may be interpreted as nonspecific, and other cutaneous and soft tissue sarcomas (e.g., angiosarcoma of the skin[38]) may be confused with KS. These lesions may be present at the initial physician's visit. They may be absent, however, or be considered benign by both patient and physician.

Diagnosis of cutaneous KS is by biopsy of the skin lesion. A sterile, sharp circular punch of at least 4 mm in diameter is recommended to obtain the specimen. The punch should be inserted through the dermis and the base of the plug should be snipped off. All specimens are studied microscopically. Histologically, KS may be confused with the hypertrophic type of lichen planus, the lepromatous type of Hansen's disease, ulcerated lesions of late syphilis, subungal melanoma, and the histological capillary nodules of stasis dermatitis.[39]

Because of the potential (although yet unproven) transmissibility of KS, physician self-protection is mandatory. Specimens of blood, secreta, excreta, and biopsy should be handled carefully by the physician using adequate glove and gown protection, as detailed in Chapter 3.

THERAPY

Therapy of KS, especially in the current epidemic of cases involving homosexual men, is experimental. No therapeutic regimen can claim success of any magnitude. There have been some reported limited successes with certain treatment schedules, but in many cases clinical trials are still under way and final results are not yet available. The following descriptions of various therapeutic modalities are based primarily on discussions with investigators currently conducting clinical trials.

Interferon

Interferon seems to hold some promise, although clinical trials using this substance are ongoing. Among the limited results available are the findings in a series of four patients at Memorial Hospital/Sloan–Kettering Cancer Center in New York City, who were given 36×10^6 units of synthetic α_1 interferon daily for twenty-eight days followed by twice-weekly doses of the same size. One patient went into complete remission; a second went into partial remission; the third demonstrated a response to the therapy initially but developed new lesions during the second stage of therapy; a fourth did not respond at all. These results have been reported by Bijan Safai, M.D., who will use interferon in future clinical trials. A parallel study of 20 patients is being conducted at the University of California, Los Angeles, and at San Francisco General Hospital, under the guidance of Michael Gottlieb, M.D., and Paul A. Volberding, M.D., respectively. At these centers, α_2 interferon is being administered to all 20 patients. Dosage is 1.5 to 2.0×10^6 units per day, five days a week. Results are not yet available.

Thymosin Fraction 5

The hormone thymosin 5 is produced by the thymus gland. Its function is to induce the maturation of uncommitted lymphocytes of the bone marrow into mature T lymphocytes, thus theoretically inducing a higher helper T/suppressor T cell ratio. This immune potentiator is being tried at several centers, but no results of this mode of therapy are available at this time.

Chemotherapy

It is unfortunate that patients with KS who are treated with chemotherapeutic drugs may show good response to the antineoplastic agents only to experience the occurrence of OIs (e.g., PCP, CMV pneumonitis, cryptococcosis). Combinations of bleomycin sulfate, vinblastine sulfate, and doxorubicin hydrochloride are currently being tried. These agents, however, further depress the already weak immune system. In a recent study of T-lymphocyte populations of patients with KS and OI, antitumor chemotherapy was shown to lower further the helper/suppressor ratio in KS patients in the direction of the extremely low ratios seen in OI patients.[17] VP-16213 (Etoposide) is an experimental substance being used at New York University Medical Center that functions similarly to an alkaloid chemotherapeutic agent but has less marrow-suppressive side effects. Fewer OIs have been reported in patients receiving this drug, even those with lymph node involvement and mucocutaneous lesions. Final results of the use of this substance are not yet available, but results of studies of less immunosuppressive anticancer agents may yet offer some hope for the future.

Treatment of Lymphadenopathy Syndrome

For patients who present with chronic lymph node involvement in the neck, groin, and armpits, opinions vary as to the proper course of action. The conservative approach is to follow the patient closely on an outpatient basis at least every two months and more often if the patient presents with any other symptoms. Since biopsy of the swollen lymph glands most often results in a diagnosis of benign reactive hyperplasia, many physicians believe it is physically and psychologically detrimental to put the patient under these added stresses when little may be learned. In many instances, the patient's lymph status returns to normal after six to twelve months.[18] An opposing school of thought considers that at least a portion of patients with lymphadenopathy will go on to develop KS, lymphoma, or some other life-threatening disease. These practitioners believe that chronic lymphadenopathy present for three to six months requires biopsy to assess the status of the lymph system. This approach is probably wise if the patient has other symptoms of AIDS. Only by adequate individualized evaluation can this decision be made. Obviously, more specific prognostic markers that can distinguish between "benign" and "progressive" lymphadenopathy in this population need to be developed.

Donald I. Abrams, M.D., is currently studying a large group of patients with lymphadenopathy syndrome at the Cancer Research Institute of the University of California at San Francisco. A majority of his patients have stool examinations positive for one or more enteric protozoans. Treatment of parasites, regardless of their classifications as nonpathogens, has resulted in clinical improvement in a number of patients. This suggests that all newly diagnosed patients with lymphadenopathy have serial stool specimens examined for ova and parasites and that aggressive therapy be instituted if the results are positive. Collection of specimens and therapy are discussed in Chapters 7–9.

Hospitalization

The decision to hospitalize the patient must be made on an individual basis. Some physicians prefer to have the patient in-house at least while therapy is being administered. There is no reason for the patient with KS to be hospitalized if he can function as an outpatient. The patient usually is not able to work and complains of chronic fatigue, thus making his outpatient status dependent on the presence of a significant other to care for him. Hospitalization is probably indicated once the patient's symptoms and disease progress to the point where he is incapacitated and requires professional nursing care usually not available in the home setting.

Two schools of thought prevail as to the use of isolation or enteric nursing techniques. Some hospitals, such as the University of California Medical Center, do not use isolation techniques but rather the same kind of precautions necessary when caring for the patient with hepatitis. These include separate dishes, a private bathroom, and adequate protection of the staff when handling any patient specimens. Others, such as San Francisco General Hospital, place the patient in isolation, particularly in the terminal stages of the disease.[40] This nursing approach has a great psychological impact on the patient, but the hospitals who deem isolation procedures necessary do so in consideration of the possible transmissibility of the disease, as well as to reduce the chance of nosocomial OI.

COUNSELING THE PATIENT WITH KAPOSI'S SARCOMA

Whether hospitalized or not, the patient should be introduced to one of the support groups or organizations available in his area. Support groups formed particularly to aid the victims of KS should be contacted if the patient is in an area where they are located. These include the Shanti Project, Berkeley, California; the KS Foundation of San Francisco; the Gay Men's Health Crisis of New York City; and the AIDS Action Project of the Howard Brown Memorial Clinic of Chicago. The patient finds support from these groups and from others with the disease, so that he need not go through this tragic experience alone. Trained professionals and volunteers are available who use the already established techniques of cancer patient support.

All AIDS patients must be advised of the possible dangers to themselves and partners of any sexual activities. If in a monogamous relationship, the patient may be counseled to confine sexual contacts to this partner once that person has been informed of the potential risks. Intimacy between the patient and his significant other should not be discouraged, even if specific sexual practices are, and the partner should be included in support sessions with the patient in those sessions arranged particularly for the families and friends of the victim. The assignment of a "buddy" to KS patients without a significant other has been found to be extremely beneficial in helping such patients cope with the extreme stress involved with the disease and the diagnostic and treatment processes.

The association of AIDS with intravenous drug use and manual–anal intercourse suggests that percutaneous and/or mucocutaneous routes of infection play a role in the etiology of this syndrome. Therefore, the KS patient should be especially warned about the risk of further deterioration of his cellular immune system if he engages in either of these activities. In addition, the advocacy of extreme care to avoid even minor cuts, bruises, or scratches and immediate attention to any wounds would appear advisable.

COUNSELING THE ASYMPTOMATIC PATIENT

With the recognition of this epidemic in homosexual men, a large number of asymptomatic men are seeking medical attention to discover if they are candidates for AIDS or to have the physician examine their skin for real or imagined "spots" or lesions. Usually the physician can tell the patient what these "spots" or lesions are at first examination and can allay his fears. It is also an opportunity for the physician to caution the patient concerning his general health. We advocate advising the patient to lessen or eliminate his sexual encounters of an anonymous variety and to be more selective in those he does choose, to eat a balanced diet, to get adequate sleep, to eliminate or cut down drastically the recreational use of drugs (including marijuana, nitrites, and cocaine), and to practice the tenets of good hygiene.

Although this advice may seem puritanical to many physicians and to the patients as well, and may carry the taint of homophobia to some, we do know that evidence is accumulating that the life-style of homosexual men does play a role in the epidemics of AIDS, as already explained. Naturally, the utmost consideration of the patient's feelings must prevail in the offering of this advice, and it most probably will be a challenge to the physician not to sound judgmental. However, the patient must be told—especially after it is ascertained in the taking of the sexual practices history (Chapter 2) that the patient is in the high-risk category of having multiple anonymous sexual partners—that he has a high chance of contacting *any* STD and that to lessen this risk he should find an alternative to his present sexual habits. For the patient with lymphadenopathy syndrome, this advice becomes especially important, particularly if the physician has chosen the conservative approach of wait-and-see. With this patient, it is imperative that he change whatever aspects of his life-style are necessary to accommodate good diet, adequate sleep, and elimination of casual sexual encounters. With this patient, there can be no doubt that failure to do so may result in further progression to fatal opportunistic infection(s).

Currently, symposia, workshops, and rap sessions are scheduled in many major cities for homosexual men who wish to know more about these diseases. The concern of the gay community is, of course, justified, and, as homosexual men become more aware of the inherent dangers of certain aspects of their life-styles, it is assumed that they will correct their problems with the support of the health care profession. Since there is little good news to tell patients concerning the treatment of AIDS and the OIs and malignancies that can accompany these diseases, it is wise to be overcautious and to present the consequences of "unwellness." It is to be hoped that this approach will be enough to reach any intelligent person. It is also a time for physicians to relate the hazards of contracting the more prevalent STDs, which may suppress the immune system, and the patient's future jeopardy for contracting AIDS. This is a golden opportunity for the physician to practice patient education, which is our strongest available means of preventing KS and fatal OIs.

REFERENCES

1. Kaposi M: Idiopathisches multiples Pigmentsarkom des Haut. *Arch Dermatol Syphilol* 4:265–273, 1872.
2. Urmocher C, Myskowski P, Ochoa M, et al: Outbreak of Kaposi's sarcoma with cytomegalovirus in young homosexual men. *Am J Med* 72:569, 1982.
3. Klepp O, Dahl O, Stenning JT: Association of Kaposi's sarcoma with prior immunosuppressive therapy: A 5-year study of Kaposi's sarcoma in Norway. *Cancer* 12:2626–2630, 1978.
4. Laor Y, Schwartz RA: Epidemiologic aspects of American Kaposi's sarcoma. *J Surg Oncol* 12:299–303, 1979.
5. Safai B, Mile V, Geraldo G, et al: Association of Kaposi's sarcoma with second primary malignancies. Possible etiopathogenic implications. *Cancer* 45:1472, 1980.
6. Centers for Disease Control: Pneumocystis pneumonia—Los Angeles. *MMWR* 30:250–252, 1981.
7. Centers for Disease Control: Kaposi's sarcoma and *Pneumocystis carinii* among homosexual men—New York City and California. *MMWR* 30:305, 1982.
8. New York City Department of Health: Acquired immunodeficiency syndrome. *City Health Information* 1:1–2, 1982.
9. Mathur V, Enlow RW, Spigland I, et al: Generalized lymphadenopathy: A prodrome of Kaposi's sarcoma in male homosexuals? in *Abstracts of the 1982 ICAAC*, 1982, p 218.
10. Jaffe H: Epidemiology of acquired immunodeficiency syndrome. Presented at the 1982 ICAAC, Miami, Oct 5, 1982.
11. Centers for Disease Control: Opportunistic infections and Kaposi's sarcoma among Haitians in the U.S. *MMWR* 30:353–361, 1982.
12. Liautand B, Laroche C, Duvivier J, et al: Le sarcome de Kaposi—Est-il fréquent en Haiti? Presented at the 18th Congrès des Médecins Francophones de l'Hémisphère Americaine, Port-au-Prince, Haiti, April, 1982.
13. Centers for Disease Control Task Force on Kaposi's Sarcoma and Opportunistic Infections: Epidemiologic aspects of the current outbreak of Kaposi's sarcoma and opportunistic infections. *N Engl J Med* 306:248–252, 1982.
14. Marmor M, Laubenstein L, William DC, et al: Risk factors for Kaposi's sarcoma in homosexual men. *Lancet* 1:1083–1087, 1982.
15. Kornfield H, Vande Stouwe RA, Lange M, et al: T-lymphocyte subpopulations in homosexual men. *N Engl J Med* 307:729–731, 1982.
16. Kalish S, Phair JP, Ostrow DG, et al: Evaluation of homosexuals not responding to hepatitis B vaccine, in *Abstracts of the 1982 ICAAC*, 1982, p 218.
17. Ammann AJ, Abrams D, Conant M, et al: Acquired immune dysfunction in homosexual men: Immunologic profiles. *J Immunology* (submitted for publication).
18. Centers for Disease Control: Persistent, generalized lymphadenopathy among homosexual males. *MMWR* 31:249, 1982.

19. Kalish SB, Ostrow DG, Phair JP, et al: The spectrum of immunological abnormalities in homosexually active males: Association of laboratory findings with prodromal symptoms of the acquired immunodeficiency syndrome (AIDS) (manuscript in preparation).
20. Wintrobe M: *Clinical Hematology,* ed 8. New York, Lea and Febiger, 1981, pp 1279–1281.
21. Ostow DG: A glossary of AIDS terms. *Homosexual Health Report* 1:10–11, 1983.
22. Centers for Disease Control: Diffuse undifferentiated non-Hodgkin's lymphoma among homosexual males—United States. *MMWR* 31:277, 1982.
23. Cooper HS, Patchefsky AS, Marks G: Cloacogenic carcinoma of the anorectum in homosexual men: An observation of four cases. *Dis Colon Rectum* 22:557–558, 1979.
24. Li FP, Osborn D, Cronin CM: Anorectal squamous carcinoma in two homosexual men. *Lancet* 1:391, 1982.
25. Minutes of a workshop on AIDS held at the CDC, Atlanta, Georgia, March 3, 1982 (unpublished).
26. Friedman-Kien AE: Disseminated Kaposi's sarcoma syndrome. *J Am Acad Dermatol* 5:471, 1981.
27. Klein G: Herpes viruses and oncogenesis. *Proc Natl Acad Sci USA* 69:1056–1064, 1972.
28. Donnenberg AD, Bell RB, Aurelian L: Immunity to herpes simplex virus II. I. Development of virus-specific lymphoproliferative and LMIF responses in HSV-2 infected guinea pigs. *Cell Immunol* 56:526–539, 1980.
29. Drew WL, Conant MA, Miner RC, et al: Cytomegalovirus and Kaposi's sarcoma in young homosexual men. *Lancet* 1:125–127, 1982.
30. Drew WL, Mintz L, Minet RC, et al: Prevalence of cytomegalovirus in homosexual men. *J Infect Dis* 143:188, 1981.
31. Ostrow DG: Kaposi's sarcoma and acquired immunodeficiency syndrome: An overview. *Homosexual Health Report* 1:13, 1982.
32. Safai B, Good RA: Kaposi's sarcoma: A review of recent developments. *Clin Bull* 10:62, 1982.
33. Hymes KB, Cheung TL, Greene JB, et al: Kaposi's sarcoma in homosexual men: A report of 8 cases. *Lancet* 2:598, 1981.
34. Hardy MA, Goldforb P, Levine S, et al: De novo Kaposi's sarcoma in renal transplant. *Cancer* 38:144–148, 1976.
35. Anderson KV: Tumors of the skin, in Rook A, Wilkinson DS, Ebling FJB (eds): *Textbook of Dermatology,* Oxford, Blackwell, 1972, vol 2, p 1998.
36. Finkbeiner WE, Egbert BM, Groundwater JR, et al: Kaposi's sarcoma in young homosexual men. A histopathological study with particular reference to lymph node involvement. *Arch Pathol Lab Med* 106:261–264, 1982.
37. Epstein DM, Gefter WB, Conrad K, et al: Lung disease in homosexual men. *Radiology* 143:7–20, 1982.
38. Rosai J, Sumner HW, Kostianovsky M, et al: Angiocarcinoma of the skin. A clinicopathologic and fine structural study. *Hum Pathol* 7:83–109, 1976.
39. Domonkos AN: *Andrew's Diseases of the Skin: Clinical Dermatology.* Philadelphia, Saunders, 1971, pp 712–716.
40. Schietinger H: Personal communication.

Diagnosis and Treatment of Acquired Immune Deficiency States and Opportunistic Infections

STEVE B. KALISH, DAVID G. OSTROW, and JOHN P. PHAIR

The majority of conditions presented in this monograph are concerned with the management of infections occurring in presumably immunocompetent or normal hosts. Recently, an acquired immunodeficiency syndrome (AIDS) associated with opportunistic infections (OIs), Kaposi's sarcoma (KS), and lymphoproliferative malignancies has been described in homosexually active men.[1-8] In this chapter the clinical and immunologic evaluation of patients with AIDS and the diagnosis and management of infections caused by opportunistic pathogens are discussed. Further, the current status of attempts to modulate the immune response and an approach to counseling individuals at risk are presented.

ACQUIRED IMMUNODEFICIENCY SYNDROME

Leukocytes and their interaction with humoral factors determine the status of host defenses. Dysfunction or a low number of polymorphonuclear leukocytes,

STEVE B. KALISH ● Department of Medicine, Section of Infectious Disease, Northwestern University Medical School, Chicago, Illinois 60611. DAVID G. OSTROW ● Biological Psychiatry Program, Lakeside Veterans Administration Medical Center, and Departments of Psychiatry and Community Medicine, Northwestern University Medical School, Chicago, Illinois 60611; and Howard Brown Memorial Clinic, Chicago, Illinois 60616. JOHN P. PHAIR ● Department of Medicine, Section of Infectious Disease, Northwestern University Medical School, Chicago, Illinois 60611.

lymphocytes, or macrophages is associated with increased susceptibility to specific infections. The AIDS in homosexually active males has recently been identified as a high-risk condition associated with infections by opportunistic pathogens such as cytomegalovirus (CMV), herpesvirus, fungi, and protozoa, as well as neoplastic diseases such as KS and lymphoproliferative syndromes.[1-8] The pathogens causing infection in these patients suggested a deficiency in cell-mediated immunity; laboratory investigations have confirmed these suspicions. The demonstration of cutaneous anergy, lymphopenia, altered ratio of helper to suppressor T lymphocytes, and depressed in vitro responses of peripheral blood lymphocytes to nonspecific mitogens and antigens suggest alterations in T-cell (thymus-dependent lymphocyte) function as the central defect in this syndrome.[9,10]

The mononuclear phagocytes (monocyte, macrophage) are also centrally involved in cell-mediated immune response and maintenance of host defenses against pathogens commonly infecting patients with AIDS. Phagocytosis and "preparation" of antigen by these cells play an important role in the presentation of antigen to lymphocytes, a precondition for a normal immune response. In addition, macrophage secretion of interleukin 1 (lymphocyte-activating factor) or cell-to-cell contact facilitates lymphocyte responses. In turn, T cells produce the lymphokines that amplify the host response to the infections mentioned. Lymphokines interact with nonsensitized lymphocytes and neutrophils but their major effects are reflected in activation of macrophages, the effector cells that ingest and kill intracellular pathogens.[11]

CLINICAL AND IMMUNOLOGIC EVALUATION

Initial evaluation of an individual suspected of having AIDS includes a thorough history and physical examination. A patient who is homosexually active should be closely questioned as to persistence of fever, malaise, weight loss, or skin lesions. In addition, a detailed sexual practices history should be obtained (see Chapter 2). In addition to the routine physical examination, assessment should include a careful funduscopic evaluation and a search for oral *Candida* infection, herpetic skin lesions, lymphadenopathy, and hepatosplenomegaly.

Basic laboratory investigation of host defenses includes a total peripheral white cell and differential count, determination of serum immunoglobulin concentrations, and skin testing with a battery of antigens to assess delayed hypersensitivity reactions (Table 1). This screening mechanism provides baseline information regarding the number of polymorphonuclear leukocytes and lymphocytes, the status of immunoglobulin-secreting lymphocytes (B cells), and cell-mediated immunity. T cells are detected, classically, by their ability to form rosettes with sheep erythrocytes. Approximately 75% of peripheral blood lymphocytes spon-

TABLE 1. Evaluation of Immune Function

Test	Significance	Comments
White blood cell count and differential	Detection of patients having decreased numbers of polymorphonuclear leukocytes and lymphocytes	Readily available, inexpensive, rapid screening test for identifying patients who may be at risk of acquiring AIDS. Low counts are nonspecific and may occur in malignancies or with infections unrelated to AIDS.
Quantitative serum immunoglobulins (IgG, IgA, and IgM)	Determination of antibody-producing capability	Readily available, relatively inexpensive. Elevations of different isotypes frequently occur in various forms of AIDS; nonspecific hypergammaglobulinemia results from common (usually chronic) infections and other disorders.
Delayed cutaneous hypersensitivity	In vivo measure of T-lymphocyte function in assessing cell-mediated immunity	Readily available, inexpensive screening method for assessment of cell-mediated immunity. A positive response indicates an intact system but many conditions may result in anergy.
Lymphocyte response to various mitogens and antigens	In vitro measure of T-lymphocyte function in assessing cell-mediated immunity	Expensive; available at most medical centers; nonspecific: responses depressed for weeks to months after common infection and in various disease states; should be limited to investigational use.
HLA typing (e.g., HLA DR-5)	Specific immune response genes may define immunoregulatory abnormalities	Expensive; available at most major medical centers; not sensitive or specific and should be limited to investigational use.
Lymphocyte subpopulation enumeration	Determination of inducer–helper to suppressor–cytotoxic T-cell ratio	Expensive; available at most major medical centers; may be useful in identifying patients at risk for acquiring AIDS or in following patients with this syndrome; the ratio is abnormal in numerous infections and other diseases.

taneously rosette with three or more sheep red blood cells following incubation in vitro of peripheral blood lymphocytes and the erythrocytes. More recently, T cells have been identified using a system employing mouse monoclonal antibodies directed at cell-surface antigens plus fluoresceinated goat antimouse antibody.[12] Total T cells and T-cell subsets, including suppressor (cytotoxic), helper (inducer), and killer cells, can be identified.

The functional capability of T cells in vivo can be inferred by using skin tests or, alternately, by attempting to induce contact sensitivity with agents such as dinitrochlorobenzene. There is variability in assessing skin reactions, but a positive response indicates an intact system. Anergy is less easily interpreted. Patients are commonly unable to respond because of intercurrent disease, or the tests may have been improperly performed. Finally, observer variation is great. The most readily available measure of T-cell function in vitro is the response of lymphocytes to such nonspecific mitogens as plant lectins, such specific antigens as purified protein derivative, or histocompatibility antigens (mixed lymphocyte culture). Incorporation of a radiolabeled precursor into DNA or protein following incubation with these agents is determined by scintillation counting. These tests are often difficult to interpret. Both T and B lymphocytes are known to respond to nonspecific mitogens, but B-cell proliferation requires the presence of T cells.

Functional assays of the mononuclear phagocytes in vitro are difficult and not readily available. The capacity of the reticuloendothelial system to take up particles can be assayed by scanning of the liver and spleen following intravenous injection of radionucleotide-labeled reagents.

Whether screening individuals who are asymptomatic but at potentially high risk detects those most likely to develop fulminant AIDS is unclear.[10] Preliminary studies in our laboratory at Northwestern University Medical School of 40 healthy homosexually active men indicate that skin test reactivity is commonly depressed; 16.3% are anergic to tests with five antigens and 27.9% respond to only one. In contrast, 90% of control subjects respond to two or more antigens. A low T-lymphocyte helper/suppressor ratio was equally prevalent; 17.9% of the individuals studied had ratios greater than 2 standard deviations (SDs) below the mean of age-matched healthy heterosexual males; the ratio was greater than 1 SD but less than 2 SDs below normal in another 41%. Longitudinal studies are in progress to determine if asymptomatic individuals with these alterations in immune status are at risk of developing either KS or OIs. Furthermore, the prevalence of increased infection caused by hepatitis B, hepatitis A, CMV, and other herpesviruses complicates analysis of these findings. Such viral infections are associated with profound alteration in lymphocyte function and number.[13]

In summary, individuals who have had fever unexplained by the usual causes persisting for three or more weeks, profound malaise, weight loss, lymphadenopathy, hepatosplenomegaly, or OIs should be evaluated immunologically. This assessment should include, in addition to the routine laboratory studies, skin testing, total T-cell and T-lymphocyte subpopulation enumeration, and response to mitogens (Table 1). These studies help monitor progression of the condition and are readily available at major medical centers in most urban centers. This information is useful in providing counsel to affected individuals, as discussed in a later section.

DIAGNOSIS OF OPPORTUNISTIC INFECTIONS

In light of the evidence demonstrating defective cell-mediated immunity, it is not surprising that fungi, viruses, and various mycobacterial and protozoan parasites are the predominant pathogens infecting patients with AIDS.[1-10] Other defects in cell-mediated immunity occur with many cytotoxic immunosuppressive drugs, such as those used in treating KS.[14] Bacterial infections develop late in the course of disease and are usually associated with low granulocyte counts, interrupted integument (e.g., bladder or intravenous catheters), or surgical procedures (tracheostomy, assisted ventilation, endoscopy).[15] The following section outlines a diagnostic and therapeutic approach for OIs in patients with AIDS (Table 2).

Candidal Infections

Stomatopharyngitis caused by *Candida albicans* is usually aymptomatic or may cause the throat or mouth to become red and sore with the appearance of a white or dirty gray exudate.[16] Gram's stain reveals yeasts, pseudohyphae, polymorphonuclear leukocytes, and some normal pharyngeal flora; culture grows the usual pharyngeal flora plus *Candida*.

The most common symptoms of *Candida* esophagitis are dysphagia and odynophagia.[17] The patient may initially complain of sticking of food on swallowing, which is soon followed by substernal burning pain. Occasionally symptoms may be absent and patients may not have oral thrush. Thus, the correct diagnosis requires an awareness of the increased frequency of this type of infection in patients with AIDS and a carefully obtained history. The initial diagnostic step is a barium swallow, which may reveal a "moth-eaten" appearance of the esophagus, especially in its distal third, resulting from multiple ulcerations. A similar radiographic picture may occur with herpes simplex esophagitis or bacterial ulcers.[18] In many patients with esophageal candidiasis, however, the barium swallow can be normal. Fiberoptic esophagoscopy with washings, brushings, and biopsy is the most useful method for confirming the diagnosis. Direct wet mounts, gram and methanamine silver stains, cultures, cytology of brushings or washings, and histopathology of biopsies readily identify fungi or herpes

TABLE 2. Summary of Chemotherapy for Opportunistic Infections[a]

Pathology	Site	Recommended therapeutic regimen	Effectiveness
Candida albicans	Mouth or esophagus	Nystatin, 500,000 units gargled then swallowed after each meal and at bedtime *or*	Highly effective
		Ketoconazole, 200 mg PO once or twice daily *or*	Highly effective
		Clotrimazole oral troches, three to four times daily *or*	Highly effective
		Flucytosine (5-FC), 100 mg/kg per day PO in four divided doses *or*	Greater toxicity and less effective than other agents
		Amphotericin B, 10 to 20 mg/day IV for 10 days	Most effective agent but highly toxic
		Gentian violet, 0.1%, apply 5 ml to mouth and swallow three times daily	For adjuvant use with other agents
	Bloodstream or disseminated infection	Amphotericin B, 0.5 to 0.6 mg/kg per day IV *plus*	Synergism with the use of both agents
		Flucytosine, 100 to 150 mg/kg per day PO in four divided doses	
Cryptococcosis	Pneumonia, meningitis and disseminated infection	Amphotericin B plus flucytosine in above doses	Most effective regimen currently available
	Severe or recurrent meningitis	*Add* intraventricular amphotericin B via an Ommaya reservoir	
Mycobacterium avium-intracellulare	Pulmonary or disseminated	An aminoglycoside plus isoniazide, ethambutol, ethionamide, pyrazinamide, and cycloserine with or without rifampin	Difficult to administer but effective in 60% to 75% of patients
	Single lobe or segment of lung	Surgical resection	

Herpes simplex	Mucocutaneous	Topical acyclovir	Decreased duration of viral shedding and pain in immunosuppressed patients; no effect on incidence of recurrences
	Genital	Topical acyclovir	Decreases duration of viral shedding and time to healing only in those with true primary infection; no effect on the incidence of recurrences
	Encephalitis	Vidarabine (Vira A®, Ara-A®, adenine arabinoside), 15 mg/kg per day at 12-h IV infusion for 10 days	Proven effectiveness; potential toxicity well documented
	Mucocutaneous, genital, and encephalitis	Intravenous acyclovir	Investigational; preliminary results are promising
Herpes zoster	Mucocutaneous	Intravenous vidarabine in above doses	Effective in stopping new vesicle formation in localized and disseminated disease
		Intravenous acyclovir; intravenous interferon	Investigational; effective in decreasing cutaneous spread when given early
Cytomegalovirus	Dissemination	Intravenous interferon	Investigational; proven effective when used prophylactically in renal transplant recipients
Pneumocystis carinii	Lung	Trimethoprim (TMP), 20 mg/kg per day IV plus sulfamethoxazole (SMZ), 100 mg/kg per day IV in four divided doses for at least 10 days	Regimen of first choice
		Pentamidine, 4 mg/kg per day IM for 12 to 14 days	Effective in patients failing to respond to TMP-SMZ
	Prophylaxis	TMP, 5 mg/kg per day, and SMZ, 20 mg/kg per day PO	Effectiveness in preventing Pneumocystis infection demonstrated in childhood leukemia

(Continued)

TABLE 2 (Continued)

Pathology	Site	Recommended therapeutic regimen	Effectiveness
Toxoplasma gondii	Central nervous system	Pyrimethamine, 100- to 200-mg PO loading dose followed by a maintenance dose of 1 mg/kg per day for at least 1 month *plus* Sulfadiazine, 50-mg/kg PO loading dose followed by 100 mg/kg per day divided into four hourly doses for at least 1 month	Effectiveness and optimal duration of therapy currently unknown
Cryptosporidium	Gastrointestinal	Supportive therapy; correct immunosuppression	No known effective therapy

[a] For a discussion of agents modulating immune responsiveness, see the text.

inclusions and determine bacterial invasion. Aspergillus esophagitis, which has also been described in patients with AIDS,[2] can be diagnosed by this method.

Bloodstream invasion and dissemination of *Candida* may arise from ulcerated esophageal plaques and in patients requiring an indwelling intravenous catheter for nutritional support or antibiotic therapy.[19] Blood cultures are positive in less than 50% of cases and may take days to weeks before growth is seen. Attempts to diagnose invasive candidiasis by various serologic methods have been unsuccessful, although recent studies measuring the metabolite arabinitol show some promise.[20]

Cryptococcal Meningitis

Meningitis with *Cryptococcus neoformans* may be difficult to detect because of its highly variable clinical course.[21,22] Most patients have a headache that is usually frontal or temporal; however, the diagnosis of cryptococcal meningitis should be strongly suspected if the headache is predominantly occipital. Nuchal rigidity, cranial nerve palsies, and papilledema are seen in a minority of cases, and fever is often minimal or absent. Slowed mentation, personality changes, and disturbances of thought processes in patients with AIDS should lead to an examination of the cerebrospinal fluid (CSF). About 15% of patients with cryptococcal meningitis have no symptoms referable to the central nervous system.

In addition to routine studies including cell count, protein, glucose, Gram's stain, and cultures for bacteria, fungi, and mycobacteria, the CSF should be analyzed for cryptococcal antigen and an India ink preparation should immediately be made. A mild to moderate lymphocytic pleocytosis with low glucose and moderately elevated protein represents the typical findings. In about 50% of cases the India ink preparation is positive: A clear halo caused by the polysaccharide capsule is seen surrounding the yeast. On Gram's stain, the fungi appear as irregularly stippled gram-positive organisms with a faintly gram-negative capsule. CSF cultures yield positive results in more than 90% of cases but visible growth may not be apparent for several days to several weeks. The latex agglutination test for cryptococcal capsular antigen is highly reliable; false-negative results seldom occur when controls for antiglobulin (rheumatoid factors) are included.[22]

Cryptococcosis: Pneumonia and Disseminated Disease

Patients with AIDS have also been reported with *Cryptococcus neoformans* pneumonia. As with meningitis, pulmonary involvement may be difficult to detect. The patient may develop cough and fever or an infiltrate may be seen on chest radiographs in the absence of symptoms.[23] Fever is usually minimal or absent and pleuritic pain infrequent. Chest X ray commonly reveals an acute diffuse interstitial pneumonia which progresses to an alveolar pattern. A rapidly progressing focal infiltrate or single or multiple nodules with or without cavitation may also be seen. Pleural effusions rarely occur.

Isolation of *Cryptococcus* from the sputum usually represents colonization rather than progressive pulmonary disease. However, recovery of this organism from the respiratory tract of a patient in whom the diagnosis of AIDS is established or suspected should suggest possible pulmonary *Cryptococcus*. Lung biopsy is the best method to establish a definitive diagnosis when cultures and India ink preparation of any pleural effusion are negative. Blood cultures are rarely positive but the diagnosis is highly suspect when circulating cryptococcal antigen is found in the serum in the absence of a positive rheumatoid factor. In disseminated disease, urine cultures may show *C. neoformans* and urine and spinal fluid may contain cryptococcal antigen.

THERAPY OF FUNGAL INFECTIONS

The number of drugs currently available for treating fungal infections is increasing.[24] The usefulness of many of these agents, however, is limited by the minimal efficacy of some and the toxicity of others. Before beginning treatment, the patient should be fully evaluated to define the extent of infection, and the potential benefits of therapeutic intervention must be considered and weighed against the toxicity of the drug selected. Deciding whether to treat and which agent to use may be extremely difficult. Although general guidelines are suggested below, no general rules exist for complex cases; each patient must be evaluated on an individual basis.

Nystatin, a topical polyene antibiotic, or ketoconazole, an imidazole derivative, are effective agents for the treatment of oral or esophageal candidiasis.[25,26] Nystatin has been proven a safe and effective drug that is not absorbed from the intestine. Although primarily fungistatic, this agent does not induce resistance in *Candida* despite prolonged therapy. The usual dosage is 500,000 units (5 ml) four times a day, after each meal and at bedtime, for seven to fourteen days. The medicine should be gargled like mouthwash for several minutes then swallowed.

Ketoconazole is given as a single oral dose of 200 rng or 400 mg daily. It is usually well tolerated but may cause occasional mild gastrointestinal disturbances and elevation of liver enzymes; several cases of hepatitis have recently been reported.[27] Since ketoconazole degrades extensively in vivo, the dosage does not need to be modified in patients with renal insufficiency. Ketoconazole is considered a safe and effective drug and has been approved by the Food and Drug Administration only for the treatment of systemic candidiasis, chronic mucocutaneous candidiasis, and oral thrush, as well as other fungal infections.

It is not currently approved for use in the treatment of candidal esophagitis. Nevertheless, several recent studies demonstrate its effectiveness in treating this condition,[27] and some investigators may prefer ketoconazole as the initial antifungal agent. We have failed with ketoconazole to cure candidal esophagitis that subsequently responded to nystatin. Clotrimazole, another imidazole derivative, is safe and effective therapy for oral and esophageal candidiasis when given as 10-mg oral troches three to four times a day.[28] However, this form of clotrimazole is currently unavailable.

Flucytosine (5-FC), a synthetic oral antibiotic agent, has been used successfully in a few cases of esophageal candidiasis; however, it has greater toxicity and is less effective than the previously mentioned agents.[24] Approximately 80% to 90% of this agent is excreted unchanged in the urine, requiring that the creatinine clearance be monitored and the dosage reduced in patients with impaired renal function. Adverse effects include nausea, vomiting, diarrhea, thrombocytopenia, neutropenia, and liver function abnormalities. Of particular concern is the high degree of primary resistance and the observation that initially sensitive *Candida* species acquire resistance during the course of therapy. The dosage for treating oral or esophageal candidiasis is 100 to 150 mg/kg per day in four divided doses. Recent in vitro data demonstrate a synergistic interaction of ketoconazole and 5-FC against various *Candida* species, including some with resistance to 5-FC.[29] Lack of adequate clinical trials currently precludes recommendation of this regimen.

Patients failing to respond to the previously described antifungal agents and those with suspected systemic candidiasis should be treated with intravenous amphotericin B. In addition to its in vitro and in vivo activity against most fungi that cause systemic mycoses, amphotericin B can markedly enhance humoral immunity and augment cell-mediated immunity.[24] Dosage recommendations are not well defined because of toxicity and a lack of reliable data regarding the appropriate length of therapy for many fungal infections.[30] Most patients require six to twelve weeks of treatment. An initial test dose of 1 mg in 50 ml to 150 ml of 5% dextrose in water is infused over a period of thirty minutes. Depending on the presence and severity of any reactions, the subsequent daily doses are increased by 5-mg increments given in 500 ml of 5% dextrose in water over two to six hours until a maximum daily dose of 0.5 to 0.6 mg/kg per day is achieved. Patients with oral or esophageal candidiasis should be treated with 10 to 20 mg/day for ten days; the dose may be increased if the medication is tolerated and the patient fails to improve. The synergistic interaction of amphotericin B and 5-FC against *C. neoformans* and *Candida* species has led most investigators to recommend their simultaneous use in treating disseminated or deep-seated infection (e.g., meningitis, pneumonia) with either of these organisms. The results of a randomized controlled study have clearly demonstrated that low-dose amphotericin B (0.3 mg/kg per day) and 5-FC (150 mg/kg per day) is more effective than amphotericin B alone (0.4 mg/kg per day) in treating cryptococcal meningitis.[31] Serum 5-FC concentrations should be measured when combined therapy is administered and the dose of 5-FC adjusted so that serum concentrations remain below 100 μg/ml. In severe or recurrent cases of cryptococcal meningitis, administration of intraventricular amphotericin B via an Ommaya reservoir is often required to achieve a cure.[21]

Chills, fever, and hypotension are common adverse reactions occurring with amphotericin B. Control may require the addition of 25 mg to 50 mg of hydrocortisone to the infusion bottle with or without 25 mg to 50 mg of diphenhydramine or meperidine. Premedicating the patient with 650 mg of aspirin may also be useful.

Dose-dependent renal damage is the most important toxic effect of the agent.[24] Early, reversible nephrotoxicity is related to the daily dose; late, more permanent nephrotoxicity correlates with the total dose received.[30] For this reason baseline and twice-weekly blood urea nitrogen (BUN) and creatinine levels are indicated during therapy. If the serum creatinine rises above 3.0 mg/dl, or the BUN over 40 mg/dl, the dosage should be lowered. Monitoring of amphotericin B toxicity also requires measurement of the hematocrit, serum potassium, and carbon dioxide and urinalysis before treatment is initiated and twice weekly during therapy. Phlebitis may be prevented by the addition of 1000 units of heparin to each infusion.

Miconazole, an imidazole derivative, should not be considered a first-line antifungal agent and should be used only when therapy with amphotericin B fails.[24] A five-week course of a 5% oral suspension was effective in treatment of a case of oral–esophageal candidiasis; the intravenous administration of 200 mg to 600 mg of miconazole every eight hours has been reported as curing a case of systemic candidiasis. Reported success in the treatment of cryptococcal meningitis awaits confirmation and evaluation with controlled studies.[32] The drug must be administered over sixty minutes to avoid cardiac arrhythmias; pruritus, anemia, and hyponatremia are relatively common adverse effects.

Adjuvant therapy with gentian violet in conjunction with any of the above regimens has also been used for oral thrush. Five milliliters of a 0.1% solution is used to paint the mouth and is swallowed three times daily.

MYCOBACTERIAL INFECTIONS

Another group of pathogens affecting patients with AIDS are various mycobacterial species, particularly strains of atypical mycobacteria. Members of the avium-intracellulare group appear to be isolated most often.[33,34] Compared with infections caused by most other atypical mycobacteria or with tuberculosis, infections caused by organisms of the *Mycobacterium avium-intracellulare* complex are much less responsive to standard antituberculosis chemotherapy.[35,36]

Treatment requires an intensive six- or seven-drug regimen consisting of one of the aminoglycosides plus isoniazide, ethambutol, ethionamide, pyrazinamide, cycloserine, and, optionally, rifampin. Although this type of regimen is extremely difficult to administer, a success rate of 60% to 75% has been reported. Infections with *M. avium-intracellulare* result in a wide spectrum of subclinical and clinical diseases, however, and patients with AIDS who develop this mycobacterial infection should be aggressively treated. Patients with adequate pulmonary function and disease involving only a single lobe or segment of lung can safely undergo surgical resection even while sputum cultures remain positive.[37]

VIRAL INFECTIONS

Disorders of cell-mediated immunity are frequently associated with infection by members of the herpesvirus group (herpes simplex, CMV, Epstein–Barr virus, and varicella zoster) and less often with infection by adeno- and other viruses. Patients with AIDS appear to be at great risk for severe, disseminated infection owing to CMV and herpes simplex.[9,10] CMV may cause a variety of clinical syndromes, including pneumonitis, hepatitis, mononucleosis, retinitis, gastrointestinal bleeding, and possibly encephalitis. Since elevated antibody titers and isolation of the virus from various sites (such as urine) occur in the absence of disease,[38] the most reliable marker for invasive infection is histopathology obtained by biopsy. Alternatively, demonstration of a rising titer of anti-CMV antibody, or an IgM antibody response in the appropriate clinical setting, strongly suggests CMV infection. Isolation of CMV often requires weeks and thus is of little clinical value.[39]

Infection with herpes simplex may result in widespread involvement of the liver, lungs, adrenals, gastrointestinal tract, central nervous system, and skin. Esophagitis with herpes simplex frequently coexists with and may be difficult to differentiate from *Candida* esophagitis.[18] The diagnosis of herpes is dependent upon the specific cytopathic changes in cell culture, which are usually seen within twenty-four to forty-eight hours, and the demonstration of characteristic multinucleated giant cells by cytological and histological techniques in various tissues. Serologic techniques are rarely of value.[39]

Only a few antiviral agents are currently available. Vidarabine (adenine arabinoside) is presently the only approved drug in the United States for systemic therapy of herpes simplex encephalitis. Initial reports suggest that intravenous acyclovir may be at least as effective but have less toxicity than vidarabine. Currently, topical acyclovir is approved for use in the treatment of mucocutaneous herpes simplex type 1 infection in immunosuppressed patients and for the treatment of initial herpes type 2 (genital) infection in healthy hosts. Double-blind placebo-controlled studies have shown intravenous acyclovir to be effective in both the prophylaxis and treatment of herpes simplex in recipients of bone marrow transplants.[40,41] Unfortunately, several recent reports have demonstrated recovery of resistant herpes simplex from patients treated with acyclovir, suggesting that widespread use may limit its future effectiveness.[42,43] Despite isolated case reports suggesting that acyclovir may be useful in treating CMV pneumonia in adults, there are presently insufficient data to support this claim.[44]

Experimental studies have demonstrated the effectiveness of human leukocyte interferon against CMV when used prophylactically in renal transplant recipients.[45] Other studies in compromised patients have shown intravenous interferon to be effective in decreasing the cutaneous spread of segmental herpes zoster when given early after the onset of lesions and continued for seven to eight days.[46] Recently a child with prolonged CMV and Epstein–Barr virus infection was successfully treated with oral bovine transfer factor.[47]

PROTOZOAL INFECTIONS: *PNEUMOCYSTIS CARINII*

Pneumocystis carinii is a protozoal organism originally recognized in malnourished children but now diagnosed most commonly in immunocompromised hosts.[48,49] Patients with AIDS appear highly susceptible to infection with *Pneumocystis,* which has a mortality rate of over 50% in this group.[50] Patients most commonly present with dyspnea and fever. The majority of patients are tachypnic, and cough, which is usually nonproductive, is present in about 50% of patients. The typical radiologic pattern, a diffuse bilateral alveolar infiltrate, is nonspecific, like the signs and symptoms. Since patients with AIDS are susceptible to a wide variety of unusual and often fatal pulmonary infections, rapid correct etiologic diagnosis is essential. Most authorities recommend a transtracheal aspiration or either fiberoptic bronchoscopy with brushing or transbronchial biopsy as the initial diagnostic step. Sputum cultures alone are only rarely helpful in making the diagnosis of *Pneumocystis* infection. An open lung biopsy should be performed when these procedures fail to establish a diagnosis. In addition to routine Gram's stain, acid-fast smear, and bacterial, fungal, and mycobacterial cultures, specimens should be stained with Giemsa's, toluidine blue, Gram–Weigert's, and Gomori's methenamine silver nitrate stains. Serologic tests are less reliable in establishing a diagnosis; when positive or when titers increase during recovery, they are suggestive of *Pneumocystis* infection. An indirect immunofluorescent antibody assay is available through the Centers for Disease Control.[48] In a highly suspect patient with a normal chest X ray, a gallium scan may reveal increased uptake over the lungs; however, this is not specific for *Pneumocystis* infection.[51]

Once the diagnosis of *Pneumocystis* is established, treatment with trimethoprim–sulfamethoxazole (TMP-SMZ) is started immediately. Many clinicians prefer to initiate therapy intravenously because of possible inadequate oral absorption of this agent in a critically ill patient. Patients who are intubated, those who have undergone tracheostomy, and those with an altered mental status may not be able to take the oral forms of TMP-SMZ. Intravenous therapy is preferred because of the recommendation of some authorities to monitor closely serum TMP or SMZ levels when the oral form is used[52]; serum levels of these drugs are not obtainable in most hospitals. However, serum drug levels should be obtained in *any* patient who fails to respond within seventy-two to ninety-six hours or in patients with compromised renal function.[53]

The dosage of TMP is 20 mg/kg of body weight and that for SMZ is 100 mg/kg of body weight administered intravenously or orally in four equally divided doses for at least ten days. Peak serum levels of TMP or SMZ after either oral or intravenous therapy should be 5 μg/ml and 100 μg/ml, respectively. Refractory cases of severe pneumonia requiring twice the optimal serum drug concentration to achieve cures have been reported.[54] Side effects include skin rash, nausea, and vomiting; hematologic toxicity is observed infrequently. In our experience, patients with AIDS treated with TMP-SMZ frequently develop a rash or other allergic manifestations.[55] In addition, a large number of these patients fail to respond to TMP-SMZ.[56]

Pentamidine in a dose of 4 mg/kg per day given intramuscularly for twelve to fourteen days should be substituted following TMP-SMZ failure.[48,53] Total dose should usually not exceed 60 mg/kg. In the United States, this agent is available only from the Parasitic Diseases Drug Service of the Centers for Disease Control (telephone number 404-329-3670). Side effects are frequent and include azotemia, hypoglycemia, glucosuria, various hematologic and cutaneous abnormalities, sterile abscesses at the site of injection, nausea and vomiting, and, infrequently, shock.[55] More recently, cases of acute pancreatitis have been associated with pentamidine therapy.[57]

The high rate of recurrent *Pneumocystis* in patients with AIDS has led many investigators to recommend long-term prophylaxis in nonallergic patients, with oral TMP-SMZ following the first episode of infection.[1,9] Successful chemoprophylaxis for cancer patients at high risk for *P. carinii* pneumonitis has been achieved with 5 mg/kg per day TMP and 20 mg/kg per day SMZ.[58] Unfortunately, the frequent occurrence of adverse reactions in patients with AIDS has limited the usefulness of prophylaxis with this agent.

TOXOPLASMOSIS

Toxoplasma gondii, the other major protozoan parasite infecting patients with AIDS,[7,9,56] primarily invades the central nervous system, resulting in a diffuse encephalopathy, meningoencephalitis, or an enlarging central nervous system mass. Focal signs, seizures, and impaired consciousness are common in central nervous system infection.[21,48] Examination of the CSF usually shows a mild lymphocytic pleocytosis with slightly elevated protein. The organism is rarely isolated from the CSF. Results of serologic tests may be suggestive of infection, especially with a rising titer of IgM antibody in serial specimens. Unfortunately, most of the commonly available serodiagnostic methods reflect IgG antibody, which may remain elevated for years after acute infection. Several recently developed experimental serodiagnostic techniques show promise.[48] If lesions are accessible and there are no contraindications, a brain biopsy may result in a definitive diagnosis. Susceptible patients, however, are often treated on the basis of suggestive clinical findings and a positive serology.

Therapy should be initiated with a loading dose of 100 mg to 200 mg PO of pyrimethamine followed by a maintenance daily dosage of 1 mg/kg per day. In addition, sulfadiazine is given in a loading dose of 50 mg/kg PO followed by 100 mg/kg per day divided into four hourly doses. Megaloblastic bone marrow changes should respond to folinic acid, which does not inhibit the action of pyrimethamine on *T. gondii*. Patients should be treated with both agents for at least one month, but the optimal duration of therapy is currently unknown.

CRYPTOSPORIDIUM

A number of patients with AIDS have developed severe diarrhea and vomiting as a result of infection with *Cryptosporidium,* a coccidian parasite.[33] Previously, only a few reports of human infection with this organism had been published[59–61]; most occurred in immunocompromised hosts. One patient in whom no underlying disease could be detected at autopsy succumbed to simultaneous infection with cryptosporidiosis and disseminated toxoplasmosis. There is no known effective treatment for this infection. Some patients have responded when their immunosuppression was corrected; three patients without underlying diseases responded to supportive therapy. One patient failed to respond to adequate doses of metronidazole or TMP-SMZ, and two patients failed a trial of pyrimethamine and sulfadiazine.

MODULATION OF IMMUNE STATUS

Immunologic reconstitution of patients with deficiency of cell-mediated immunity remains a formidable challenge. In children with pure thymic defects or severe combined immunodeficiency disease (SCID), transplantation of immunologically competent cells has resulted in reversal of the defect.[62] Grafting of fetal thymus of less than fourteen weeks gestation to prevent graft-versus-host reactions has been successful in children with thymic aplasia. Bone marrow transplantation has been successful in some children with SCID, but graft-versus-host reactions remain a problem.[62] Administration of transfer factor to children with cellular immune defects and immunodeficiency with Wiskott–Aldrich syndrome has resulted in control of infection in some individuals.[62] No studies of the effect of transfer factor in persons with AIDS have been published. Another humoral factor, thymosin, is a thymic protein hormone deficient in children with thymic aplasia and SCID. Administration of thymosin has restored some T-lymphocyte functions in these children[63] but has failed to alter the immunodeficiency of aged individuals.[64] Attempts to arrest the terminal course of disseminated CMV infections in patients with severe AIDS with thymosin have been unsuccessful. In an animal model, thymosin was successful in increasing resistance to infection with *Candida albicans*.[65] Experimental interest in the immunopotentiating effects of the Bacillus Calmette–Guérin vaccine, bacterial endotoxins, and such agents as levamisole, nonsteroidal antiinflammatory drugs, isoprinosine, lithium, and thymopoietin continues.

COUNSELING THE PATIENT WITH AIDS

Physicians with large numbers of homosexually active men in their practices, especially in New York and California, are having to counsel increasing numbers of individuals who either have one or more of the conditions described in this and the preceding chapter or fear developing AIDS. The reported numbers of persons suffering from KS, *Pneumocystis carinii* pneumonia, or other severe OIs are still increasing, and several recent samplings of cellular immune status among otherwise healthy homosexually active men in New York and Chicago[66,67] suggest that altered immune status is a widespread phenomenon. A sizeable proportion, variously estimated to be from 10% to 50%, of homosexual males with multiple sexual partners may be at risk for acquiring OIs, KS, and lymphoproliferative diseases. Because of the high mortality rates and difficulty of treating these diseases, effective preventive measures must be sought and promoted for individuals at risk. At present, preventive measures are limited to behavioral modification designed to decrease exposure to potential immunosuppressive agents.

Many patients and physicians will experience difficulty in talking about avoiding agent(s) whose identity is unknown at this time. Especially when talking about individual sexual behavior, statements such as "there's no idea what is causing the problem, so what can I possibly do about it" are commonplace. A common denial mechanism is to assume that unknown threats are nonexistent or attack only others; understanding that such statements and attitudes on the part of patients are attempts to deny and control considerable amounts of anxiety is the first step in dealing with the problem. Patient concerns in this area fall into two general categories: Those with AIDS are concerned about recurrent infections and the potential social stigma of being labeled a victim or "carrier." Conversely, relatively healthy patients express concern that their sexual activities or drug use will result in AIDS or an associated malignant or infectious disease.

While there are many obvious gaps in current knowledge concerning AIDS, several facts should be stressed when talking to patients about this problem. First, there is epidemiologic evidence of clustering of cases, suggesting that the underlying etiologic process is an infectious agent(s),[68] the most likely candidate being an immunosuppressive virus.[13] Second, once cellular immunity has been destroyed, it is a relatively irreversible condition, and a person suffering from one OI is at high risk for other infections or neoplasms. Third, sex with multiple partners—particularly anonymous partners and "orgy room sex" such as is available at gay bathhouses, "backroom bars," movie houses, and bookstores—carries the greatest degree of risk for contacting such agent(s). Finally, while drug use may not be a primary pathological agent, the use during sex of recreational drugs—such as marijuana, volatile nitrites, methylenedioxyamphetamine, cocaine, and others—may increase the extent of immunologic damage sustained.

Having established a common "data base" as previously outlined, the counseling of patients can be relatively straightforward. Persons already diagnosed as having AIDS need watchful medical surveillance and should definitely be warned about the danger of exposure to any pathogen, whether the route be sexual, occupational, intravenous, or through close contact with others. While there is no evidence to indicate a "carrier" state for the potential etiologic agent(s) for AIDS, and thus no reason to stigmatize persons with this condition, there is considerable evidence that continued promiscuous sexual activity is inadvisable for these persons.

The psychological consequences of being told that one suffers from AIDS are enormous. There are reports of individuals attempting suicide upon being told that they had an altered immune system. Obviously, anyone dealing with these problems should be able to provide psychological support and counseling to patients with a life-threatening medical condition. In cities with the largest number of AIDS patients, such as New York, San Francisco, and Los Angeles, self-help groups and specialized counseling referral networks have been established for AIDS patients. In other cities, such as Chicago and Atlanta, the local gay community sexually transmitted disease (STD) clinics and health professional organizations act as referral sources for AIDS patients. However, it is recommended that the physician involved in the primary treatment of AIDS patients also be involved in supportive counseling of patients. Oftentimes the AIDS patient feels beleaguered by an endless set of specialists, researchers, and interviewers attempting to treat or find out about his condition. Knowing that one individual is the primary person responsible for his care and is coordinating the activity of any specialists involved can be extremely helpful for the patient.

As for counseling the potential patient, the "at-risk" individual, the situation is somewhat less straightforward. Advising a reduction in the number of sexual partners, particularly in anonymous and group sex situations, is easier said than done. Advising more frequent STD examinations and including a careful physical examination for thrush, lymphadenopathy, splenomegaly, herpes zoster, or disseminated herpes simplex can be of both practical and educational value. Many patients will have lymphadenopathy when examined. The possible relationship of chronic lymphadenopathy to AIDS is discussed in Chapter 16. Some STD clinics with large numbers of homosexually active patients have considered adding specialized tests of immune function to their laboratory procedures. While there is little agreement at this time as to which of these relatively expensive diagnostic procedures are of value in the routine screening of STD patients, routine blood cell counts, including a differential count, can be useful in detecting lymphopenia. Patients with unexplained lymphopenia, lymphadenopathy, disseminated herpes, or other signs of deficient function should be referred for specialized immunologic evaluation. The development of close ties between gay community STD clinics, individual doctors practicing in the area, and specialists in the diagnosis and treatment of immunologic deficiency states can be of immense benefit to patients at risk for developing AIDS.

In New York, Chicago, San Francisco, Los Angeles, Washington, D.C., and elsewhere, the response of the gay community to discussions of these "new" diseases has been overwhelming. Obviously, there is a great deal of interest, desire for further information, and fear about the subject of AIDS, OIs, and neoplastic conditions in this community. Not only are patients scared and frustrated over the lack of definitive information, but practitioners are experiencing similar reactions, coupled with a sense of inability to offer meaningful practical advice to patients. A conservative and optimistic approach, stressing the concepts of preventive holistic health care and reduction of individual risk for acquiring STDs of any kind, appears to be most sensible. As stated in the introductory chapters of this book, an increased awareness of those aspects of patients' behavior that place them at risk for disease acquisition plus a nonjudgmental concern by the physician are the means by which the STD epidemic related to homosexual activity can be reduced.

REFERENCES

1. Gottlieb MS, Schroff R, Schanker HM, et al: *Pneumocystis carinii* pneumonia and mucosal candidiasis in previously healthy homosexual men: Evidence of a new acquired cellular immunodeficiency. *N Engl J Med* 305:1425–1431, 1981.

2. Masur H, Michelis MA, Greene JB, et al: An outbreak of community-acquired *Pneumocystis carinii* pneumonia: Initial manifestation of cellular immune dysfunction. *N Engl J Med* 305:1431–1438, 1981.
3. Siegal FP, Lopez C, Hammer GS, et al: Severe acquired immunodeficiency in male homosexuals, manifested by chronic perianal ulcerative herpes simplex lesions. *N Engl J Med* 305:1439–1444, 1981.
4. Hymes KB, Greene JB, Marcus A, et al: Kaposi's sarcoma in homosexual men—A report of eight cases. *Lancet* 2:598–600, 1981.
5. Friedman-Kien AE, Laubenstein LJ, Rubinstein P, et al: Disseminated Kaposi's sarcoma in homosexual men. *Ann Intern Med* 96:693–700, 1982.
6. Mildvan D, Mathur U, Enlow RW, et al: Opportunistic infections and immune deficiency in homosexual men. *Ann Intern Med* 96:700–704, 1982.
7. Follansbee SE, Busch DF, Wofsy CB, et al: An outbreak of *Pneumocystis carinii* pneumonia in homosexual men. *Ann Intern Med* 96:705–713, 1982.
8. Gerstoft J, Malchow-Moller A, Bygbjerg I, et al: Severe acquired immunodeficiency in European homosexual men. *Br Med J* 285:17–19, 1982.
9. Durack DT: Opportunistic infections and Kaposi's sarcoma in homosexual men. *N Engl J Med* 305:1465–1467, 1982.
10. Fauci AS: The syndrome of Kaposi's sarcoma and opportunistic infections: An epidemiologically restricted disorder of immunoregulation. *Ann Intern Med* 96:777–779, 1982.
11. Haynes BF, Katz P, Fauci AS: Immune responses of human lymphocytes *in vitro*, in Schwartz RA (ed): *Progress in Clinical Immunology*. New York, Grune & Stratton, 1980, pp 23–106.
12. Reinherz EL, Kung PC, Goldstein G, et al: Separation of functional subsets of human T cells by a monoclonal antibody. *Proc Natl Acad Sci USA* 76:4061–4065, 1979.
13. Notkins AL, Mergenhagen SE, Howard RJ: Effect of virus infections on the function of the immune system. *Annu Rev Microbiol* 24:525–528, 1976.
14. Fauci AS, Haynes BF, Katz P: Drug-induced T and B lymphocyte and monocyte dysfunction, in Grieco MH (ed): *Infections in the Abnormal Host*. New York, Yorke Medical Books, 1980, pp 163–182.
15. Armstrong D: Infections in patients with neoplastic disease, in Verhoef J, Peterson PK, Quie PG (eds): *Infections in the Immunocompromised Host—Pathogenesis, Prevention and Therapy*. New York, Elsevier/North-Holland, 1980, pp 129–158.
16. Armstrong D: Fungal infections in the compromised host, in Rubin RH, Young LS (eds): *Clinical Approach to Infection in the Compromised Host*. New York, Plenum Medical, 1981, pp 195–228.
17. Sheft DJ, Shrago G: Esophageal moniliasis: The spectrum of disease. *JAMA* 213:1859–1862, 1970.
18. Shortsleeve MJ, Gauvin GP, Gardner RC, et al: Herpetic esophagitis. *Radiology* 141:611–617, 1981.
19. Stone HH, Kolb LD, Currie CA, et al: *Candida* sepsis: Pathogenesis and principles of treatment. *Ann Surg* 179:697–711, 1974.
20. Eng RHK, Chmel H, Buse M: Serum levels of arabinitol in the detection of invasive candidiasis in animals and humans. *J Infect Dis* 143:677–683, 1981.
21. Armstrong D, Wong B: Central nervous system infections in immunocompromised hosts. *Annu Rev Med* 33:293–308, 1982.
22. Armstrong D: Central nervous system infections in the compromised host, in Rubin RH, Young LS (eds): *Clinical Approach to Infection in the Compromised Host*. New York, Plenum Medical, 1981, pp 163–194.
23. Sen P, Louria DB: Higher bacterial and fungal infections, in Grieco MH (ed): *Infections in the Abnormal Host*. New York, Yorke Medical Books, 1980, pp 326–359.

24. Medoff G, Kobayashi GS: Strategies in the treatment of systemic fungal infections. *N Engl J Med* 302:145–155, 1980.

25. Kantrowitz PA, Fleischli CJ, Butler WT: Successful treatment of chronic esophageal moniliasis with a viscous suspension of nystatin. *Gastroenterology* 57:424–430, 1969.

26. Petersen EA, Alling DW, Kirkpatrick CH: Treatment of chronic mucocutaneous candidiasis with ketoconazole: A controlled clinical trial. *Ann Intern Med* 93:791–795, 1980.

27. Graybill JR, Drutz DJ: Ketoconazole: A major innovation for treatment of fungal disease. *Ann Intern Med* 93:921–923, 1980.

28. Kirkpatrick CH, Alling DW: Treatment of chronic oral candidiasis with clotrimazole troches. *N Engl J Med* 299:1201–1203, 1978.

29. Beggs WH, Sarosi GA: Combined activity of ketoconzaole and 5-fluorocytosine on potentially pathogenic yeasts. *Antimicrob Agents Chemother* 21:355–357, 1982.

30. *Med Lett* 24:36–38, 1982.

31. Bennett JE, Dismukes WE, Duma RJ, et al: A comparison of amphotericin B alone and combined with flucytosine in the treatment of cryptococcal meningitis. *N Engl J Med* 301:126–131, 1979.

32. Bennett JE, Remington JS: Miconazole in cryptococcosis and systemic candidiasis: A word of caution. *Ann Intern Med* 94:708–709, 1981.

33. Gottlieb MS, Schroft R, Fligiel S, et al: Gay-related immunodeficiency (GRID) syndrome: Clinical and autopsy observations. *Clin Res* 30:349A, 1982.

34. Fainstein V, Bolivar R, Mavligit G, et al: Disseminated infection due to *Mycobacterium avium-intracellulare* in homosexual men with Kaposi's sarcoma. *J Infect Dis* 145:586, 1982.

35. Lester TW: Drug-resistant and atypical mycobacterial disease: Bacteriology and treatment. *Arch Intern Med* 139:1399–1401, 1979.

36. Davidson PT, Khanijo V, Goble M, et al: Treatment of disease due to *Mycobacterium intracellulare*. *Rev Infect Dis* 3:1052–1059, 1981.

37. Corpe RF: Surgical management of pulmonary disease due to *Mycobacterium avium-intracellulare*. *Rev Infect Dis* 3:1064–1067, 1981.

38. Drew WL, Mintz L, Miner RC, et al: Prevalence of cytomegalovirus infection in homosexual men. *J Infect Dis* 143:188–192, 1981.

39. Hirsch MS: Herpes group virus infection in the compromised host, in Rubin RH, Young LS (eds): *Clinical Approach to Infection in the Compromised Host*. New York, Plenum Medical, 1981, pp 389–415.

40. Wade JC, Newton B, McLaren C, et al: Intravenous acyclovir to treat mucocutaneous herpes simplex virus after marrow transplantation: A double-blind study. *Ann Intern Med* 96:265–269, 1982.

41. Straus SE, Smith HA, Brickman C: Acyclovir for chronic mucocutaneous herpes simplex virus infection in immunosuppressed patients. *Ann Intern Med* 96:270–277, 1982.

42. Crumpacker CS, Schnipper LE, Marlowe SI, et al: Resistance ot antiviral drugs of herpes simplex virus isolated from a patient treated with acyclovir. *N Engl J Med* 306:343–346, 1982.

43. Burns WH, Santos GW, Seral R, et al: Isolation and characterization of resistant herpes simplex virus after acyclovir therapy. *Lancet* 1:421–423, 1982.

44. Ashraf MH, Campalani GC, Qureshi SA, et al: Acyclovir in treatment of cytomegalovirus pneumonia after cardiac transplantation. *Lancet* 1:173–174, 1982.

45. Cheeseman SH, Rubin RH, Stewart MD, et al: Controlled clinical trial of human leukocyte interferon in renal transplantation. I. Effects of cytomegalovirus and herpes simplex virus infections. *N Engl J Med* 300:1345–1349, 1979.

46. Merigan TC: Interferon therapy in human viral infections and malignant disease, in: Stiehm ER (moderator): Interferon: Immunobiology and Clinical Significance. *Ann Intern Med* 96:80–93, 1982, pp 88–90.

47. Jones JF, Jeter WS, Fulginiti VA, et al: Treatments of childhood combined Epstein–Barr virus/ cytomegalovirus infection with oral bovine transfer factor. *Lancet* 2:122–124, 1981.
48. Ruskin J: Parasitic diseases in the compromised host, in: Rubin RH, Young LS (eds): *Clinical Approach to Infection in the Compromised Host.* New York, Plenum Medical, 1981, pp 269–334.
49. Hughes WT: *Pneumocystis carinii* pneumonia. *N Engl J Med* 297:1381–1383, 1977.
50. Centers for Disease Control: Update on Kaposi's sarcoma and opportunistic infections in previously healthy persons—United States. *MMRW* 31:294, 300–301, 1982.
51. Turbiner EH, Yeh SDJ, Rosen PP, et al: Abnormal gallium scintigraphy in *Pneumocystis carinii* pneumonia with a normal chest radiograph. *Radiology* 127:437–438, 1978.
52. Young LS: Trimethoprim-sulfamethoxazole in the treatment of adults with pneumonia due to *Pneumocystis carinii. Rev Infect Dis* 4:608–613, 1982.
53. Sattler FR, Remington JS: Intravenous trimethoprim-sulfamethoxazole therapy for *Pneumocystis carinii* pneumonia. *Am J Med* 70:1215–1221, 1981.
54. McKenna F, Davison AM, Giles GR: Response of *Pneumocystis carinii* pneumonia only after high-dose cotrimoxazole. *Lancet* 1:174, 1982.
55. Lawson DH, Paice BJ: Adverse reactions to trimethoprim-sulfamethoxazole. *Rev Infect Dis* 4:429–433, 1982.
56. Centers for Disease Control Task Force on Kaposi's Sarcoma and Opportunistic Infections: Epidemiologic aspects of the current outbreak of Kaposi's sarcoma and opportunistic infections. *N Engl J Med* 306:248–252, 1982.
57. Murphey SA, Josephs AS: Acute pancreatitis associated with pentamidine therapy. *Arch Intern Med* 141:56–58, 1981.
58. Hughes WT, Kuhn S, Chaudhary S, et al: Successful chemoprophylaxis for *Pneumocystis carinii* pneumonitis. *N Engl J Med* 297:1419–1426, 1977.
59. Stemmermann GN, Hayashi T, Glober GA, et al: Cryptosporidiosis: Report of a fatal case complicated by disseminated toxoplasmosis. *Am J Med* 69:637–642, 1980.
60. Tzipori S, Angus KW, Gray EW, et al: Vomiting and diarrhea associated with cryptosporidial infection. *N Engl J Med* 303:818, 1980.
61. Fletcher A, Sims TA, Talbot IC: Cryptosporidial enteritis without general or selective immune deficiency. *Br Med J* 285:22–23, 1982.
62. Ammann AJ, Fudenberg HH: Immunodeficiency diseases, in: Fudenberg HH, Stites DP, Caldwell JL, et al (eds): *Basic and Clinical Immunology,* ed 2. Los Altos, California, Lange Medical Publications, 1978, pp 391–421.
63. Wara DW, Ammann AJ: Activation of T-cell rosettes in immunodeficient patients by thymosin. *Ann NY Acad Sci* 249:310–314, 1975.
64. Quinti I, Pandolfi F, Fiorilli M, et al: T dependent immunity in aged humans. I. Evaluation of T-cell subpopulation before and after short term administration of a thymic extract. *J Gerontol* 36:674–679, 1981.
65. Bistoni F, Marconi P, Frati L, et al: Increase of mouse resistance to *Candida albicans* infection by thymosin. *Infect Immun* 36:609–614, 1982.
66. Kalish SB, Ostrow DG, Phair JP, et al: The spectrum of immunological abnormalities in homosexually active males: Association of laboratory findings with prodromal symptoms of the acquired immunodeficiency syndrome (AIDS) (manuscript in preparation).
67. Wallace JI, Coral FS, Rimm IJ, et al: T-cell ratios in homosexuals. *Lancet* 1:908, 1982.
68. Centers for Disease Control: A cluster of Kaposi's sarcoma and *Pneumocystis carinii* pneumonia among homosexual male residents of Los Angeles and Orange Counties, California. *MMWR* 31:305–307, 1982.

VII

A Special Consideration

Medical Consequences of the Inhalation of Volatile Nitrites

KENNETH H. MAYER

Amyl and butyl nitrite have had legitimate medical indications for their use for over a century, but in the last two decades they have become an increasingly popular means for getting high, and have currently come to be frequently scrutinized as the cause of or a cofactor in a plethora of somatic disorders. The compounds are liquids at room temperature that rapidly evaporate and decompose unless kept cool, sealed, and protected from excess light exposure. Their volatile properties allow for sniffing to be the route of intoxication. They are touted as a means to alter consciousness and heighten sexual arousal and as adjuvants in achieving a euphoric state. The use of these substances has increased markedly over the past two decades, becoming a $20-million-a-year industry with an estimated cadre of over 5 million regular users.[1] A nationwide survey in 1978 of graduating high school students revealed that one in nine had contact with this class of drugs.[2]

Amyl nitrite was first reported to be efficacious in the relief of angina pectoris in 1867 by a Scottish medical student who noted that the vapors caused facial flushing secondary to vascular dilation, findings which the young researcher extrapolated to the coronary circulation.[3] Amyl nitrite has traditionally been sold in boxes of cloth-covered ampules, which are crushed to afford ease of inhalation. The street name for this class of drugs, "poppers," was derived from the sound made when the glass capsules were squeezed. Subsequently, sublingual nitroglycerin was found to be more reliable and convenient in the management of angina, and amyl nitrite drifted into obscurity, except as a diagnostic aid in

KENNETH H. MAYER • Departments of Medicine, and Microbiology and Molecular Genetics, Harvard Medical School, and Fenway Community Health Center, Boston, Massachusetts 02115.

elucidating the nature of specific cardiac murmurs. Until 1960, it was a controlled substance. The period of decontrol lasted less than a decade, as awareness of the drug's abuse potential grew.

The limited accessibility of amyl nitrite led to the widespread use of butyl nitrite in the 1970s, which was available over the counter as a "room freshener." Butyl nitrite, possessing a four-carbon alkyl chain versus the three-carbon chain of amyl nitrite, is somewhat more labile, and is therefore merchandised as a faster "rush." The distinction between the nitrites is blurred, since investigators have found multiple preparations that are combinations of volatile nitrites but are marketed generically as one compound or the other.[4] Current preparations are generally sold in opaque vials that contain 10 ml to 30 ml of these substances, under numerous trade names that often have a sexual connotation. The ease with which these products may be obtained in bookstores, bathhouses, and bars is currently being challenged by physicians, particularly in the gay community.[5]

Many of the immediate physiological responses to inhaled nitrites are well known; the primary mode of action is the relaxation of vascular smooth muscle by the nitrite ion. The subsequent acute preload reduction (i.e., vascular dilation) results in a compensatory tachycardia, which allows a stable cardiac output.[6] Orthostatic symptoms, dizziness, syncope, palpitations, and headache are well known sequelae. Secondary autonomic augmentation can result in diaphoresis, nausea, tremulousness, anxiety, weakness, and an urge to defecate or urinate.[7]

Symptoms from nitrite inhalation usually can be relieved by having the affected person lie down. Any position that increases blood flow to the brain (e.g., feet higher than the head) helps to attenuate dizziness, and, if the patient becomes unconscious, this maneuver facilitates awakening as rapidly as possible. Whatever the source of the syncope, in the acute phase, the health care practitioner must pay attention to the adequacy of respiration and tissue perfusion by noting the patient's breathing patterns, skin color and temperature, and pulse rate and rhythm. What might seem to be a simple nitrite-induced blackout could be an incipient arrest, although nitrites have not been implicated in serious acute cardiac disturbances. If a nitrite user complains of persistent lightheadedness, increasing fluid intake may also help cerebral perfusion and diminish persistent symptoms. The administration of nasal flow oxygen may also be of benefit. In general, the most useful "cure" for acute nitrite-related symptoms is to decrease dosage size and frequency; time tends to alleviate most of the common side effects.

Other medical problems that are believed to be associated with nitrite use include transient electrocardiographic abnormalities, including ST-segment depression and T-wave inversions,[8] although the clinical significance of these findings is not totally certain. One might presume that the acute hemodynamic changes elicited by these agents would relatively counterindicate their use in persons with uncontrolled angina (particularly the vasospastic syndromes) unless carefully monitored, as well as in persons with aortic stenosis. Likewise, their propensity to exacerbate vascular headaches would suggest that persons who suffer from migraines would be wise to avoid nitrites. These drugs have been shown to increase intraocular, as well as intracranial, pressure, so the drug class should be avoided by persons with glaucoma or increased intracranial pressure of any etiology.[9]

Nitrites have been alleged to exacerbate asthma; however, the reports have not been substantiated to date, and the concomitant use of cigarettes and marijuana may obfuscate a clear delineation of the problem. The frequent use of alcohol and exposure to other hepatotoxins and hepatotrophic viruses among nitrite users do not facilitate the clarification of whether these hepatically excreted substances may be responsible for either cholestatic or hepatocellular patterns of liver dysfunction. Since interactions among multiple agents are possible, the clinician might best advise a patient who has hepatitis to abstain from using these drugs.

A clear-cut liability of nitrite use is the potential for chemical burns to occur if the liquid comes in contact with the skin, as well as the development of contact and hypersensitivity dermatoses.[10] The management of these problems often requires formal dermatologic consultation, as the clinical presentations of these disorders may be protean. The resultant lesions have varied from vesicular to purulent to diffusely maculopapular in configuration, underscoring the need for obtaining a good clinical history. Another potential problem that can affect the skin, and occasionally the viscera, relates to the high degree of flammability of these agents. The possibilities for burns are enhanced by the fact that the places in which these drugs are used may often be cramped, with many cigarette (or marijuana) smokers in close proximity.

Nitrite-mediated conversion of hemoglobin to methemoglobin was useful in the Vietnam era in treating cyanide poisoning; however, methemoglobinemia may result in cyanosis, exertional dyspnea, tachycardia, anorexia, nausea, and lethargy if the intoxication occurs rapidly.[11,12]

Stupor may generally be seen at levels greater than 55% and death at over 70% in otherwise healthy individuals. A recent report[13] described clinically significant methemoglobinemia (18%) after nitrite inhalation in a patient who was found to have a rare partial deficiency of NADH-methemoglobin reductase. However, six normal controls did not develop levels greater than 8% after twelve minutes of continuous inhalation. Several recent reports have noted clinically significant methemoglobinemia after butyl nitrite ingestion,[14,15] including one fatality.[16] The possibility of chronic subclinical methemoglobinemia in long-term users and potential sequelae remain to be delineated. If a person with a history of recent prolonged nitrite use is noted to be cyanotic, inordinately lethargic, or short of breath, methemoglobinemia should be suspected, and early administration of oxygen is appropriate. Most urban toxicology laboratories can run methemoglobin levels, and, if there is clinical suspicion of nitrite ingestion, starting intravenous methylene blue is indicated. This management should only be undertaken in an intensive care unit setting.

The National Institute of Drug Abuse noted thirteen emergency room admissions resulting from the ill effects of nitrite use in 1976, and its network processed 84 related complaints that year.[1] If viewed in the context of over 5 million users, what is known about volatile nitrites does not appear to pose a major health hazard.

It has been widely assumed that nitrite use has been particularly prevalent within the gay community. One recent study in the psychiatric literature[17] attempted to evaluate patterns of nitrite use among homosexual men by examining responses to a standard questionnaire. The authors found that no respondent used nitrites on a daily basis, and only 5% of the respondents acknowledged using the drug more than three times a week. They also noted that regular users had an increased incidence of sexually transmitted diseases, sexual promiscuity, alcoholism, and being assaulted, but the stratification of frequent users versus nonusers was distorted by a lack of controls for salient demographic factors.

Nitrite inhalation has been postulated to be a risk factor for the development of the acquired immunodeficiency syndrome (AIDS) among homosexual men, either alone or in combination with one or more infectious agents,[13] but corroborative laboratory data are still scant. Italian scientists have shown that volatile nitrites can be mutagenic in bacteria,[14] but extrapolation to mammalian cells may not be appropriate. Researchers at Purdue University have studied the acute and chronic effects of isobutyl nitrite on mice and have found that the methemoglobinemia that is induced is irreversible, suggesting that chronic use may produce progressive tissue hypoxia, which could lead to end organ impairment.[15,16] The investigators noted that mice sacrificed in the experiments often had blanched livers, corroborating their concerns. In the course of the experiments, one of the mice developed a thymoma, a tumor often associated with immunologic disturbances in humans, although this neoplasm is not rare in that murine strain.

The Centers for Disease Control and the National Institute for Occupational Safety and Health are currently engaged in a collaborative study regarding the effects of nitrite inhalation in laboratory mice on cell-mediated immunity. However, the rigorous nature of these studies means that definitive data will probably not be available until later in 1983. If the work goes well, the investigators are considering infecting the mice with cytomegalovirus and then exposing them to nitrites. This is a combination that would not be uncommon among homosexually active men, and it is therefore being scrutinized as contributory to the newly emergent syndrome.

In a recent study,[13] homosexual male nitrite users ($N = 9$, including two patients undergoing treatment for Kaposi's sarcoma) were compared with non-users ($N = 7$) regarding the ratio of helper T lymphocyte to suppressor T lymphocyte cells, one parameter of cell-mediated immunity. The users were found to be more immunocompromised. However, the study was flawed by the small sample size and the presence of confounding variables, e.g., other intercurrent illness and stresses that could alter these ratios were not controlled with sufficient rigor.

The jury is really still out regarding the ultimate toxicity of chronic volatile nitrite inhalation, but this begs the issue. Currently many well-documented, if uncommon, deleterious side effects are seen with these drugs. There are no urgent medical indications for nitrite use. The questions that are being raised because of the seriousness of the AIDS are of sufficient magnitude to suggest that concerned clinicians discourage the use of these agents until sufficient data exonerate them. This approach borders on the puritanical and does not have substantive scientific underpinnings, but the current stressful situation mandates erring on the side of caution.

REFERENCES

1. Reed D: The multi-million dollar mystery high. *Christopher Street* 2:21–27, 1979.
2. Johnson L, Bachman J, O'Malley P: *1979 Highlights: Drugs and the Nation's High School Students; Five-Year National Trend.* Rockville, Maryland, National Institute on Drug Abuse, 1979, pp 1–235.
3. Brunton T: On the use of nitrite of amyl in angina pectoris. *Lancet* 2:97–98, 1867.
4. Ostrow D: Kaposi's sarcoma: An interview with Dr. James Curran, CDC Kaposi's task force director. *Homosexual Health Reports* 1:3–8, 1982.
5. Alfred R: Dateline San Francisco—Popper Safety. *Out Magazine,* April 8, 1982, p 5.
6. Nickerson M: Vasodilator drugs, in Goodman LS, Gilman A (eds): *The Pharmacologic Basis of Therapeutics,* ed 5. New York, Macmillan, 1975, pp 727–743.
7. Louria F: Hazards of sniffing amyl nitrite during sexual intercourse. *JAMA* 236:1622, 1976.
8. Nickerson M, Parker JO, Lowry TP, et al: *Isobutyl Nitrite and Related Compounds.* San Francisco, Pharmex, 1979, pp 1–64.
9. Huff B: Amyl nitrite, in *Physician's Desk Reference,* ed 33. Oradell, New Jersey, Medical Economics Company, 1979, p 995.
10. Fisher AA: Personal communication.
11. Sharp CW, Brehm ML: *Review of Inhalants: Euphoria to Dysfunction.* Rockville, Maryland, National Institute on Drug Abuse, 1978, pp 1–312.
12. Jaffe E: Methemoglobinemia and sulfhemoglobinemia, in Beeson P, McDermott W, Wyngaarden JB (eds): *Cecil–Loeb Textbook of Medicine.* Philadelphia, WB Saunders, 1979, pp 1780–1782.

13. Goedert JJ, Neuland CY, Wallen WC, et al: Amyl nitrite may alter T lymphocytes in homosexual men. *Lancet* 2:412–415, 1982.
14. Fain N: Is it safe to sniff: The controversy over poppers and other inhalants. *Advocate*, August 5, 1982, pp 22–24.
15. Maickl RP, McFadden DP: Acute toxicology of butyl nitrites and butyl alcohols. *Res Commun Clin Pathol Pharmacol* 26:75–83, 1979.
16. Maickl RP: Personal communication.
17. Sigell LT: Popping and snorting volatile nitrites: A current fad for getting high. *Ann Int Med* 64:460–470, 1966.

Sexually Transmitted Diseases
Treatment Guidelines, 1982

U.S. Department of Health and Human Services, Public Health Service, Centers for Disease Control, Center for Prevention Services, Venereal Disease Control Division, Atlanta, Georgia 30333.

Abridged from *Morbidity and Mortality Weekly Report* (Supplement) 31(2S):35S–60S, August 20, 1982.

These guidelines may differ in the treatment of some disease entities as they present in homosexually active men. Please consult individual chapters.

These guidelines for treatment of sexually transmitted diseases (STD) were established after careful deliberation by a group of experts* and staff of the Centers for Disease Control (CDC). Commentary received after dissemination of preliminary documents to a large group of physicians was also considered. Certain aspects of these guidelines represent the best judgment of experts. The guidelines should not be construed as rules, but rather as a source of guidance within the United States. This is particularly true for topics that are controversial or based on limited data.

Chlamydia trachomatis Infections

Infections caused by *Chlamydia trachomatis* are the most prevalent sexually transmitted diseases in the United States today. The importance of serious complications related to chlamydial infections has been established. Diagnosis and treatment of these infections are frequently based on the clinical syndrome since chlamydial cultures often are unavailable. The following guidelines are for *culture-proven* infections caused by non-lymphogranuloma venereum (LGV) strains of *C. trachomatis*. For approaches to the treatment of common chlamydial infections when cultures are not available, see Common STD-Associated Syndromes.

Uncomplicated Urethral, Endocervical, or Rectal Infection in Adults

Drug Regimens of Choice

Tetracycline hydrochloride (HCl): 500 mg, by mouth, 4 times a day for at least 7 days

OR

Doxycycline: 100 mg, by mouth, twice a day for at least 7 days

Alternative Regimens
(for patients in whom tetracyclines are contraindicated or not tolerated)

Erythromycin: 500 mg, by mouth, 4 times a day for at least 7 days

Sulfonamides are also active against *C. trachomatis*, but have not been extensively studied.

Management of Sexual Partners
All persons exposed to *C. trachomatis* infection should be examined for STD and promptly treated for exposure to *C. trachomatis* with one of the above regimens.

Follow-up
Posttreatment cultures are advisable. Positive cultures may not be detectable until 3-6 weeks after treatment; when they are positive, patients should be treated again with one of the above regimens.

---
*GL Mandell, MD, School of Medicine, University of Virginia; ER Alexander, MD, Health Science Center, University of Arizona; KA Arndt, MD, Beth Israel Hospital, Boston; RE Berger, MD, VA Medical Center, Seattle; CR Dawson, MD, The Proctor Foundation, University of California, San Francisco; R Dolin, MD, College of Medicine, University of Vermont; SK Dritz, MD, City and County Department of Health, San Francisco; KK Holmes, MD, PhD, School of Medicine, University of Washington; FN Judson, MD, Department of Health, Denver; WM McCormack, MD, Downstate Medical Center, Brooklyn; PB Mead, MD, College of Medicine, University of Vermont; GB Miller Jr, MD, Virginia Department of Health; MF Rein, MD, School of Medicine, University of Virginia; RB Rothenberg, MD, New York State Department of Health; D Satcher, MD, PhD, Morehouse School of Medicine, Atlanta; J Schachter, PhD, School of Medicine, University of California, San Francisco; MR Spence, MD, Johns Hopkins Hospital.

Gonococcal Infections

The following guidelines for the treatment of gonococcal infection in the United States take into account several observations: the increasing incidence of infections due to penicillinase-producing *N. gonorrhoeae* (PPNG), unpublished reports of the emergence of tetracycline-resistant gonococci in several geographic areas, the high frequency of coexisting chlamydial and gonococcal infections, and increased recognition of the serious complications of chlamydial and gonococcal infections. In addition, new antimicrobials, in particular new cephalosporins, that may prove to be effective in treating gonococcal infection are becoming available in the United States. Therefore, these guidelines do not attempt to be a comprehensive list of all possible treatment regimens. Rather, they seek to provide guidance for regimens that meet general criteria of efficacy, safety, ease of administration, and cost.

Uncomplicated Infection in Adults

Recommended Regimens
(the order of presentation does *not* indicate preference)

Tetracycline HCl: 500 mg, by mouth, 4 times a day for 7 days (total dose 14.0 g). Other tetracyclines are not more effective than tetracycline HCl. All tetracyclines are ineffective as a single-dose therapy. Doxycycline hyclate 100 mg by mouth, twice a day for 7 days may be substituted for tetracycline.

Advantage	*Disadvantages*
1. Effective against coexisting chlamydial infections	1. Requires compliance with multiple doses
	2. May encourage the emergence of tetracycline-resistant strains if the regimen is not strictly followed
	3. Ineffective against anorectal gonococcal infections in men

OR

Amoxicillin/ampicillin: Amoxicillin, 3.0 g, or ampicillin, 3.5 g, either with 1.0 g probenecid by mouth

Advantage	*Disadvantages*
1. Single-dose treatment	1. Ineffective against chlamydial infections
	2. Ineffective against anorectal and pharyngeal gonococcal infections

OR

Aqueous procaine penicillin G: 4.8 million units injected intramuscularly (IM) at 2 sites, with 1.0 g of probenecid by mouth

Advantage	*Disadvantages*
1. Single-dose therapy	1. Injection
	2. Possible procaine reaction
	3. Possible penicillin anaphylaxis
	4. Ineffective against chlamydial infections

An important concern in the treatment of gonorrhea is coexisting chlamydial infection, which has been documented in up to 45% of gonorrhea patients for whom adequate chlamydial cultures are done. Patient compliance can also be a problem with multiple-day tetracycline/doxycycline regimens for gonococcal infections, as can the potential selection of tetracycline-resistant isolates when incomplete doses are taken. To address these concerns, a single-dose regimen could be administered just before the tetracycline/doxycycline regimen. On theoretical grounds, this combined regimen (outlined below) is very attractive, but its efficacy and side effects have not been evaluated. CDC intends to undertake such an evaluation and encourages others to do the same.

The combined regimen includes:

Amoxicillin/ampicillin: Amoxicillin 3.0 g or ampicillin 3.5 g, either with 1.0 g probenecid by mouth

PLUS

Tetracycline HCl:500 mg, by mouth, 4 times a day for 7 days (total dose 14.0 g) Doxycycline hyclate 100 mg, by mouth, twice a day for 7 days may be substituted for tetracycline HCl.

Advantages	*Disadvantage*
1. Provides adequate single-dose treatment for gonorrhea	1. Efficacy and side effects of this specific combined regimen have not been evaluated.
2. Effective against chlamydial infections	

Special Note:

Tetracycline or aqueous procaine penicillin G (APPG) is the preferred therapy for pharyngeal gonococcal infection. Pharyngeal infection is not effectively treated by either the amoxicillin or ampicillin regimens.

A homosexual man with uncomplicated gonococcal infection should be treated with aqueous procaine penicillin G 4.8 million units, plus 1.0 g of probenecid. If he is allergic to penicillin, use spectinomycin 2.0 g, IM, in 1 injection. Both of these regimens provide adequate treatment for urethral and anorectal gonococcal infection. However, spectinomycin is ineffective in the treatment of pharyngeal gonococcal infection.

Other Considerations

Patients other than homosexual men who are allergic to penicillins or probenecid should be treated with oral tetracycline or doxycycline as above. Penicillin-allergic patients who cannot tolerate tetracyclines may be treated with spectinomycin HCl, 2.0 g, IM, in 1 injection.

Patients with incubating syphilis (seronegative without clinical signs of syphilis) are likely to be cured by all the above regimens except spectinomycin. All patients treated for gonorrhea should have a serologic test for syphilis.

Patients with gonorrhea who also have syphilis or are established contacts of syphilis patients should be given additional treatment appropriate to the stage of syphilis. (See Syphilis, p.50S.)

Treatment of Sexual Partners

Men and women exposed to gonorrhea should be examined, cultured, and treated at once with one of the regimens above.

Follow-Up

Follow-up cultures should be obtained from the infected site(s) 4-7 days after completion of treatment. In addition, cultures should be obtained from the rectum of all women who have been treated for gonorrhea.

Treatment Failures

The patient in whom gonorrhea persists after treatment with one of the non-spectinomycin regimens above should be treated with 2.0 g of spectinomycin IM. (See PENICILLINASE-PRODUCING *NEISSERIA GONORRHOEAE*) Recurrent gonococcal infections after treatment with the recommended schedules may be due to reinfection and indicate a need for improved contact tracing and patient education. Since PPNG infection is a cause of treatment failure, posttreatment isolates should be tested for penicillinase production.

Drugs Not Recommended

Although long-acting forms of penicillin (such as benzathine penicillin G) are effective in the treatment of syphilis, they have NO place in the treatment of gonorrhea. Oral penicillin preparations such as penicillin V are not recommended for the treatment of gonococcal infection.

Penicillinase-Producing *Neisseria gonorrhoeae*

Patients with proven PPNG infection or who are likely to have acquired gonorrhea in areas of high PPNG prevalence and their sexual partners should receive spectinomycin 2.0 g, IM, in a single injection. Tetracycline may be added to treat coexistent chlamydial infection. Patients with positive cultures after spectinomycin therapy should be treated with cefoxitin 2.0 g, IM, in a single injection plus probenecid 1.0 g, by mouth; OR cefotaxime 1.0 g, IM, in a single injection without probenecid. A daily single dose of 9 tablets of trimethoprim/sulfamethoxazole (80 mg/400 mg) for 5 days should be used to treat pharyngeal gonococcal infection due to PPNG. Spectinomycin and cefoxitin are ineffective in pharyngeal infections.

Disseminated Gonococcal Infection

Treatment Schedules

Hospitalization is usually indicated, especially for those who cannot reliably comply with treatment, have uncertain diagnosis, or have purulent joint effusions or other complications.

There are several, acceptable treatment schedules for the gonococcal arthritis-dermatitis syndrome. These include the following:

Aqueous crystalline penicillin G: 10 million units, intravenously (IV), per day until improvement occurs, followed by amoxicillin 500 mg or ampicillin 500 mg, by mouth, 4 times a day to complete at least 7 days of antibiotic treatment

OR

Amoxicillin/ampicillin: amoxicillin 3.0 g or ampicillin 3.5 g, by mouth, each with probenecid 1.0 g, followed by amoxicillin 500 mg or ampicillin 500 mg, by mouth, 4 times a day for at least 7 days

OR

Tetracycline HCl: 500 mg, by mouth, 4 times a day for at least 7 days. Tetracycline HCl should not be used for complicated gonococcal infection in pregnant women.

OR

Cefoxitin/cefotaxime: cefoxitin 1.0 g or cefotaxime 500 mg, either given 4 times a day IV for at least 7 days (treatment of choice for disseminated infections caused by PPNG)

OR

Erythromycin: 500 mg, by mouth, 4 times a day for at least 7 days

Special Considerations
Open drainage of joints other than the hip is not indicated. Intraarticular injection of antibiotics is unnecessary.

Meningitis and Endocarditis
Meningitis and endocarditis caused by the gonococcus require high-dose IV penicillin therapy. Optimal duration of therapy is unknown, but most authorities treat patients for a month. Therapy of penicillin-allergic patients must be individualized.

Gonococcal Ophthalmia in Adults
Adults with gonococcal ophthalmia should be hospitalized and treated with aqueous crystalline penicillin G 10 million units, IV, daily for 5 days. For PPNG, use cefoxitin 1.0 g or cefotaxime 500 mg, IV, 4 times a day. Eyes should be irrigated immediately with saline or buffered ophthalmic solutions and then at least at hourly intervals as long as necessary to eliminate discharge. Cases must have careful ophthalmic follow-up to deal with ocular complications.

Common STD-Associated Syndromes
Several, often serious, clinical syndromes are associated with STD. Some are more clearly defined than others. The following guidelines outline approaches to the initial treatment of these conditions *when complete bacteriologic evaluation is not possible* or while the physician awaits the results of specific laboratory tests.

Nongonococcal Urethritis
Urethritis not associated with *N. gonorrhoeae* is usually caused by *C. trachomatis* or *Ureaplasma urealyticum.* Nongonococcal urethritis (NGU) requires prompt antimicrobial treatment of the patient and evaluation and treatment of sexual partner(s).

Drug Regimens of Choice

Tetracycline HCl : 500 mg, by mouth, 4 times a day for at least 7 days

OR

Doxycycline : 100 mg, by mouth, twice a day for at least 7 days

Alternative Regimen
(for patients in whom tetracyclines are contraindicated or not tolerated)

Erythromycin : 500 mg, by mouth, 4 times a day for at least 7 days

Management of Sexual Partners
All persons who are sexual partners of patients with NGU should be examined for STD and promptly treated with one of the above regimens.

Follow-up
Patients should be advised to return if symptoms persist or recur.

Persistent or Recurrent NGU
Recurrent NGU may be due to failure to treat the sexual partner(s). Patients with persistent or recurrent objective signs of urethritis after adequate treatment of the patient and partner(s) warrant further evaluation for less common causes of urethritis.

Acute Epididymo-orchitis

Acute epididymo-orchitis has 2 forms: a sexually transmitted form usually associated with urethritis and commonly caused by *C. trachomatis* and/or *N. gonorrhoeae* and a non-sexually transmitted form associated with urinary tract infections caused by Enterobacteriaceae or *Pseudomonas.* Urine should be examined by Gram stain and culture to exclude bacteruria in all patients, including those with urethritis. Testicular torsion is a surgical emergency that should be considered in all cases.

Sexually Transmitted Epididymo-orchitis

Sexually transmitted epididymo-orchitis occurs in young adults and is associated with presence of urethritis, absence of underlying genitourinary pathology, and absence of gram-negative rods on Gram stain of urine.

Drug Regimens of Choice

Tetracycline HCl : 500 mg, by mouth, 4 times a day for at least 10 days

OR

Doxycycline : 100 mg, by mouth, twice a day for at least 10 days

Alternative Regimens

Alternative regimens have not been well studied. The following regimens can be considered in patients who cannot tolerate tetracycline:

Gonococcal urethritis and epididymitis:

Amoxicillin : 500 mg, by mouth, 3 times a day for at least 10 days
(For epididymitis caused by PPNG, clinical experience is limited, but a 10-day course of therapy with oral trimethoprim/sulfamethoxazole or parenteral cefotaxime, cefoxitin, or spectinomycin can be used.)

Nongonococcal urethritis and epididymitis:
Erythromycin : 500 mg, by mouth, 4 times a day for at least 10 days

Management of Sexual Partners

Sexual partners of patients with sexually transmitted acute epididymo-orchitis should be examined for STD and promptly treated with a regimen effective against uncomplicated gonococcal and chlamydial infection.

Adjuncts to Therapy

Bed rest and scrotal elevation until fever and local inflammation have subsided are recommended.

Follow-up

Failure to improve within 3 days requires reevaluation of diagnosis/therapy and consideration for hospitalization. Persistence of swelling for longer than 1 month should lead to evaluation for tumor.

Non-Sexually Transmitted Acute Epididymo-orchitis

Management includes prompt administration of broad-spectrum antimicrobial therapy. Choice of therapy is initially dictated by the severity of infection and later by results of urine culture and sensitivity tests. Evaluation for underlying urinary tract disease is indicated. Adjuncts to therapy and follow-up are the same as for sexually transmitted epididymo-orchitis.

Trichomoniasis

Recommended Regimen
   Metronidazole : 2.0 g, by mouth, in a single dose

Alternative Regimen
   Metronidazole may be administered in a dosage of 250 mg, by mouth, 3 times a day for 7 days.

Asymptomatic Women
   Asymptomatic women with trichomoniasis should be treated the same as symptomatic women.

Management of Sexual Partners
   Male sexual partners of women with trichomoniasis should be treated with metronidazole 2.0 g, by mouth, in a single dose and examined for coexistent STD.

Follow-up
   Tests of cure should be sought whenever possible. Resistance of *Trichomonas vaginalis* to metronidazole has been observed, but is rare.

Trichomoniasis in Pregnancy
   Metronidazole is contraindicated in the first trimester of pregnancy and should be avoided throughout pregnancy. Clotrimazole 100 mg, intravaginally, at bedtime for 7 days may produce symptomatic improvement and some cures. Other local treatments may be used for symptomatic relief but have low cure rates. Lactating women may be treated with metronidazole 2.0 g, by mouth, in a single dose, but breast-feeding should be interrupted for at least 24 hours after therapy.

Neonatal Trichomonal Infections
   Infants with symptomatic trichomoniasis or with persistent urogenital trichomonal colonization beyond the fourth week of life can be treated with metronidazole 10-30 mg/kg daily for 5-8 days.

Genital Herpes Simplex Virus Infections

   Genital herpes infection is a viral disease that may be chronic and recurring and for which there is no known cure.

First Clinical Episode

   A careful history should be obtained to establish that this is the patient's first disease episode.

Clinicians may elect to use :
   Acyclovir ointment 5%: Apply sufficient quantity to adequately cover all lesions every 3 hours, 6 times a day for 7 days. Therapy should be initiated as early as possible following onset of signs and symptoms.
   This treatment reduces viral shedding and the duration of disease in patients with primary initial infection who are treated within 6 days of the onset of symptoms; however, it does not prevent recurrences.
   Acyclovir has not been tested in pregnant or lactating women.

Recurring Disease

There is no effective treatment to prevent recurrences of genital herpes infection or to shorten their duration.

Patients should be told about the natural history of genital herpes infection and advised to abstain from sexual contact while lesions are present. The risk of transmission of the herpes virus during asymptomatic periods is unknown. Some consultants recommend that asymptomatic patients use condoms, but their efficacy is unproved. Women with genital herpes infection should be advised to have yearly Pap tests. Early in pregnancy, women should inform their clinician of their history of genital herpes infection.

Ano-Genital Warts *(Condylomata acuminata)*

The treatment of ano-genital warts has not been well studied. No treatment is completely satisfactory. Ano-genital warts have recently been linked to the development of cancer. For these reasons, atypical or persistent warts should be biopsied. A Pap smear is recommended for all women with ano-genital warts. Women with cervical warts should not be treated until the result of the Pap smear is available to guide therapy. While podophyllin is widely used in the treatment of ano-genital warts, some consultants feel that cryotherapy, when available, may be preferable to podophyllin.

External Genital/Perianal Warts

Podophyllin: 10%-25% in compound tincture of benzoin. Apply carefully to wart, avoiding normal tissue. Wash off thoroughly in 1-4 hours. If the wart does not regress after 4 weekly applications, alternative treatments may be used.

Podophyllin should not be used during pregnancy.

Alternative therapies:
  Cryotherapy (e.g., liquid nitrogen, solid carbon dioxide)
  Electrosurgery
  Surgical removal (scissor or curette)

Urethral/Meatal Warts

Accessible meatal warts: May be treated with the regimen below:

Podophyllin: 10%-25% in compound tincture of benzoin (see above). Great care should be taken to ensure that the treated area is dried before contact with normal mucosa is allowed.

Alternative therapies:
  Same as for external genital/perianal warts

Urethral Warts: Intraurethral warts should be suspected in men with recurrent meatal warts. Urethroscopy is necessary to diagnose this condition. Intraurethral 5% 5-fluorouracil or thiotepa may be effective in this condition, but neither has been adequately evaluated. Podophyllin should not be used.

Anorectal Warts

Many consultants avoid the use of podophyllin for anorectal warts.

Podophyllin: 10%-25% in compound tincture of benzoin may be used to treat anorectal warts accessible by anoscope. Extreme care must be taken to avoid exposure of normal mucosa to podophyllin. Allow the treated area to dry before removal of the anoscope.

Alternative therapies :
Same as for external genital/perianal warts
Patients with extensive or proximal anorectal warts should be referred for proctologic evaluation

Oral Warts

Oral warts should be treated with:
Cryotherapy (e.g., liquid nitrogen, solid carbon dioxide)
Electrosurgery
Surgical removal (scissor or curette)

Syphilis

Early Syphilis

Recommended Regimen
Early syphilis (primary, secondary, latent syphilis of less than 1 year's duration) should be treated with:

Benzathine penicillin G : 2.4 million units total, IM, at a single session

Pencillin-Allergic Patients

Patients who are allergic to penicillin should be treated with:

Tetracycline HCl : 500 mg, by mouth, 4 times a day for 15 days

Tetracycline appears to be effective, but has been evaluated less extensively than penicillin. Patient compliance with this regimen may be difficult, so care should be taken to encourage optimal compliance.
Penicillin-allergic patients who cannot tolerate tetracycline should have their allergy confirmed. For these patients there are 2 options:
1. If compliance and serologic follow-up can be assured, administer erythromycin 500 mg, by mouth, 4 times a day for 15 days.
2. If compliance and serologic follow-up cannot be assured, the patient should be managed in consultation with an expert.

Syphilis of More Than One Year's Duration

Recommended Regimen
Syphilis of more than 1 year's duration, except neurosyphilis (latent syphilis of indeterminate or more than 1 year's duration, cardiovascular, or late benign syphilis) should be treated with:

Benzathine penicillin G : 2.4 million units, IM, once a week for 3 successive weeks (7.2 million units total)

The optimal treatment schedules for syphilis of greater than 1 year's duration have been less well established than schedules for early syphilis. In general, syphilis of longer duration requires more prolonged therapy.

Therapy is recommended for established cardiovascular syphilis. Antibiotics may not reverse the pathology associated with this disease, however.

Pencillin-Allergic Patients

There are no published clinical data that adequately document the efficacy of drugs other than penicillin for syphilis of more than 1 year's duration. Cerebrospinal fluid examinations should be performed before therapy with these regimens.

Patients who are allergic to penicillin should be treated with:

Tetracycline HCl: 500 mg, by mouth, 4 times a day for 30 days. Patient compliance with this regimen may be difficult, so care should be taken to encourage optimal compliance.

Penicillin-allergic patients who cannot tolerate tetracycline should have their allergy confirmed. For these patients there are 2 options:

1. If compliance and serologic follow-up can be assured, administer erythromycin 500 mg, by mouth, 4 times a day for 30 days.
2. If compliance and serologic follow-up cannot be assured, the patient should be hospitalized and managed in consultation with an expert.

Cerebrospinal Fluid Examination

Cerebrospinal fluid (CSF) examination should be done for patients with clinical symptoms or signs consistent with neurosyphilis. This examination is also desirable for other patients with syphilis of greater than 1 year's duration to exclude asymptomatic neurosyphilis.

Neurosyphilis

Published studies show that a total dose of 6.0-9.0 million units of penicillin G over a 3- to 4-week period results in a satisfactory clinical response in approximately 90% of patients with neurosyphilis. This information must be considered along with the observation that regimens employing benzathine penicillin or procaine penicillin in doses under 2.4 million units daily do not consistently provide treponemicidal levels of penicillin in CSF, and with the knowledge that several case reports show the failure of such regimens to cure neurosyphilis.

Drug Regimens

Potentially effective regimens, none of which have been adequately studied, include:

Aqueous crystalline penicillin G: 12-24 million units, IV, per day (2-4 million units every 4 hours) for 10 days, followed by benzathine penicillin G, 2.4 million units, IM, weekly for 3 doses

OR

Aqueous procaine penicillin G: 2.4 million units, IM, daily plus probenecid 500 mg, by mouth, 4 times a day, both for 10 days, followed by benzathine penicillin G 2.4 million units, IM, weekly for 3 doses

OR

Benzathine penicillin G: 2.4 million units, IM, weekly for 3 doses

Penicillin-Allergic Patients

Patients with histories of allergy to penicillin should have their allergy confirmed and managed in consultation with an expert.

Syphilis in Pregnancy

Evaluation of Pregnant Women
All pregnant women should have a nontreponemal serologic test for syphilis, such as the VDRL or RPR test, at the time of the first prenatal visit. The treponemal tests such as the FTA-ABS test should not be used for routine screening. For women suspected of being at high risk for syphilis, a second nontreponemal test should be done during the third trimester, and the cord blood should be tested for syphilis antibody.
Seroreactive patients should be expeditiously evaluated. This evaluation should include a history and physical examination, as well as a quantitative nontreponemal test and a confirmatory treponemal test.
If the FTA-ABS test is nonreactive and there is no clinical evidence of syphilis, treatment may be withheld. Both the quantitative nontreponemal test and the confirmatory test should be repeated within 4 weeks. If there is clinical or serologic evidence of syphilis or if the diagnosis of syphilis cannot be excluded with reasonable certainty, the patient should be treated as outlined below.
Patients for whom there is documentation of adequate treatment for syphilis in the past need not be treated again unless there is clinical or serologic evidence of reinfection such as dark-field-positive lesions or a 4-fold rise in titer when a quantitative nontreponemal test is used.

Recommended Regimens
For patients at all stages of pregnancy who are not allergic to penicillin, penicillin should be used in dosage schedules appropriate for the stage of syphilis as recommended for the treatment of nonpregnant patients.

Penicillin-Allergic Patients
For patients at all stages of pregnancy who have documented allergy to penicillin:
1. If compliance and serologic follow-up can be assured, administer erythromycin in dosage schedules appropriate for the stage of syphilis as recommended for the treatment of nonpregnant patients. Infants born to mothers treated during pregnancy with erythromycin for early syphilis should be treated with penicillin.
2. If compliance and serologic follow-up cannot be assured, the patient should be hospitalized and managed in consultation with an expert.
Tetracycline is not recommended in pregnant women because of potential adverse effects on the fetus.

Follow-up
Pregnant women who have been treated for syphilis should have monthly quantitative nontreponemal serologic tests for the remainder of the current pregnancy. Women who show a 4-fold rise in titer should be treated again. After delivery, follow-up is as outlined for nonpregnant patients.

Follow-up After Treatment and Re-Treatment

All patients with early syphilis and congenital syphilis should be encouraged to return for repeat quantitative nontreponemal tests at least 3, 6, and 12 months after treatment. For these patients quantitative nontreponemal tests will decline to nonreactive or to reactive with a low titer within a year following successful treatment with benzathine penicillin G. Titers decline more slowly with serologic tests for patients treated for disease of longer duration. Patients with syphilis of more than 1 year's duration should also have a repeat serologic test 24 months after treatment. Careful follow-up serologic testing is particularly important in patients treated with antibiotics other than penicillin. Examination of CSF should be planned as part of the last follow-up visit after treatment with alternative antibiotics.

All patients with neurosyphilis must be carefully followed with periodic serologic testing, clinical evaluation at 6-month intervals, and repeat CSF examinations for at least 3 years

The possibility of reinfection should always be considered when patients with early syphilis need to be treated a second time. A CSF examination should be performed before re-treatment unless reinfection and a diagnosis of early syphilis can be established.

Re-treatment should be considered when:

1. Clinical signs or symptoms of syphilis persist or recur
2. There is a 4-fold increase in titer with a nontreponemal test
3. A nontreponemal test showing a high titer initially fails to show 4-fold decrease within a year

Patients should be re-treated according to the schedules recommended for syphilis of more than 1 year's duration. In general, a patient should be re-treated only once since patients may maintain stable, low titers when nontreponemal tests are used or may have irreversible anatomical damage.

Epidemiologic Treatment

Persons who have been exposed to infectious syphilis within the preceding 3 months and other persons who on epidemiologic grounds are at high risk for early syphilis should be treated as for early syphilis. Every effort should be made to determine if such persons have syphilis.

Haemophilus ducreyi Infection (Chancroid)

Chancroid may be a more common cause of genital ulcers than presently recognized. The diagnosis is best made by isolation of *Haemophilus ducreyi* from ulcers and/or fluctuant nodes on appropriate selective medium.

Drug Regimens

Erythromycin : 500 mg, by mouth, 4 times a day

OR

Trimethoprim/sulfamethoxazole: double-strength tablet (160/800 mg), by mouth, twice a day

Therapy should be continued for a minimum of 10 days and until ulcers and/or lymph nodes have healed.

Lesion Management

Fluctuant lymph nodes should be aspirated through healthy adjacent normal skin. Incision and drainage or excision of nodes will delay healing and are contraindicated.

Apply compresses to ulcers to remove necrotic material.

Sexual Partners

Treat sexual partners with a 10-day course of one of the above regimens.

Note : Antimicrobial susceptibility testing should be done on *H. ducreyi* isolated from patients who do not respond to the recommended therapies.

Lymphogranuloma venereum:
Genital, Inguinal, or Anorectal

Infection with a lymphogranuloma venereum (LGV) serotype of *C. trachomatis* should be treated in the following way.

Drug Regimen of Choice

Tetracycline HCl: 500 mg, by mouth, 4 times a day for at least 2 weeks

Alternative Regimens

The following drugs are active against LGV serotypes *in vitro* but have not been evaluated extensively in culture-confirmed cases.

Doxycycline: 100 mg, by mouth, twice a day for at least 2 weeks

OR

Erythromycin: 500 mg, by mouth, 4 times a day for at least 2 weeks

OR

Sulfamethoxazole: 1.0 g, by mouth, twice a day for at least 2 weeks. Other sulfonamides can be used in equivalent dosage.

Lesion Management

Fluctuant lymph nodes should be aspirated as needed through healthy adjacent normal skin. Incision and drainage or excision of nodes will delay healing and are contraindicated. Late sequelae such as stricture and/or fistula may require surgical intervention.

Scabies
Adults and Older Children

Treatment

Lindane (1%): 1 oz of lotion, or 30 g of cream applied thinly to all areas of the body from the neck down and washed off thoroughly after 8 hours. *Not recommended for pregnant or lactating women.*

Alternative Therapies

Crotamiton (10%): applied to the entire body from the neck down nightly for 2 nights and washed off thoroughly 24 hours after the second application

OR

Sulfur (6%) in petrolatum: applied to the entire body from the neck down nightly for 3 nights. Patients may bathe before reapplying the drug and should bathe 24 hours after the final application.

Contacts

Sexual contacts and close household contacts should be treated as above.

Special Considerations

Pruritus may persist for several weeks after adequate therapy. A single re-treatment after 1 week may be appropriate if there is no clinical improvement. Additional weekly treatments are warranted only if live mites can be demonstrated.

Clothing or bed linen that may have been contaminated by the patient within the past 2 days should be washed and/or dried by machine (hot cycle in each) or dry cleaned.

Pediculosis Pubis

Drug Regimens

Lindane (1%) lotion or cream: applied in a thin layer to the infested and adjacent hairy areas and thoroughly washed off after 8 hours; or **lindane (1%) shampoo**: applied for 4 minutes and then thoroughly washed off. *Not recommended for pregnant or lactating women.*

OR

Pyrethrins and piperonyl butoxide (nonprescription): applied to the infested and adjacent hairy area and washed off after 10 minutes.

Re-treatment is indicated after 7 days if lice are found or eggs are observed at the hair-skin junction. Clothing or bed linen that may have been contaminated by the patient within the past 2 days should be washed and/or dried by machine (hot cycle in each) or dry cleaned.

Contacts

Sexual contacts should be treated as above.

Special Considerations

Pediculosis of the eyelashes should be treated by the application of occlusive ophthalmic ointment to the eyelid margins twice daily for 10 days to smother lice and nits. Lindane or other drugs should not be applied to the eyes.

Enteric Infections

Treatment of proctitis and enterocolitis should be based on etiologic diagnosis. Appropriate gastroenterologic work up should be pursued in all cases. Asymptomatic, infected individuals for whom anal-oral contact is a sexual practice should be treated in accordance with recommendations for symptomatic individuals, as should persons whose work or social situation is associated with a likelihood of transmission (e.g., food handlers, hospital workers, day-care-center employees, etc.). Sexual partners at risk for fecal-oral transmission should be evaluated. Sexual transmission does not preclude the possibility of nonvenereal transmission as well. Careful attention to hand washing and other hygienic practices is strongly urged.

Campylobacter jejuni

The drug of choice for symptomatic enterocolitis or proctitis is:

Erythromycin: 500 mg, by mouth, 4 times a day for 7 days

Shigella Species

Antibiotic choice must be based on the sensitivity pattern of the isolate. Immediate treatment, when required, may be based on local sensitivity patterns. Current national sensitivity patterns suggest that the drug of choice is:

Trimethoprim/sulfamethoxazole: double-strength tablet (160/800 mg), by mouth, twice daily for 7 days

An alternative is ampicillin 500 mg, by mouth, 4 times a day for 7 days, although the variability of regional sensitivity of shigellae to ampicillin must be considered. Amoxicillin is *not* an acceptable substitute.

Nontyphoidal *Salmonella* Species

Treatment for asymptomatic carriage or uncomplicated symptomatic infection is not generally recommended. Sexual partners should be evaluated.

Amebiasis

Laboratory diagnosis may be complicated by prior use of antidiarrheal agents and antibiotics such as tetracycline or erythromycin.

Symptomatic Patients

In symptomatic patients the regimen of choice consists of a systemic drug plus a lumenal amebicide:

Metronidazole: 750 mg, by mouth, 3 times a day for 5-10 days

PLUS EITHER

Iodoquinol (diiodohydroxyquin): 650 mg, by mouth, 3 times a day for 20 days; OR **diloxanide furoate:** 500 mg, by mouth, 3 times a day for 10 days*

An alternative would be to use metronidazole alone followed sequentially by one of the lumenal amebicides if clinical cure is not achieved.

The regimen of second choice is:

Paromomycin: 25-30 mg/kg/day in 3 divided doses for 7 days.*

This drug is used alone. Although primarily a lumenal amebicide, it has been noted to have superficial tissue effect.

Severe disease or extraintestinal illness should prompt appropriate medical consultation and referral.

Asymptomatic Cysts Passers

For asymptomatic passers of amebic cysts, the lumenal amebicides alone are sufficient (iodoquinol 650 mg, by mouth, 3 times a day for 20 days, or diloxanide furoate 500 mg, by mouth, 3 times a day for 10 days).

Giardiasis

The drug of choice for symptomatic and asymptomatic infection is:

Quinacrine: 100 mg, by mouth, 3 times a day for 7 days

An alternative therapy is:

Metronidazole: 250 mg, by mouth, 3 times a day for 7 days

---

*available through CDC

In the case of coexistent symptomatic amebiasis and giardiasis, metronidazole in the higher dose may be preferred (see Amebiasis).

As with other protozoal pathogens, initial treatment of asymptomatic carriers is indicated. Re-treatment of recurrences, either from relapse or reinfection, depends on individual and epidemiologic circumstances.

> Note: Chlamydial and gonococcal rectal infections are discussed in the sections dealing with those organisms. Presently, there is no specific treatment for proctitis associated with herpes simplex virus infection.

Index

Abrasions, physical, and sexual practices, 14
Acquired immune deficiency syndrome
  (AIDS), 213–234
  and hepatitis B vaccine, 130
  immunologic evaluation, 214–217
  and Kaposi's sarcoma, 198
  patient counseling, 229–231
  precautions in handling patients, specimens,
    32–34
  T lymphocytes, 214ff
  See also Opportunistic infections
Acyclovir (Zovirax®)
  for cytomegalovirus, 218, 225
  for herpes simplex, 179, 219, 251
  for herpes zoster, 218
AIDS: *see* Acquired immune deficiency
  syndrome
Amebiasis, 87–98
  and anilinction, 15
  clinical aspects, 89
  control, 97
  diagnosis, 90–92, 94–95
    anoscopy, 91
    sigmoidoscopy, 91
    stool examination, 90
  diet, 89
  epidemiology, 87
  and Kaposi's sarcoma, 202
  patient education, 96, 97
  postamebic colitis, 96
  prevention, 96
  testing frequency for, 24

Amebiasis (*cont.*)
  transmission, 88
  treatment, 92
American Medical Association, study of
  physician education, 8
American Psychiatric Association, and
  homosexuality, 8
American Venereal Disease Association, viii
Aminophylline, and Mycolog® cream
  dermatitis, 187
Amoxicillin
  for disseminated gonorrhea, 65, 248
  for epididymitis, 250
  for gonococcal urethritis, 250
  for gonorrhea, 65, 246, 247
Amphotericin B
  for *Candida albicans,* 218
  for cryptococcosis, 218
  for fungal infections, 223
Ampicillin
  for disseminated gonorrhea, 248
  for gonorrhea, 65, 246, 247
  for rectal trauma, 155
Amyl nitrite: *see* Nitrites, amyl, butyl
Anal fissure, 144–145
  clinical aspects, 144
  diagnosis, 144
  treatment, 145
Anal intercourse
  and anal fissure, 145
  and gonorrhea, 57
  and hemorrhoids, 143